Inflammatory Bowel Disease and Irritable Bowel Syndrome

Inflammatory Bowel Disease and Irritable Bowel Syndrome

Edited by Drake Baldwin

hayle
medical

New York

Hayle Medical,
750 Third Avenue, 9th Floor,
New York, NY 10017, USA

Visit us on the World Wide Web at:
www.haylemedical.com

ISBN: 978-1-63241-610-0

Cataloging-in-Publication Data

Inflammatory bowel disease and irritable bowel syndrome / edited by Drake Baldwin.
    p. cm.
Includes bibliographical references and index.
ISBN 978-1-63241-610-0
1. Inflammatory bowel diseases. 2. Irritable colon.
3. Intestines--Diseases. 4. Gastroenteritis. I. Baldwin, Drake.
RC862.I53 I54 2019
616.344--dc23

Table of Contents

Preface

Inflammatory bowel disease (IBD) and irritable bowel syndrome (IBS) are two of the most common gastrointestinal disorders. A group of inflammatory conditions associated with the colon and small intestine is termed as inflammatory bowel disease. The two main types of inflammatory bowel disease include Crohn's disease and ulcerative colitis. A group of symptoms like, abdominal pain and changes in the pattern of bowel movements comes under the broad term, irritable bowel syndrome. There are four main types of IBS, namely, constipation-predominant (IBS-C), diarrhea-predominant (IBS-D), with alternating stool pattern (IBS-A) and pain-predominant. This book unravels the recent studies related to inflammatory bowel disease and irritable bowel syndrome. It consists of contributions made by international experts. Those in search of information to further their knowledge will be greatly assisted by this book.

This book is a result of research of several months to collate the most relevant data in the field.

When I was approached with the idea of this book and the proposal to edit it, I was overwhelmed. It gave me an opportunity to reach out to all those who share a common interest with me in this field. I had 3 main parameters for editing this text:

1. Accuracy – The data and information provided in this book should be up-to-date and valuable to the readers.

2. Structure – The data must be presented in a structured format for easy understanding and better grasping of the readers.

3. Universal Approach – This book not only targets students but also experts and innovators in the field, thus my aim was to present topics which are of use to all.

Thus, it took me a couple of months to finish the editing of this book.

I would like to make a special mention of my publisher who considered me worthy of this opportunity and also supported me throughout the editing process. I would also like to thank the editing team at the back-end who extended their help whenever required.

Editor

Cytokines in Inflamed Mucosa of IBD Patients

Tsvetelina Velikova, Dobroslav Kyurkchiev,

Ekaterina Ivanova-Todorova, Zoya Spassova,

Spaska Stanilova and Iskra Altankova

Abstract

Cells of the innate and the adaptive immune system have been identified as the key players in inflammatory bowel disease (IBD) pathogenesis, and the cytokines are central components of the inflammatory pathways that take place in the gut mucosa during the active and chronic phases of IBD. The effector cell response is largely determined by the type of cytokines that predominate in the intestinal mucosa. Here we describe the main cytokine players in intestinal inflammation during IBD—related to innate immune responses (tumor necrosis factor α—TNFα), TNF-like cytokine 1A, IL-8), and related to adaptive immune responses—Th1 (IL-1β, IL-18, IFNγ, IL-12), Th2 (IL-4, IL-5, IL-13, IL-11, IL-33), Th17 (IL-17A, IL-17F, IL-21, IL-22, IL-25, IL-27), cytokines required for Th17 development (IL-6, TGFβ, IL-23), anti-inflammatory cytokine IL-10 and Tregs along with IL-2. Recently described innate lymphoid cells (ILCs) could also be potential sources of IFN-γ, TNF, IL-5, IL-13, IL-17, and IL-22. The effects of cytokines in the gut are described in conjunction with the clinical implication and available biologic therapy. The data in the literature and our own results make us believe that in order to achieve immune homeostasis in the gut, pro-inflammatory and anti-inflammatory responses that define the mucosal cell immunophenotype should achieve balance.

Keywords: IBD, cytokines, mucosal inflammation, Th17, Tregs

1. Introduction

Both ulcerative colitis (UC) and Crohn's disease (CD), usually referred to as inflammatory bowel disease (IBD), are examples of complex disorders, which include inflammatory and autoimmune features with prominent intestinal immune dysregulation. Cells of the innate and the adaptive immune system have been identified as the key players of IBD. Cytokines are central components of the inflammatory pathways that take place during the active and chronic phases of IBD. However, a clear picture of these processes is still missing. Since the inflammation is located in the intestinal mucosa, the latter is the main source of biomarkers in IBD allowing various immunological pathways to be explored in the gut. Thus, the determination of cytokine expression profile could help to elucidate the local immune responses during intestinal inflammation. Expression of IBD-related proteins such as cytokines, chemokines, adhesion molecules, and their corresponding cellular and soluble receptors has revealed their significant role in the pro- and anti-inflammatory processes in the inflamed gut mucosa. Indeed, the implication of some cytokines in the immunopatho-genesis of IBD is investigated intensively and proved in experimental models of intestinal inflammation. Lack of enough investigation in humans, however, predetermines the need for further studies since it is proved that the common clinical phenotype of colitis may result from largely diverse genetic or immunological backgrounds.

2. Intestinal inflammation and cytokines

Since the pathogenesis of IBD is related to both dysregulated innate and adaptive immune pathways, which contribute to the aberrant intestinal inflammatory response in genetically susceptible individuals, the main focus of research attempts is directed to the initiation, perpetuation, and cessation of gut inflammation associated with IBD [1].

Cytokines are abundantly produced by the cells of the gut-associated immune system maintaining lymphocyte homeostasis under both steady-state and inflammatory conditions. These small, cell-signaling protein molecules act in a paracrine, autocrine, or endocrine manner, coordinate the communication between immune and non-immune cells of the intestinal compartment, and modify acute and chronic inflammatory responses at both local and systemic levels [2]. Moreover, elevation of pro-inflammatory cytokines is considered to be associated with the severity of gut inflammation [3]. Therefore, it is no surprise that cytokines have been a major therapeutic management of IBD [4].

It is believed that dysregulated immune mechanisms are related to T cells in the gut in IBD pathogenesis. Unregulated T lymphocytes activities can lead to autoimmunity, especially during inflammation when they can cause excessive tissue damage [5]. The ability of CD4+ T helper (Th) cells to alter the magnitude and outcome of the intestinal tissue-damaging inflammatory responses is mostly dependent on the production of distinct profiles of cyto-kines. Traditionally, the lesions in CD patients have been associated with a predominant activation of Th1 cells and production of large quantities of IFNγ under the stimulus of IL-12 through STAT4 signaling. By contrast, the lesions in UC patients were believed to be driven by Th2 cytokines, such as IL-4 and IL-13, through STAT6 activation. In the mouse model of IBD, CD3+ (T cell) depletion results in dramatic reduction of the gross pathology, neutrophil influx, and expression of pro-inflammatory cytokines and chemokines [6]. The cytokine expression pattern that strictly follows the polarization model of Th1 versus Th2, however, does not appear to be fully applicable in IBD. Nearly 20 years ago, Mosmann and Coffman concluded their paradigm with the prediction: "… further divisions of helper T cells may have to be recognized before a complete picture of helper T cell function can be obtained" [7, 8]. Indeed, several recent studies had led to the identification of more complex networks of cytokine interaction in IBD tissue, thus shedding light on the role of a distinct subset of T cells in the pathogenesis of IBD—Th17 cells. On the other hand, another T cell subpopulation, namely T regulatory cells (Tregs), is implicated in gut homeostasis and tolerance induction, and it is believed that Th17 and Tregs are in a mutually polarizing relationship [9]. An overview of the main cells and cytokines involved in intestinal inflammation is presented in **Figure 1**.

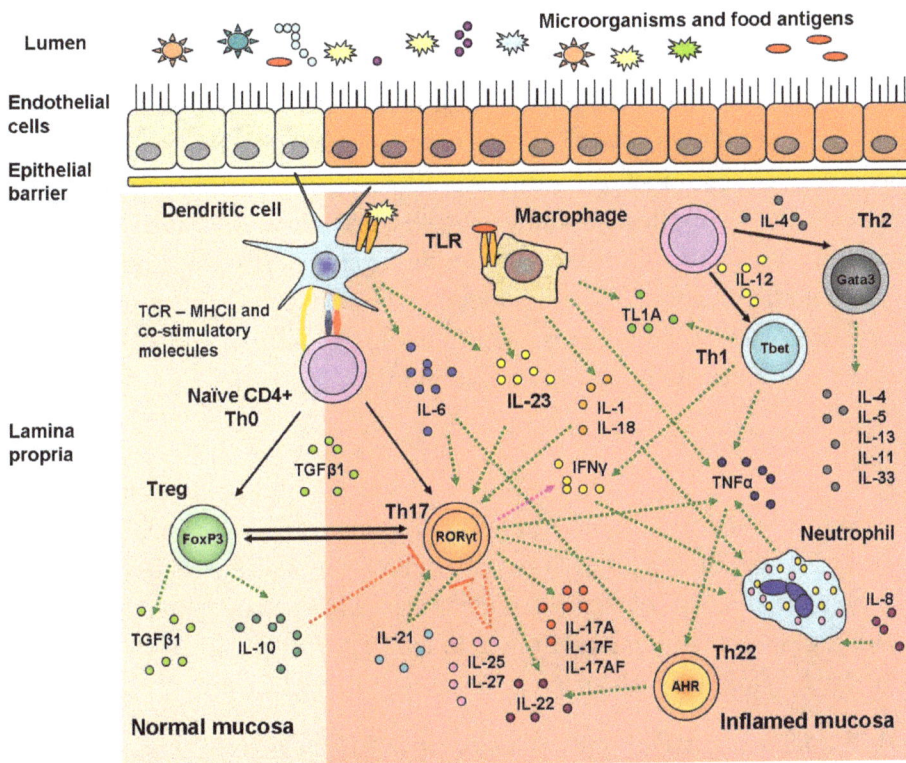

Figure 1. T-helper cells and cytokines interactions in normal and inflamed mucosa of IBD patients. The fate of naïve T cell depends on the interactions with the antigen-presenting cells (i.e. dendritic cells, macrophages) and the secreted cytokines. In normal mucosa, the abundant TGFβ1 directs naïve Th0 cells to Treg differentiation which secrete IL-10 and TGFβ1. "Danger" signals through TLR activation (on antigen-presenting cells), followed by secretion of IL-6, IL-23, IL-1, etc., with the simultaneous presence of TGFβ1, all favor the development of Th17 cells. The latter secrete many cytokines, for example, IL-21 acts as an autocrine positive regulator but IL-25 and IL-27 inhibit Th17 cells in autocrine manner. Th17 cells could also secrete IL-17 cytokines, TNFα, and in special circumstances—IFNγ; thus, Th17 cells play an intermediate role between innate and adaptive immune response, especially during inflammation in the intestinal mucosa. The balance between Th17 cells and Tregs is desired to maintain the immune homeostasis in the gut. However, Tregs and Th17 cells can convert into each other demonstrating same plasticity, depending on the cytokine milieu. Nevertheless, there are other players in the inflamed mucosa such as Th1, Th2, and Th22 cells. Legend: black arrow—cell differentiation; green arrow—secretion; pink arrow—possible secretion; red arrow—inhibition; TCR—T cell receptor; TLR—Toll-like receptor; MHCII—major histocompatibility complex—Class II; TL1A—TNFα-like 1 A.

Thus, the effector response is largely determined by the combination of cytokines that predominate in the intestinal mucosa, and it defines the mucosal T cell immunophenotype in each case [2].

2.1. Innate immune response and related cytokines

Dendritic cells (DCs), macrophages, epithelial cells, and myofibroblasts are able to recognize pathogen-associated molecular patterns (PAMPs) through their pattern-recognition receptors including Toll-like and NOD-like receptors. This recognition results in nuclear factor (NF)-kB activation with gene transcription and production of pro-inflammatory cytokines, such as IL-1 and TNFα, ensuring an effective innate response against microbial antigens. That also triggers antigen presentation, maturation, and up-regulation of co-stimulatory molecules which lead to efficient adaptive immunity involving T cell activation [10]. There is evidence for down-regulated protein level of TLR-3 in IBD, whereas TLR-2 and TLR-4 are up-regulated in intestinal mucosa of active IBD [11]. A specific mutation in NOD2 gene induces loss of NF-kB function during TLR-2 activation with a subsequent increased risk of infection with commensal bacteria and increased susceptibility to the ileal form of CD [12]. Recent studies suggest that increased mucosal permeability in the intestinal mucosa during IBD flare allows infiltration of a large number of granulocytes into the colonic mucosa. These leukocytes are activated, have a prolonged survival time, and release various pro-inflammatory cytokines (e.g. IL-1β, IL-6, TNFα, IL-18), which exacerbate and maintain the inflammation in the gut [13].

2.1.1. TNFα

TNFα links the innate and the adaptive immune responses and has crucial importance in the pathogenesis of IBD by inducing the differentiation of stromal cells into myofibroblasts and promoting their production of matrix metalloproteinases. The latter induce enterocyte apoptosis and digestion of gut basement membrane [10]. TNFα also exerts its pro-inflammatory effect through cytokines such as INFγ, IL-1β, and IL-6 [12].

TNFα is a well-established inflammatory mediator in CD whereas contradictory reports exist in UC [12]. There is a lack of studies on the mucosal expression of TNFα and the prediction of the clinical course, and only a few reports announced the predictive value of mucosal TNFα concentrations and the response to therapy in IBD patients. In fact, increased levels of TNFα and IL-15 have been previously reported in intestinal biopsies from IBD patients in remission without biopsy alterations [14]. Interestingly, the presence of TNFα in non-affected areas of IBD mucosa may not be sufficient to trigger mechanisms of mucosal damage. In preliminary reports, normalizing of mucosal TNFα seemed to predict a longstanding remission after stopping of anti-TNFα therapy in UC [12].

Certain TNFα polymorphisms (i.e. TNFα-308 A allele) are associated with increased serum levels of TNFα and therefore with higher susceptibility of IBD [15].

2.1.2. TNF-like cytokine 1A

TNF-like cytokine 1A (TL1A) is a novel member of TNF superfamily of proteins, produced by endothelial cells, macrophages, lamina propria T cells and plasma cells, monocytes, and monocyte-derived DCs [16]. Association with its functional receptor provides co-stimulatory signals for activation of T lymphocytes, leading to cell proliferation, cytokine secretion, and amplification of pro-inflammatory pathways, as well as induction of apoptosis in target cells [2]. Several studies have clearly demonstrated that TL1A and its receptor are up-regulated at mucosal protein and mRNA levels in IBD patients. TL1A is localized in the lamina propria and shows preferential expression on plasma cells and mucosal DCs. Of great importance is the fact that TL1A was shown to increase IL-13 secretion by natural killer T (NKT) cells, which are considered to be central to the mucosal injury that takes place in UC pathogenesis. Furthermore, TL1A induces IFNγ secretion in synergy with stimulation via TCR or IL-12/IL-18 [2]. TL1A expression is induced by TNFα and IL-1α as well and since the latter are abundantly expressed in the inflamed mucosa of UC patients, they may provide a strong stimulus for enhanced TL1A expression. On the other hand, several microorganisms were shown directly to stimulate TL1A secretion by DCs via TLR-signaling (TLR-4), LPS-induced and NFkB-dependent pathway [16]. Moreover, there is an inhibitory component of the TL1A receptor which could augment pro-inflammatory pathways at the intestinal mucosa by rendering activated lymphocytes resistant to apoptosis. Thus, increased expression of this inhibitory TL1A receptor may offer a survival advantage to effector lymphocytes, preventing their elimination and perpetuating tissue injury [2].

2.1.3. IL-8

IL-8, as a member of the CXC chemokines family, is not only a strong chemoattractant for neutrophils, monocytes, etc. but also triggers the secretion of superoxide anions and lysosomal enzymes in neutrophils, thus contributing to the tissue damage during inflammation. IL-8 mRNA expression in the inflamed mucosa is shown to be significantly higher than the level in non-inflamed mucosa of IBD patients or in the normal mucosa of non-IBD patients [13].

2.2. Th1 profile-related cytokines

Th1 cells are an essential part of the adaptive immune response, mainly against intracellular microorganisms and protozoa. The master transcription factors for Th1 definition are STAT4 and T-bet. Th1 cells in gut mucosa which are induced by increased levels of IL-12 and IL-18 are thought to cause intestinal inflammation in CD patients via production of high amounts of IFNγ. The latter induces enterocyte apoptosis and triggers the release of TNFα by activated mucosal macrophages. Th1 cells by themselves appear as an important source of TNFα [10].

2.2.1. IFNγ

IFNγ is a mediator of intestinal inflammation in CD, but contradictory reports exist for UC. However, increased levels of IFNγ have been observed in the inflamed mucosa from UC patients too. IFNγ levels also correlated with the clinical activity but not with the endoscopic score in UC, whereas no correlation to the clinical activity was observed in CD patients [12].

2.2.2. IL-12

The role of IL-12 in intestinal inflammation will be discussed later along with IL-23.

2.2.3. IL-1

IL-1 exists in two forms, IL-1α and IL-1β, encoded by different genes but exhibit almost identical functions [16]. The major sources of IL-1 are activated myeloid cells and its production can be induced by bacterial lipopolysaccharide, TNFα, IFNα, IFN-β, IFN-γ, as well as IL-1. IL-1 was found to promote Th17 development in the presence of IL-6 and TGFβ, and also to potentiate their actions in humans but not in mice. Moreover, it has been reported that IL-1 can increase their effect on Th17 definition. However, the mechanism through which IL-1 influences Th17 differentiation is not fully determined yet [17]. Some suggestions include that IL-1β or IL-1α cooperates with IL-23 to enhance IL-17 production independent of TCR stimulation. Additionally, IL-1 may suppress the inhibitory effect which IL-2 exerts on Th17 cell production through induction of IL-1R, IL-23R, and transcription factor RORγt [16].

IL-1β was shown to be increased in CD and UC patients, whereas the IL-1-receptor/IL-1β ratio was negatively associated with the IBD activity. When comparing the IBD patients with controls, a significant variation in genotype frequency of the IL-1β promoter polymorphism was found. Higher levels of the pro-inflammatory cytokine IL-1β would be expected to increase the likelihood of developing IBD since higher levels of such cytokines occur in this disease [15].

2.2.4. IL-18

IL-18 is another member of the IL-1 pro-inflammatory cytokine family. IL-18 is an epithelial-derived cytokine that has been proposed to promote barrier function in the intestine, but its effects on intestinal T cells are poorly understood. Although IL-18 is mainly responsible for inducing IFNγ production and Th1 differentiation, this cytokine might be involved in Th17 cell definition as well. Antigen-presenting cells express IL-18R on their surface and its binding with the cytokine is required for generation of Th17 cells through an IL-23-dependent mechanism. Moreover, IL-18 synergizes with IL-23 in the induction of Th17 cell [16] However, there are more reliable proofs about the involvement of IL-18R in Th17 cell definition, but not for IL-18 itself. Probably this action might be fulfilled through binding of an unknown alternative ligand, distinct from IL-18, to the receptor [17]. In contrast, Maloy et al. [18] demonstrated that during steady state, intestinal epithelial cells constitutively secrete IL-18, which acts directly on IL-18R1-expressing CD4+ T cells to limit colonic Th17 cell differentiation. In addition, they found that IL-18R1 signaling was critical for Tregs-mediated control of intestinal inflammation, though IL-18R1 is not required for Tregs development [18]. Thus, since IL-18 may regulate differentially homeostatic and inflammatory subsets of T cells, this finding has potential for treatment of IBD and other chronic inflammatory disorders.

IL-18 was found elevated in the inflamed colonic mucosa of UC and CD patients and poly-morphisms in the IL-18R1-IL-18RAP locus are associated with IBD susceptibility [18]. More-over, the local expression of IL-18 has been shown to be associated with the grade of inflammation [19].

2.3. Th2 profile-related cytokines

Th2 cells, another important part of the adaptive immune system, are mainly involved in the effector responses against extracellular parasites, including helminths, as well as in allergy pathogenesis. They are defined by the transcription factors STAT6 and GATA3 [7]. The importance of Th2 response in IBD is still under debate. In UC, the inflammatory response is less skewed along specific pathways, even though there is enhanced production of IL-4, IL-5, and IL-13, cytokines made by Th2 cells, unlike CD where Th1 activation has been mainly employed in pathogenesis [20].

2.3.1. IL-13

IL-13 exerts the potential to increase intestinal permeability and induce both enterocyte differentiation and apoptosis. IL-13 is released mainly by Th2 cells but another source of that cytokine is NKT cells. NKT cells express surface CD161 but not invariant T cell receptor, which is a well-established characteristic of this population. They produce IL-13 in response to stimulation of antigen-presenting cells expressing surface CD1d. Most probably, these atypical NKT cells are stimulated to produce IL-13 in the colonic mucosa by flora-derived microbial products [2]. This was observed in patients with UC, but not in CD patients. Further studies revealed that CD161-expressing NKT cells showed IL-13-dependent cytotoxic activity against colon epithelial cells [2]. Moreover, IL-13 independently exerts harmful effects on epithelial barrier function, such as derangement of tight junction integrity, decreased restitution velocity, etc. [2]. Therefore, blockade of IL-13 downstream signaling may be an effective anti-inflam-matory approach in UC which requires further investigations.

2.3.2. IL-11

IL-11 is a member of the IL-6 cytokine family and exerts pleiotropic effects on various cell types as it acts synergistically with other cytokines such as IL-3 and IL-4, thus it has been implicated in Th2-mediated sensitization and inflammation. IL-11 also prevents cell death and inhibits inflammation at sites of tissue injury. IL-11 mediates anti-inflammatory effects by down-regulation of LPS-induced NFkB activation, thus preventing transcription of inflammatory genes [12]. This may be implemented in IBD therapy, but still needs additional verification.

2.3.3. IL-33

IL-33 is the latest identified member of the IL-1 family of cytokines. mRNA and protein expression of IL-33 was detected in normal colonic cells both at the surface epithelium and in crypts, as well as in inflamed bowel onto lamina propria mononuclear cells (CD11b+ mono-cytes/macrophages and CD19+ B cells), endothelial cells, and subepithelial myofibroblasts.

During active intestinal inflammation, IL-33 actively participates in the epithelial-immune cell crosstalk that takes place in IBD mucosa. IL-33 expression is augmented under stimulation with IL-1β and TNFα, two cytokines that are enriched at the inflamed mucosa and are of pathogenic relevance in UC, as well as after TLR-3 and TGFβ signals [2].

Regarding mucosal expression, up-regulation of IL-33 appears to be specific for UC, as it was not observed in CD colonic inflammation [2]. Moreover, IL-33-expressing myofibroblasts were absent in fissuring areas in patients with colonic CD. Therefore, these observations may provide information of distinctive pathway between the two forms of IBD [2].

IL-33 was shown also to induce particularly the expression of Th2 effector molecules IL-5 and IL-13. Given the central role of IL-13 in UC, IL-33 may be involved in UC pathogenesis through the induction of IL-13 secretion. It has been proposed that IL-33 may function as "alarmin" for the gut-associated immune system activating toward intestinal inflammation or perpetuating the ongoing one [2].

2.4. Prerequisite cytokines for Th17 development

To emphasize the importance of Th17 in intestinal inflammation, here we start with the description of the prerequisite cytokines for the development of Th17 cells from naïve T cells.

2.4.1. TGFβ1

Transforming growth factor β (TGFβ) is a potent cytokine with multi-faceted regulatory and inhibitory activities and has two forms—TGFβ1 and TGFβ2. TGFβ1 is a pleiotropic cytokine best known for its potential to induce peripheral tolerance in the absence of IL-6 [12]. One of the mechanisms by which TGFβ1 is able to maintain tolerance is to support the survival of naturally occurring FoxP3+ Tregs (nTregs) in thymus. In addition, along with IL-2 and retinoic acid, TGFβ1 promotes the differentiation of induced Tregs (iTregs). Another mechanism of TGFβ-induced tolerance is to suppress the innate immune cells such as DCs and NK cells [5].

TGFβ1 also regulates the development of resident macrophages in the normal intestine, which possess some unusual features such as constitutive production of IL-10 and TNFα, refractory to TLR stimulation, high expression of MHCII and CXCR1, and avid phagocytic activity. Thus, this is another mechanism through which TGFβ1 favours local homeostasis [21].

TGFβ1 plays an important role under inflammatory conditions. In the presence of IL-6, TGFβ1 drives the differentiation of Th17 cells which promotes further inflammation and augmentation of ongoing autoimmune conditions. In addition, TGFβ1 in combination with IL-4 promotes the differentiation of IL-9-producing and IL-10-producing T cells, which surprisingly lack suppressive function and also promote tissue inflammation [12]. Increased protein levels of TGFβ1 are found in the mucosa of both CD and UC patients, whose levels correlated with the severity of disease in CD but not in UC patients [5, 12]. We also found significantly higher gene and protein levels of TGFß1 in the inflamed mucosa of CD patients alone [22]. This is not surprising since the tissue remodeling properties of TGFβ1 are well-established. Interestingly, TGFβ1 orchestrates the differentiation of both Tregs and Th17 cells in a concentration-dependent manner—low doses induce Th17 cell differentiation while higher doses inhibit Th17 cell development and promote Tregs [5, 11].

2.4.2. IL-6

IL-6 is a pleiotropic cytokine with regulatory effects on inflammation development. In addition to its stimulatory effects (i.e. induction of acute phase proteins), IL-6 also has inhibitory functions (i.e. cessation of the antiviral antibody response after certain immunizations). Recent studies have demonstrated that IL-6 has a crucial role in the regulation of the balance between Th17 cells and Tregs [23]. IL-6 activates a receptor complex consisting of IL-6R and the signal transducing subunit gp130 which activates downstream STAT1 and STAT3. STAT3 regulates IL-6-induced expression of RORγt and RORα, the crucial transcription factors for Th17 cells. In contrast to STAT3 activation, STAT1 inhibits the development of Th17 cells. Although IL-6 activates both STAT1 and STAT3, it has been demonstrated that in Th17 cell activation, they play two different roles—STAT3 maintains while STAT1 suppresses it [23]. Furthermore, STAT family members activated by various cytokines provide both positive and negative regulation for Th17 development (i.e. IL-27 inhibits Th17 differentiation through STAT1) [23]. TGFβ1 can induce gene activation of both FoxP3 and RORγt, but FoxP3 is able to associate with RORγt, thus inhibiting its transcriptional activation. Nevertheless, in the presence of IL-6 this inhibition is abrogated, so IL-6 could act as a potent promoter of Th17 instead of Tregs differentiation. All facts taken together, IL-6 appears as the main partner of TGFβ in priming naïve T cells to IL-17 production, playing a pivotal role in Th17 polarization and initiation of inflammatory immune response. Currently, it is also accepted that IL-6 is able to induce expression of IL-23R in T cells, making them responsive to IL-23 which sustains the Th17 phenotype [17].

Increased levels of IL-6 and its soluble receptor are up-regulated in active CD patients, and mucosal IL-6 levels were correlated with the degree of clinical activity in CD and UC [12]. In consent with these findings, in a group of 37 IBD patients, we also found both mRNA transcripts of TGFβ1 and IL-6 up-regulated in patients' mucosa compared to the mucosa of non-IBD persons, along with increased IL-17 mRNA in inflamed tissue [22, 24].

Several polymorphisms regarding the IL-6 gene are described to be also associated with susceptibility to IBD development, such as IL-6 174 [15].

Although anti-IL-6 antibodies therapy has become a novel therapeutic strategy for some inflammatory and autoimmune disease, including CD, IL-6 inhibitory treatment acts primarily on initial CD4+ T cells response including Th17 differentiation, rather than on the effector phase [23]. However, it still remains controversial whether this antibody can inhibit Th17 differentiation in a manner that is clinically meaningful.

2.4.3. IL-23

IL-12 and IL-23 share the common p40 subunit, but whereas IL-12 drives the classical Th1 response characterized by IFNγ production, IL-23 maintains an IL-17-secreting T cell population. Th1 responses may develop normally in the absence of IL-23, but in IBD patients, their manifestations require the presence of IL-23. The systemic inflammatory response and the elevated concentrations of pro-inflammatory cytokines in the serum are driven by IL-12 while the local intestinal inflammation and production of IL-17 in the intestinal mucosa are controlled by IL-23 [11, 12, 25].

IL-23 is crucial in orchestrating the crosstalk between innate and adaptive immunity with a key role in driving early responses to microbes. In a recent study, Kamada et al. showed that IL-23 is secreted preferentially by a subset of sentinel mucosal cells expressing both macrophage (i.e. CD14, CD33, CD68) and DC markers (i.e. CD205, CD209) [26]. These cells are present in a large number in CD-involved tissue and produce IL-12 and IL-23 in response to environmental danger signals [8, 26]. The presence of pathogens or pathogen-related products (such as lipopolysaccharide) can strongly influence the production of IL-12 and/or IL-23 depending on the microbial agent. This happens within a few hours after exposure and these early events in pathogen encounter are likely to shape subsequent responses toward IL-12 or IL-23 expression [8]. It was shown that some of the pathogenic functions of IL-23 in the gut are mediated by atypical T cell populations, such as γδT cells, invariant NK cells, and innate lymphoid cells, inducing them to secrete Th17-related cytokines and contributing to intestinal inflammation [10]. IL-23 might be also closely associated with the neutrophil influx [12].

The precise function of IL-23 in Th17 regulation is still not entirely clear, although there are a lot of speculations. IL-23 failed to induce the differentiation of naïve T cells into Th17 cells due to lack of IL-23R on naïve T cells [16]. It was subsequently demonstrated that IL-23R is not expressed on naïve T cells. Instead, IL-23 acts as a survival signal for Th17 cells by the mechanism probably similar to TNFα [23, 27].

The synthesis of the common p40 subunit for both IL-12 and IL-23, and the functional heterodimeric IL-23 is enhanced in the gut of CD patients [11]. Along with other authors' findings, we detected up-regulated mRNA levels of IL-23 in inflamed mucosa, as well as significantly increased serum level of IL-23 among IBD patients in comparison with non-IBD persons [24], and we suggest that anti-IL-23 therapy could be beneficial for IBD patients.

Identification of multiple single nucleotide polymorphisms (SNPs) in the IL-23 receptor gene that has been associated with both UC and CD suggested that the IL-23 axis might play a central role in chronic inflammation. IL-23R SNPs that influence IBD susceptibility have provided a new picture of the way the local immune response can promote intestinal tissue damage [11]. Small differences in cytokine levels as a result of gene polymorphisms may have an important effect on the inflammatory response and thus, influence the pathophysiology of IBD [15]. Interestingly, one of these polymorphisms, Arg381Gln, confers protection against developing CD [20]. Nonetheless, the mechanism through which these SNPs confer either risk or protection from IBD remains unknown [15].

2.5. Th17 cells and produced cytokines

The discovery of an IL-23-dependent T cell population that produces IL-17 but not IFNγ or IL-4 suggested there is an additional Th cell subset. Th17 cells have derived their name from their ability to produce IL-17, also termed IL-17A. Th17 cells also produce other cytokines including IL-17F, IL-21, IL-22, TNFα, and IL-6 [17, 23]. However, analysis at the single cell level has revealed that not all Th17 cells secrete the whole spectrum of cytokines, probably reflecting the heterogeneity of this cell's subset [25]. The IL-17 cytokine family also includes IL-17B, IL-17C, IL-17D (IL-27), IL-17E (IL-25), and IL-17A/F (**Figure 1**). The cytokines IL-27 and IL-25 have lowest protein homology to IL-17A. They are not produced by Th17 cells but act as negative regulators on the Th17 subset development. IL-27 is structurally related to IL-6 and is able to attenuate chronic inflammation by promoting IL-10 production [17]. In line with this, IL-27 and IFNγ are responsible for the inhibition of Th17 development in a STAT1-dependent manner [23], as described above. Another negative regulator of Th17 cells is IL-25, identified as a genetic homologue of IL-17, produced by Th2 and mast cells. IL-25 is involved in the expression of the Th2 cytokines IL-5 and IL-13, thus, favors Th2 responses. IL-25 deficiency is involved in pathologic inflammation, associated with increased expression of IL-17 and IL-23 [17].

CCR6, presented not only on Th17 cells, but also on Tregs, B cells, neutrophils and immature DC, plays a critical role in the migration of these cells to the sites of inflammation. TGFβ1 was shown to be the main factor for induction of CCR6 mRNA expression in Th17 cells and DCs [19]. IL-17-producing Th memory cells selectively express both CCR6 and CCR4, unlike Th cells producing IFNγ or both IFNγ and IL-17 which express CCR6 and CXCR3 [16]. Indeed, CCR4 is important for homing to the gut, where most RORγt+IL-17+ T cells are found [16].

The relationship among Th1, Th2, and Th17 cells is complex and still not clear. Th1- and Th2-related cytokines inhibit Th17 cell differentiation while IL-17 is not able to suppress Th1 or Th2 cells, or does it weakly. The suppression of IFNγ and IL-4 or their absence represents a way by which TGFβ1 could promote Th17 cell development. TGFβ1-driven Th17 cell differentiation can also occur in the absence of IFNγ and IL-4 [11]. In parallel with these findings, it was reported that IL-17-producing cells could be generated independent of the specific cytokines and transcription factors required for Th1 and Th2 differentiation [17]. Moreover, Th17 cells could develop from naïve T cells only in the combined presence of IL-6 and TGFβ1 [12, 20]. Thus, TGFβ induction of Th17 cells and also of Tregs, which are usually contradictory acting, is dependent on the presence of IL-6. This explains the apparent discrepancy of TGFβ1 involvement in both anti- and pro-inflammatory events in the intestine mucosa [17].

2.5.1. IL-17

IL-17 is an effector cytokine in gut immunity, which may have either pro-inflammatory or tissue-protective effects in the mucosa depending on the experimental or clinical model used. On one hand, IL-17 contributes to the mucosal barrier function by several mechanisms which, upon activation, result in a mucosal immune response toward pathogens [6]. IL-17 also promotes tight junction formation and increases trans-epithelial resistance in polarized intestinal epithelial cells by stimulating the production of antimicrobial peptides such as lipocalin-2, β-defensins, and calprotectin. This suggests that the latter are involved in the maintenance of immunological homeostasis and/or in the control of specific inflammatory pathways [19]. Thus, the Th-17-related cytokines mediate protective effects in host gut against various bacteria and fungi, particularly at mucosal surfaces [10, 11]. Interestingly, pathogens that have evolved to take advantage of various aspects of the mucosal response gain an edge over the resident commensal bacteria and colonize the gut with priority. Despite that Th17 responses appear to be detrimental by promoting pathogen colonization of the mucosa, in the end, they result in decrease in bacterial dissemination from the mucosa that protects the host by inducing slight inflammation [6]. In line with this, it was shown that Th17 cells are constitutively present in the human and mouse intestinal mucosa and that Th phenotype is driven by the commensal bacteria in the gut. Additionally, stimulation of DCs with TLR ligands (e.g. fungal Dectin-1) induces synthesis of IL-6, TNFα, and IL-23 that promotes the differentiation of Th17 cells [11]. From this point of view, blocking Th-17 cytokines could have more deleterious than beneficial effects for the host [25].

On the other hand, IL-17 might mediate tissue inflammation by triggering several inflammatory pathways and by inducing various pro-inflammatory cytokines (e.g. IL-1, IL-6, TNFα, G-CSF, GM-CSF), chemokines (e.g. IL-18, CXCL-1, CXCL8, MIP-1), and enzymes (COX-2, matrix metalloproteinases). Both IL-17 and IL-22 stimulate granulopoiesis by inducing expression of the granulocyte colony stimulating factor (G-CSF) and IL-17A which rapidly recruits neutrophils to the inflammatory site. This mechanism has important evolutionary significance [25]. The neutrophil response gains time for the induction of the following antimicrobial Th1-IFNγ response which takes several days to develop. Once the appropriate immune effector functions occur, the IL-12/IFNγ axis becomes the dominant pathway in host defence. This is important for initial control of the infection, but if the IL-23/IL-17 immune pathway becomes dysregulated, there is a danger of autoimmune pathology development, such as IBD. These observations, including the fact that T-bet is expressed at lower level in Th17 cells, led McKenzie et al. to favour the hypothesis of a common lineage precursor of Th1 and Th17 cells [8]. Furthermore, the tissue localization and timing of IL-12 versus IL-23 responses explain the idea that IL-12/IFNγ axis is involved in systemic inflammatory conditions (such as lupus), whereas the IL-23/IL-17 axis appears to regulate tissue-specific disorders (such as IBD) [8].

Another layer of complexity to the mucosal existence of Th17 cells is other cell types, which can secrete IL-17-related cytokines: γδT cells (secreting IL-17 in response to IL-23), NK, NKT cells (able to produce IL-17 and IL-22), and DCs (can secrete IL-22 in response to bacterial infection). Paneth cells, which are common in the ileum, also secrete IL-17A [6, 19]. As all these cells express the IL-23 receptor, the secretion of IL-23 by DCs comprises a trigger which potentiates early T cell activation and adaptive immunity development [6]. Thus, it appears that early activation of both adaptive and atypical innate-like T cells can lead to the expression of IL-17 and IL-22. However, dysregulated production of IL-17, IL-22, and TNFα in local tissue can result in chronic immune-mediated tissue destruction [8].

Studies in murine models of IBD strongly suggest that Th17 cells and their related cytokines contribute to tissue-damaging immune responses in the gut [25]. Up-regulation of Th17-related cytokines, however, does not represent a specific hallmark of IBD in humans, as increased levels of IL-17A and other Th17-related-markers have been seen in patients with rheumatoid arthritis, multiple sclerosis, psoriasis, etc. [11]. Immunohistochemistry studies have shown that in active UC, the IL-17-expressing cells were located mainly within the lamina propria, while in active CD, these cells were scattered throughout the submucosa and muscularis propria of the gut. Corresponding with this, it was shown that RNA transcripts for IL-17A and IL-17F were up-regulated in the inflamed mucosa of UC and CD patients [3, 11, 22, 28]. Both IL-17 and IL-23 are correlated to the severity of UC [12]. More recently, Annunziato et al. demonstrated that the number of IL-17-producing T cells is higher in CD than in normal gut mucosa, and some of these cells also produce IFNγ [29].

Th17 cells have shown possession of functional plasticity. Some of the IL-17A-producing cells simultaneously express IFNγ (**Figure 1**). Majority of IL-17/ IFNγ-producing cells express CD161, a well-known marker of NKT cells, also identified recently on IL-17-producing memory T cells [11]. Th17 cells can be converted into Th1 cells if they receive appropriate stimuli, such as IL-12 which enhances the expression of Th1-related markers (i.e. T-bet and IFNγ) and down-regulates RORγt and IL-17. Additionally, recent studies have shown that treatment of intestinal lymphocytes with IL-23 can facilitate the production of either IL-17A or IFNγ in UC or CD, respectively [11].

This is in consent with the demonstration that some of the pathogenic effects of IL-23 in the gut are linked to the ability of this cytokine to turn on IFNγ production. Switching from IL-17A to IFNγ production occurs if Th17 cells are activated by a lack of TGFβ1 [25]. Th17 cells and their possible conversion to Treg direction is going to be described later.

This very complex and non-equivocal relationship of both pro-inflammatory and tissue-protective effects of IL-17 in the gut may explain the unsuccessful anti-IL-17 therapy in CD patients [10].

2.5.2. IL-21

IL-21, an IL-2-related cytokine produced by Th17 cells in response to IL-6, increases the expansion of this cell subtype by a positive autoregulatory feedback loop. IL-21, which is up-regulated in inflamed IBD mucosa, induces Th1 and Th17 immune responses in the mucosa [10], but a mixture of both Th1 and Th17 cytokines is needed to promote full pathology in the gut. In this context, a promising inducer could be IL-21, whose activity seems to be necessary for expanding both Th1 and Th17 cell responses in the intestine. [25]. As we have already noticed, IL-21 is overproduced in the gut mucosa of IBD patients, but the vast majority of IL-21-producing CD4+ T cells co-express IFNγ but not IL-17A. This fact suggests that Th1 but not Th17 cells are the major sources of IL-21 in the human gut [11]. There is evidence that IL-21 also enhances the expression of Th1-related transcriptional factors and IFNγ production in NK cells [11].

IL-21, like IL-17, stimulates gut fibroblasts to produce tissue-degrading matrix-metalloprotei-nases and enhances the secretion of chemoattractants (i.e. MIP-3α) by epithelial cells [10, 11]. IL-21, like IL-6, could also initiate Th17 differentiation together with TGFβ1 [23], even in the absence of IL-6 [16, 17]. IL-21 enhances the expression of IL-23R in Th17 cells, through a process that is dependent on STAT3 and RORγt, making these cells responsive to IL-23. IL-21 as well exerts additional biological functions that could contribute to its pro-inflammatory effect in the gut like inhibition of the peripheral differentiation of Tregs and making CD4+ T cells resistant to Treg-mediated immune suppression [11].

2.5.3. IL-22

IL-22 is a member of the IL-10 cytokine family and a Th17-related cytokine but it appears to be differentially regulated. IL-22 provides signals through a heterodimer comprising IL-22R and IL-10Rβ. The IL-22 receptor is highly expressed in tissues such as epithelial cells of the gastrointestinal tract. Via STAT3 signaling pathway, the activation of proliferative and/or anti-apoptotic programs starts, and this allows maintenance of epithelial barriers of the gut [5]. Most of the Th17 cytokines are highly dependent on the transcription factor RORγt for their expression, unlike IL-22 whose expression is dependent on the transcription factor aryl hydrocarbon receptor [5]. Th22 cells are another Th subpopulation characterized by the expression of this transcription factor and secretion of mainly IL-22 [5].

IL-22 has a dual functional nature in modulating the responses during tissue remodeling. IL-22 promotes induction of acute inflammatory proteins, mucins, and antimicrobial peptides (i.e. β-defensins), which are important for tissue integrity during inflammation. This mechanism ensures proper organ function and escape of potentially harmful effects by restricting the passage of luminal commensal flora and food antigens to the lamina propria [5, 25, 30]. It is important to point out that this process depends on the inflammatory context (the overall cytokine milieu and the tissues involved). Thus, IL-22 is important for control of pathogenic bacteria that need to translocate through host epithelial barriers to disseminate, especially in the gastrointestinal tract [5]. IL-22 also enhances intestinal barrier integrity by stimulating epithelial cell growth, goblet cell restitution, and mucus production, thus contributing to the healing of damaged tissue.

On the other hand, IL-22 can cause further inflammation by stimulating colonic fibroblasts to secrete inflammatory cytokines (e.g. TNFα, IL-8, IL-11, and leukaemia inhibitory factor), IL-6, chemokines, and matrix metalloproteinases [11]. It is not surprising that IL-22 is highly expressed during chronic inflammation [5] in mucosal samples of patients with active CD, because of the known dysbacteriosis and expected pathological microbial agents, and to a lesser degree in patients with UC, where autoimmune phenomena are more common.

IL-22 is also expressed by innate immune cells such as CD11c+ and NK cells located in the colon. The latter cells do not secrete IFNγ and are not highly cytotoxic [30]. IL-23, a traditional activator of NK cells, induces IL-22 expression in NK cells. Unlike TGFβ and IL-10 that directly modulate the immune response, IL-22 does not have direct effects on immune cells since these cells lack the expression of IL-22R [30]. This way, TGFβ1 and IL-10 are involved in maintaining immune homeostasis under steady-state conditions instead.

IL-22 is an ideal therapeutic candidate since it specifically modulates tissue remodeling and does not have direct effects on the immune response. Treatment with recombinant cytokine or gene therapy delivery of IL-22 may alleviate tissue destruction during inflammation owing to its selective modulation of tissue responses [5].

2.6. Role of FoxP3+ Tregs and related cytokines in gut inflammation

The main function of Tregs is to modulate the adaptive immune responses, and forkhead/winged helix transcription factor forkhead box P3 (FoxP3) is the master transcription factor for Tregs [23]. Two main subpopulations of Tregs have been best described: naïve (nTregs) and inducible Tregs (iTregs). The latter is believed to be derived by peripheral transformation of naïve T cells stimulated by IL-19, vitamin D3, antigens, and TGFβ1. So far, Treg function in IBD is not completely characterized [12].

Tregs are crucially involved in the maintenance of gut mucosal homeostasis by suppressing abnormal immune responses against the commensal flora or dietary antigens. They exert their function by producing the anti-inflammatory cytokines IL-10 and TGFβ, thus preventing both the activation and the effector function of T cells. Additionally, the regulatory activities of the immune response through mediators such as IL-10 and TGFβ still need to be profiled, especially those that might take place in the unaffected areas of IBD patients [14]. A certain number of Th17 and CD4+CD25+FoxP3+ Tregs cell is presented in the intestine even in the healthy state, partly due to the presence of enteric bacteria which favor the production of both Th17 and Tregs. DCs in the intestine or mesenteric lymph nodes also actively promote the production of both cell types. However, there are points of divergence, for example, the retinoic acid produced by DCs in the intestine induces only Tregs. In spite of the essential function of IL-2 as a growth factor of effector T cells, including Tregs, IL-2 has an inhibitory effect on Th17 cell production. Furthermore, IL-2 deficiency leads to systemic autoimmune disease, partly because of its involvement in the differentiation and survival of Tregs [16]. Recent studies have revealed that IL-2 deficiency promotes differentiation of Th17 cell subset in a STAT5-dependent mechanism. At present, the recognized precise mechanism is exerted by suppression of IL-17 expression by directly binding to the IL-17 gene promoter of STAT5 [16].

The importance of Tregs in maintaining immune homeostasis was once again emphasized with the X-linked IPEX syndrome (immune dysregulation, polyendocrinopathy, enteropathy), caused by mutation of FoxP3. IPEX patients quite often complain of gastrointestinal symptoms, suggesting that Tregs dysfunction may be involved in human IBD too [31].

A significant increase in production of Tregs in active-phase IBD mucosal lesions, as well as decreased numbers of Tregs in peripheral blood of IBD patients was described [9]. However, in active IBD a reduced number of peripheral Tregs have been reported to be reverted by anti-TNF treatment [12]. Indeed, Tregs are increased in the intestinal mucosa of IBD patients in comparison with the mucosa of healthy volunteers [22, 24, 27, 32]. Tregs isolated from inflamed tissue display no obvious defect in their suppressive function, at least in vitro [9]. However, Monteleone et al. found that Tregs obtained from the active-phase IBD mucosal lesions possess an ability to suppress T cell activation [11, 25]. Since Th17 cells appear to be resistant to the Tregs-mediated immunosuppression, it is likely that during chronic inflammatory process, such as in IBD, Tregs may be dysfunctional and might augment rather than suppress Th17-mediated immune responses [11]. At first, this phenomenon was explained as a feedback loop associated with an increase in the Treg cell attracted by IL-2 which is produced locally at sites of inflammation. On the other hand, however, up-regulated Th17 cells in response to increased production of pro-inflammatory cytokines were postulated [27]. Th17 cells, but not Tregs, are induced in the presence of pro-inflammatory cytokines, in addition to TGFβ1. Thus, Treg dysfunction may not be intrinsic but rather due to extrinsic milieu of activated cells that are resistant to suppression, and pro-inflammatory settings in the affected IBD mucosa [9, 33].

Plasticity of Tregs and Th17 is further demonstrated by the possibility of conversion between both subsets [27, 33]. Hu et al. have reported that Tregs express membrane-bound TGFβ and in the presence of IL-6, they convert to Th17 cells [34]. This could be an important warning regarding cell therapy with Tregs to treat chronic immune disease, including IBD, because the "homeostatic" Tregs may convert to pathogenic Th17 cells during inflammation where IL-6 is abundant [27]. Numerous studies have shown that in inflammatory cytokine environment, Tregs can lose FoxP3 expression and acquire expression of other transcription factors that define another lineage of CD4+ T cells as well as effector function. As we have already mentioned, exposure of Tregs to IL-6 results in a partial conversion to Th17 cells. Interestingly, although most IL-17-producing cells lost FoxP3 expression, some cells express both FoxP3 and IL-17. It is unclear, however, whether the resultant cells are suppressive [9]. So, once again it must be mentioned that the Th17/Tregs balance appears to play a very crucial role in IBD development [27].

2.6.1. IL-10

IL-10 is secreted by many types of immune cells including Th2, Tregs, Tr1 (IL-10-producing FoxP3-CD4+ T cells), Th3 (TGFβ and IL-10-producing CD4+ T cells induced in oral tolerance), NKT cells, B cells, macrophages, and DCs [5]. IL-10 binds to its heterodimeric receptor, composed of unique for IL-10 subunit (IL-10Rα) and shared with IL-22 subunit (IL-10Rβ). Although not completely sufficient, STAT3 is required for the inhibitory functions of IL-10. Importantly, STAT3 induces the expression of transcription factors that regulate various cytokine signaling pathways including IL-6. IL-10 down-regulates IL-12 production and expression of co-stimulatory molecules in macrophages and DCs, thereby reducing the Th1 response generation [5].

IL-10 is a key regulator of the immune system by limiting the inflammatory responses that could otherwise cause tissue damage. IL-10 is essential for homeostasis of the immune system, especially in the gastrointestinal tract where the tolerance is most needed. Evidence for that is the highly-susceptible-to-colitis IL-10-deficient mice which develop aberrant immune responses to commensal bacteria. This colitis is more severe when combined with a deficiency in TGFβ signaling [5].

Small intestine and colonic lamina propria showed the highest frequency of IL-10-expressing cells. Recent findings show that macrophages in the lamina propria preferentially induce IL-10-producing cells while DCs promote the generation of Th17 cells. On one hand, blocking IL-10 during infection can result in more severe pathology or even fatality of the host, but on the other hand, high production of IL-10 is associated with sustained chronic infections and its blockade promotes pathogen clearance. Thus, once again, the milieu of the intestines favors the generation of IL-10-producing T cells leading to tolerance against commensal bacteria, whereas the expression of IL-10 in peripheral tissues under infectious conditions leads to suppression of the immune response [5]. In line with this, when IL-10 was previously found to be abundantly expressed by macrophages in areas of dense inflammatory infiltrate, it had been directly related to the attenuation of the mucosal inflammation [14]. Knowing nowadays about the dual role of IL-10, it is not unexpected that IL-10 is presented at a higher level in the inflamed mucosa of IBD patients [13]. These findings were confirmed by us as well [24].

Some IL-10 gene polymorphisms have been associated with susceptibility to IBD (i.e. IL-10−1082) and more significantly with UC alone. Whether the polymorphisms are directly involved in regulating cytokine production, and consequently disease pathophysiology of IBD, or serve merely as markers that are in linkage disequilibrium with susceptibility genes, is still unclear [15].

The involvement of IL-10 in the regulation of the pathogenic function of Th17 cells has been definitively demonstrated in experiments where non-pathogenic Th17 subtype expressing IL-10 is generated by IL-6 and TGFβ1, even though in the absence of IL-23. These cells also prevent the induction of the disease in an IL-10-dependent manner [35]. Even though IL-10 effectively treats colitis in mouse models and suppresses inflammatory cytokine production in vitro in intestinal cells of patients with IBD, clinical trials using recombinant IL-10 to treat IBD in humans have been largely disappointing, irrespective of the acceptable side-effect profile of the therapy [36].

2.7. Role of innate lymphoid cells in gut inflammation

Innate lymphoid cells (ILCs) are recently described cells that have been involved in both maintenance and loss of gut homeostasis. ILCs are phenotypically and functionally distinct subsets of cells that inhabit the intestinal mucosa. However, they produce cytokines associated with effector T-cell responses early in inflammatory lesions of patients with IBD [37]. The novel family of cells comprises three subsets: ILC1, ILC2, and ILC3 [38]. ILC1 express the transcription factor T-bet resembling Th1 cells with production of IFN-γ and TNF; thus, they contribute to host resistance to intestinal pathogens. ILC2 produce Th2 cytokines, such as IL-5 and IL-13, and they are dependent on the transcription factor GATA-3. ILC3 which express the transcription factor RORγt produce IL-17A and IL-22 mirroring Th17 cells [37]. ILC3 is involved in gut homeostasis by secreting IL-22 and promoting IL-10 and antimicrobial peptide production. Epithelial stress-induced ligands and inflammatory conditions may switch ILC3 to ILC1 secreting TNF and IFN-γ under the influence of IL-12. The pro-inflammatory cytokines of ILC1 and ILC3 lead mainly to epithelial apoptosis and neutrophil recruitment. ILC2 are able to contribute to IBD complications by producing the fibrogenic cytokine IL-13 [37].

Since ILCs might be substantial drivers of mucosal inflammation, targeting ILC subsets may be a new exciting treatment option for IBD patients.

3. Conclusion

From a clinical perspective, IBD is a chronic persistent disease characterized by repeated relapses and remissions. One explanation could be that memory Th cells created during the disease development persist in the body, including during remission, in a manner that is dependent on the various cytokine presentations. Effector cytokines in the mucosa may induce inflammation at the time of the initial episode and during relapses. However, the ambiguity and contradictory actions of given cytokines confound the understanding of their interactions in dynamics of the immune response, and that leads to lack of synonymous conclusions about them. There is still strong need for further investigation, particularly in the gut mucosa, to fully comprehend their roles in the complex dynamic network of the immune mediators.

Th17 cells have been shown to play a central role in murine and human IBD. Inhibition of the Th17 pathway may be a promising treatment for IBD, with respect to the role of other subsets of Th1 and Th2 cells. The data in the literature and our own experience make us believe that in order to achieve immune homeostasis in the gut, pro-inflammatory and anti-inflammatory responses that define the mucosal cell immunophenotype, should achieve balance. Thus, following the clinical periods of remissions and relapses, it is important to observe their immunological equivalents in the gut and possibly in whole blood, namely regulatory and pro-inflammatory cytokines secreted by different types of immunocompetent cells.

Acknowledgements

We would like to thank the Medical University of Sofia, Bulgaria [Grant No.22/2012] and the Medical Faculty of Trakia University, Stara Zagora, Bulgaria [Grant No.4/2012] for the financial support of our studies regarding cytokines expression in inflamed mucosa. We are also immensely grateful to Stoyanka Petrova and Radislav Nakov for coordination of the financial support for this publication. We would also like to show our gratitude to Iliya Karakolev and Kalina Toumangelova-Yuzeir for assistance with some aspects of the methodology.

Author details

Tsvetelina Velikova[1*], Dobroslav Kyurkchiev[1], Ekaterina Ivanova-Todorova[1], Zoya Spassova[2], Spaska Stanilova[3] and Iskra Altankova[4]

*Address all correspondence to: ts_velikova@abv.bg

1 Department of Clinical Laboratory and Clinical Immunology, Medical University of Sofia, University Hospital St. Ivan Rilski, Sofia, Bulgaria

2 Clinic of Gastroenterology, University Hospital St. Ivan Rilski, Medical University of Sofia, Sofia, Bulgaria

3 Department of Molecular Biology, Immunology and Medical Genetics, Medical Faculty of Trakia University, Stara Zagora, Bulgaria

4 Clinical Immunology, University Hospital Lozenets, Sofia University, Sofia, Bulgaria

References

[1] Blumberg R. Inflammation in the intestinal tract: pathogenesis and treatment. Dig Dis. 2009;27(4):455–64. DOI: 10.1159/000235851

[2] Bamias G, Kaltsa G, Ladas SD. Cytokines in the pathogenesis of ulcerative colitis. Discov Med. 2011;11(60):459–67.

[3] Fujino S, Andoh A, Bamba S, Ogawa A, Hata K, Araki Y, Bamba T, Fujiyama Y. Increased expression of interleukin 17 in inflammatory bowel disease. Gut. 2003;52(1):65–70. DOI: 10.1136/gut.52.1.65

[4] Danese S, Angelucci E. New and emerging biologics in the treatment of inflammatory bowel disease: quo vadis? Gastroenterol Clin Biol. 2009;33(Suppl. 3):S217–27. DOI: 10.1016/S0399-8320(09)73157-4

[5] Sanjabi S, Zenewicz LA, Kamanaka M, Flavell RA. Anti-inflammatory and pro-inflammatory roles of TGF-beta, IL-10, and IL-22 in immunity and autoimmunity. Curr Opin Pharmacol. 2009;9(4):447–53. DOI: 10.1016/j.coph.2009.04.008

[6] Blaschitz C, Raffatellu M. Th17 cytokines and the gut mucosal barrier. J Clin Immunol. 2010;30(2):196–203. DOI: 10.1007/s10875-010-9368-7

[7] Romagnani S. Th1/Th2 cells. Inflamm Bowel Dis. 1999;5(4):285–94.

[8] McKenzie BS, Kastelein RA, Cua DJ. Understanding the IL-23-IL-17 immune pathway. Trends Immunol. 2006;27(1):17–23.

[9] Hardenberg G, Steiner TS, Levings MK. Environmental influences on T regulatory cells in inflammatory bowel disease. Semin Immunol. 2011;23(2):130–8. DOI: 10.1016/j.smim.2011.01.012

[10] Geremia A, Biancheri P, Allan P, Corazza GR, Di Sabatino A. Innate and adaptive immunity in inflammatory bowel disease. Autoimmun Rev. 2014;13(1):3–10. DOI: 10.1016/j.autrev.2013.06.004

[11] Monteleone I, Pallone F, Monteleone G. Interleukin-23 and Th17 cells in the control of gut inflammation. Mediators Inflamm. 2009;2009:1–7. DOI: 10.1155/2009/297645

[12] Florholmen J, Fries W. Candidate mucosal and surrogate biomarkers of inflammatory bowel disease in the era of new technology. Scand J Gastroenterol. 2011;46(12):1407–17. DOI: 10.3109/00365521.2011

[13] Matsuda R, Koide T, Tokoro C, Yamamoto T, Godai T, Morohashi T, Fujita Y, Takahashi D, Kawana I, Suzuki S, Umemura S. Quantitive cytokine mRNA expression profiles in the colonic mucosa of patients with steroid naïve ulcerative colitis during active and quiescent disease. Inflamm Bowel Dis. 2009;15(3):328–34. DOI: 10.1002/ibd.20759

[14] León A, Gómez E, Garrote J, Bernardo D, Barrera A, Marcos J, Fernández-Salazar L, Velayos B, Blanco-Quirós A, Arranz E. High levels of proinflammatory cytokines, but

not markers of tissue injury, in unaffected intestinal areas from patients with IBD. Mediators of Inflamm. 2009;2009:1–10. DOI: 10.1155/2009/580450

[15] Balding J, Livingstone WJ, Conroy J, Mynett-Johnson L, Weir DG, Mahmud N, Smith OP. Inflammatory bowel disease: the role of inflammatory cytokine gene polymor-phisms. Mediators Inflamm. 2004;13(3):181–7.

[16] Martinez GJ, Nurieva RI, Yang XO, Dong C. Regulation and function of proinflam-matory TH17 cells. Ann N Y Acad Sci. 2008;1143:188–211. DOI: 10.1196/annals. 1443.021

[17] González-García C, Martín-Saavedra F, Ballester A, Ballester S. The Th17 lineage: answers to some immunological questions. Inmunología. 2009;28(1):32–45. DOI: 10.1016/S0213-9626(09)70025-3

[18] Harrison OJ, Srinivasan N, Pott J, Schiering C, Krausgruber T, Ilott NE, Maloy KJ. Epithelial-derived IL-18 regulates Th17 cell differentiation and Foxp3+ Treg cell function in the intestine. Mucosal Immunol. 2015;8:1226–36. DOI: 10.1038/mi. 2015.13

[19] Bogaert S, Laukens D, Peeters H, Melis L, Olievier K, Boon N, Verbruggen G, Vandesompele J, Elewaut D, De Vos M. Differential mucosal expression of Th17-related genes between the inflamed colon and ileum of patients with inflammatory bowel disease. BMC Immunol. 2010;11:61. DOI: 10.1186/1471-2172-11-61

[20] Sarra M, Pallone F, Macdonald TT, Monteleone G. IL-23/IL-17 axis in IBD. Inflamm Bowel Dis. 2010;16(10):1808–13. DOI: 10.1002/ibd.21248

[21] Bain CC, Mowat AM. Macrophages in intestinal homeostasis and inflammation. Immunol Rev. 2014;260(1):102–17. DOI: 10.1111/imr.12192

[22] Velikova T, Karakolev I, Spassova Z, Kyurkchiev D, Altankova I, Stanilova S. Upregu-lation of mRNA cytokine expression profile in inflamed colonic mucosa of patients with inflammatory bowel disease. Comptes rendus de l'Académie bulgare des sciences: sciences mathématiques et naturelles. 2013;66(12):1769–76.

[23] Kimura A, Kishimoto T. IL-6: regulator of Treg/Th17 balance. Eur J Immunol. 2010;40(7): 1830–5. DOI: 10.1002/eji.201040391

[24] Velikova T. Investigation of immunological parameters for intestinal inflammation in order to establish new markers for diagnosis and follow-up of Inflammatory Bowel Disease patients [dissertation]. Sofia, Bulgaria: Medical University of Sofia; 2014. 146 p. DOI: 10.13140/RG.2.1.3594.6325

[25] Monteleone I, Pallone F, Monteleone G. Th17-related cytokines: new players in the control of chronic intestinal inflammation. BMC Med. 2011;9:122. DOI: 10.1186/1741-7015-9-122

[26] Kamada N, Hisamatsu T, Okamoto S, Chinen H, Kobayashi T, Sato T, Sakuraba A, Kitazume MT, Sugita A, Koganei K, Akagawa KS, Hibi T. Unique CD14 intestinal macrophages contribute to the pathogenesis of Crohn disease via IL-23/IFN-gamma axis. J Clin Invest. 2008;118(6):2269–80. DOI: 10.1172/JCI34610

[27] Kanai T, Nemoto Y, Kamada N, Totsuka T, Hisamatsu T, Watanabe M, Hibi T. Homeostatic (IL-7) and effector (IL-17) cytokines as distinct but complementary target for an optimal therapeutic strategy in inflammatory bowel disease. Curr Opin Gastroenterol. 2009;25(4):306–13. DOI: 10.1097/MOG.0b013e32832bc627

[28] Fonseca-Camarillo G, Mendivil-Rangel E, Furuzawa-Carballeda J, Yamamoto-Furusho JK. Interleukin 17 gene and protein expression are increased in patients with ulcerative colitis. Inflamma Bowel Dis. 2011;17(10):E135–6. DOI: 10.1002/ibd.21816

[29] Annunziato F, Cosmi L, Santarlasci V, Maggi L, Liotta F, Mazzinghi B, Parente E, Filì L, Ferri S, Frosali F, Giudici F, Romagnani P, Parronchi P, Tonelli F, Maggi E, Romagnani S. Phenotypic and functional features of human Th17 cells. J Exp Med. 2007;204(8):1849–61. DOI: 10.1084/jem.20070663

[30] Brand S, Beigel F, Olszak T, Zitzmann K, Eichhorst ST, Otte JM, Diepolder H, Marquardt A, Jagla W, Popp A, Leclair S, Herrmann K, Seiderer J, Ochsenkühn T, Göke B, Auern-hammer CJ, Dambacher J. IL-22 is increased in active Crohn's disease and promotes proinflammatory gene expression and intestinal epithelial cell migration. Am J Physiol Gastrointest Liver Physiol. 2006;290(4):G827–38.

[31] Hannibal MC, Torgerson T. IPEX Syndrome [Internet]. October 19, 2004 [Updated: January 27, 2011]. Available from: http://www.ncbi.nlm.nih.gov/books/NBK1118/ [Accessed: 2/12/2016].

[32] Ban H, Andoh A, Shioya M, Nishida A, Tsujikawa T, Fujiyama Y. Increased number of FoxP3+CD4+ regulatory T cells in inflammatory bowel disease. Mol Med Rep. 2008;1(5): 647–50. DOI: 10.3892/mmr_00000006

[33] Li L, Boussiotis VA. The role of IL-17-producing Foxp3+ CD4+ T cells in inflammatory bowel disease and colon cancer. Clin Immunol. 2013;148(2):246–53. DOI: 10.1016/j.clim.2013.05.003

[34] Hu H, Djuretic I, Sundrud MS, Rao A. Transcriptional partners in regulatory T cells: Foxp3, Runx and NFAT. Trends Immunol. 2007;28(8):329-32.

[35] McGeachy MJ, Chen Y, Tato CM, Laurence A, Joyce-Shaikh B, Blumenschein WM, McClanahan TK, O'Shea JJ, Cua DJ. The interleukin 23 receptor is essential for the terminal differentiation of interleukin 17-producing effector T helper cells in vivo. Nat Immunol. 2009;10(3):314–24. DOI: 10.1038/ni.1698

[36] Kelsall B. Interleukin-10 in inflammatory bowel disease. N Engl J Med. 2009;361(21): 2091–3. DOI: 10.1056/NEJMe0909225

[37] Goldberg R, Prescott N, Lord GM, MacDonald TT, Powell N. The unusual suspects—innate lymphoid cells as novel therapeutic targets in IBD. Nat Rev Gastroenterol Hepat. 2015;12:271–83. DOI: 10.1038/nrgastro.2015.52

[38] Spits H, et al. Innate lymphoid cells—a proposal for uniform nomenclature. Nat Rev Immunol. 2013;13:145–9. DOI: 10.1038/nri3365

2

Irritable Bowel Syndrome: Functional Gastrointestinal Disease Regulated by Nervous System

Victor V. Chaban

Abstract

A functional disorder is a medical condition that impairs the normal function, but without major organic cause such as irritation or inflammation and where the organ or part of the body looks completely normal under medical examination. The accumulation of abnormalities that limit body functions is a major risk factor for patients with irritable bowel syndrome (IBS), defined as a gastrointestinal disorder with abdominal pain or discomfort that is associated with a change in bowel habit. Often, this disorder is accompanied by the concomitant decline in cognitive or motor performance. Pain that in some patients is out of proportion to identifiable pathology is the most immediate and dramatic consequence of IBS and is responsible for a highly negative impact on quality of life and substantial workforce loss. For patients with IBS, the most common comorbid diagnoses include painful bladder syndrome (PBS) or chronic pelvic pain (CPP). Cells of the affected tissues may interact in cell-to-cell manner messages through the transfer of hormones, cytokines, and other mediators that influence normal functioning. The complex interplay and balance between these diverse mediators, ageing, genetic background, and environmental factors may ultimately determine the outcome of the progression of the functional disorder. On a cellular level, these responses are highly complex, involving a vast array of enzymes and receptors of virtually every class, directing recruitment of many types of cells to recover the healthy state. Indeed, a balance between the messengers with the inherent redundancy of the different body systems makes therapeutic intervention of functional disorders a considerable challenge.

Keywords: sensory neurons, extrinsic primary afferents, nociception

1. Introduction

The response properties of pelvic extrinsic primary afferent nerves (EPANs) play an important role in etiology of irritable bowel syndrome (IBS). Hypersensitivity of visceral mechanoreceptors could result from excessive production of modulatory neurotransmitters. In addition to direct stimulation of stretch-activated channels on primary afferent neurons located in dorsal root ganglia (DRG), chemicals produced by different target cells (such as smooth muscle cells and interstitial cells of Cajal) in response to stretch or inflammation play an important role in the neuromodulation of nociception. The incidence of persistent, episodic, or chronic visceral pain is more prevalent in females, which also suggests hormonal regulation. Despite extensive research of the properties of pelvic and splanchnic afferent nerves, little is known about the mechanisms underlying normal and pathological signal transduction pathways underlying many functional diseases. Despite considerable efforts by the scientific community and the pharmaceutical industry to develop novel pharmacological treatments aimed at chronic visceral pain, the traditional approaches to identifying and evaluating novel drugs for this target have largely failed to translate into effective IBS treatments [1]. A better understanding of these processes has direct implications for the development of more effective therapies. During the last decade, we identified that DRG neurons can be affected by ATP, NO, estrogen, and other mediators producing neuronal hyper- or desensitization that may unravel the enigma of the development of chronic pelvic pain associated with IBS. Moreover, our recent data that estrogen can gate primary afferent response to modulate nociception support the idea about involvement of peripheral central system in etiology of a wide range of the functional and inflammatory gastrointestinal diseases [2].

2. Role of EPANs in the mechanisms of visceral neurotransduction and modulation

Pelvic nerve afferent fibers innervating the visceral organs of the lower colon have been well characterized (reviewed in Ref. [3]). In general, during colonic distension, a large number of pelvic EPANs show static levels of discharge. Stretches that lead to the opening of stretch-activated (SA) channels on the plasma membrane lead to the selective or nonselective opening of different cation and anion channels in nodose ganglia and DRG neurons. Thus, depending on the cell type and channel type, EPANs activation may result in hyperpolarization, depolarization, or primarily Ca^{2+} influx. The function of SA channels in the plasma membrane differs between various cell types. Influx of Ca^{2+} may repolarize the plasma membrane via activation of K_{ca} channels and inactivating of voltage-gated calcium channels (VGCCs), and thus influence adaptation rates of sensory neurons during ongoing stimulations.

The cell bodies of primary visceral spinal afferent neurons are located in the lumbosacral (L1-S1) DRGs that transmit information about chemical or mechanical stimulation from the periphery to the spinal cord. Nociceptors are small- to medium-size DRG neurons whose peripheral processes detect potentially damaging physical and chemical stimuli. Until recently, ATP release from nonneuronal cells was thought to be exclusively as result of injury. It is now clear that certain integral membrane proteins contain an ATP-binding cassette so this neurotransmitter can act as signaling molecule modulating sensory afferent nerve terminals. Six P2X receptors are expressed in DRGs. Significantly, the P2X3 receptor is found exclusively in a subset of small diameter capsaicin sensitive peripheral sensory neurons (presumably nociceptors) [4]. Today, multiple lines of evidence suggest that ATP signaling via P2X receptors contribute to different pain phenotypes, therefore P2X antagonists may be useful analgesics. The availability of P2X receptor-specific antagonists also holds the promise of revealing the cellular and molecular neurobiology underlying pain states underlying functional diseases [5]. With sufficiently high levels of ATP, P2X and SA channels (which has a greater permeability for Ca^{2+} than Na^+) would depolarize nerve terminals directly producing action potentials and leading to sensation of pain. On the other hand, the response of EPANs may be tonically inhibited by NO produced by peripheral nerve terminals. The peripheral sensitization of nerve fibers is transient depending on the duration of stimuli and the presence of visceral (colonic) inflammation.

3. Estrogen receptors and visceral nociception associated with functional diseases

Changes in pain perception and variations of symptoms throughout the menstrual cycle, as well as sexual intercourse triggering symptoms in a significant portion of females diagnosed with irritable bowel syndrome (IBS), painful bladder syndrome (PBS), chronic pelvic pain (CPP), and other function syndromes, points to a connection with sex steroids. Several lines of evidence indicate that 17β-estradiol (E2) directly influence the functions of primary afferent neurons. Both subtypes of estrogen receptors (ERα and ERβ) are present in DRG neurons including the small-diameter putative nociceptors [4]. In vitro, ATP-sensitive DRG neurons respond to E2 [6, 7], which correlated well with the idea that visceral afferents are E2 sensitive: (i) visceral pain is affected by hormonal level in cycling females; (ii) there are sex differences in the prevalence of functional disorders involving the viscera; and (iii) putative visceral afferents fit into the population of DRG neurons that are sensitive to E2 [7]. These data suggest that in addition to the CNS actions, E2 can act in the periphery to modulate nociception [6, 7]. E2 modulates cellular activity by altering ion channel opening, G-protein signaling, and activation of trophic factor-like signal transduction pathways. These effects have been ascribed to membrane-associated receptors [8]. The results from our laboratory and others indicate that E2 acts in DRG neurons to modulate L-type VGCC and through group II metabotropic glutamate receptors [6].

E2 has a significant role in modulating visceral sensitivity, indicating that E2 alterations in sensory processing may underlie sex-based differences in functional pain symptoms [9]. Indeed in most clinical studies, women report more severe pain levels, more frequent pain, and longer duration of pain than men [10]. Little is known about E2-mediated mechanisms in peripheral nervous system, but the fact that DRG neurons express ERs and respond to E2 treatment suggest that they are a potential target for mediating nociception. E2 modulation of nociceptive response depends on the type of pain, its durations, and the involvement of other nociceptive-mediated mechanisms.

E2 (both short-term and long-term exposure) significantly decreased the nociceptive signaling in viscerally labeled DRG neurons [6, 7]. Thus, in addition to central regulation, estrogen may affect nociception associated with IBS peripherally.

4. Primary afferent neurons and viscero-visceral cross-sensitization: emerging model for functional gastrointestinal disorders

Most of the current literature pertains to specific functional syndromes defined by medical subspecialties. These include: IBS (gastroenterology); CPP (gynecology); PBS (urology); fibromyalgia (rheumatology); and others. Many reports described the substantial overlaps between two or more of these syndromes [11, 12]. Moreover, clinical presentations of functional syndromes lack a specific pathology in the affected organ but may respond to a viscero-visceral cross-sensitization in which increased nociceptive input from an inflamed organ (i.e., uterus) sensitizes neurons that receive convergent input from an unaffected organ (i.e., colon or bladder). The site of visceral cross-sensitivity is unknown.

Recent studies from our laboratory demonstrated that hormonal modulation of visceral inputs of primary afferent nociceptors located in the dorsal root ganglia (DRG) is responsible for changes observed in the perception of pain during the etiology of functional pain syndromes [2]. Individuals suffering from CPP frequently have pain emanating from several visceral organs. Viscero-somatic and viscero-visceral hyperalgesia and allodynia lead to the perception of pain spreading from an initial site to adjacent areas. Patients with CPP may at first have only one source of pain in the pelvis, but numerous mechanisms involving the central and peripheral nervous systems may result in the development of painful sensations in adjacent organs, such as IBS being associated with lower colonic pain.

5. Summary

Similar to other chronic diseases, a multicomponent conceptual model of IBS, which involves physiologic, cognitive and behavior factors will be necessary for developing new therapies. The different systems such as neuroendocrine regulation, pain modulation, and autonomic response will affect ascending aminergic systems (**Figure 1**).

From a public health perspective, a substantial impact on our knowledge of nociceptive diseases such IBS will help achieve a deeper understanding of data presented in clinical aspects of these symptoms. Only a thorough understanding of the mechanism implicated in these phenomena can truly contribute to the designing of new and more efficient therapies.

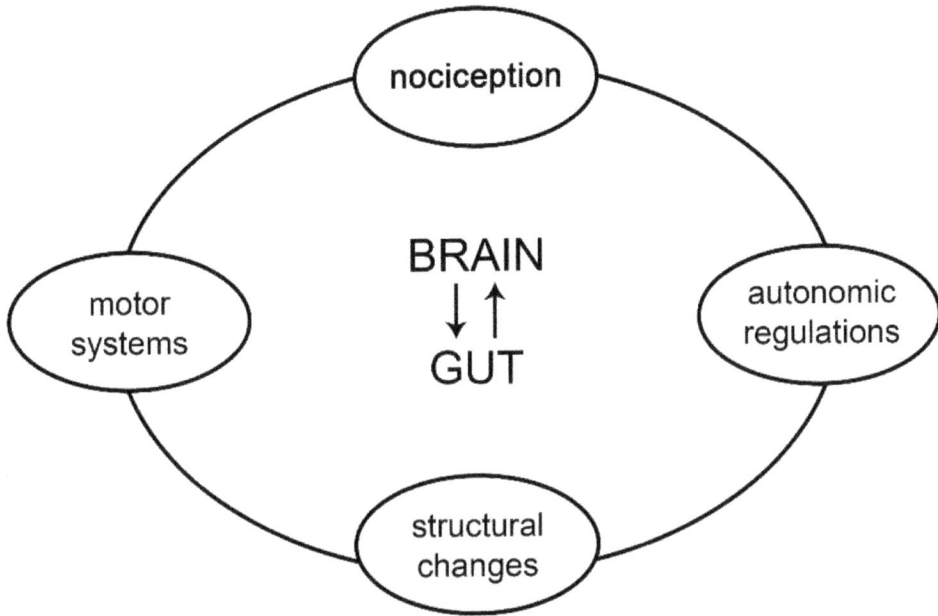

Figure 1. Different regulatory mechanisms involved in irritable bowel syndrome.

Author details

Victor V. Chaban

Address all correspondence to: victorchaban@cdrewu.edu

Department of Internal Medicine, Charles R. Drew University of Medicine and Science, Los Angeles, USA; Department of Medicine, University of California, Los Angeles, USA

References

[1] Holschneider DP, Bradesi S, Mayer EA. The role of experimental models in developing new treatments for irritable bowel syndrome. Expert Review of Gastroenterology and Hepatology, 2011, 5 (1): 43–57.

[2] Chaban V. Unraveling the enigma of visceral pain. Nova Publishers, N.Y. 2016. 77 p. ISBN: 978-63489-430-8. Library of U.S. Congress Control Number: 2015951299.

[3] Mayer EA, Labus JS, Tillisch K, Cole SW, Baldi P Towards a systems view of IBS. Nature Review Gastroenterology and Hepatology 2015, 12 (10): 592–605.

[4] Kobayashi K, Yamanaka H, Noguchi K. Expression of ATP receptors in the rat dorsal root ganglion and spinal cord. Anatomical Science International 2013, 88 (1): 10–16.

[5] Toulme E, Tsuda M, Khakh BS, Inoue K. On the role of ATP-Gated P2X receptors in acute, inflammatory and neuropathic pain. In: Kruger L, Light AR, Editors. Translational pain research: from mouse to man. CRC Press/Taylor & Francis. Chapter 10. Frontiers in Neuroscience. 2010.

[6] Chaban V et al. Estradiol attenuates the adenosine triphosphate-induced increase of intracellular calcium through group II metabotropic glutamate receptors in rat dorsal root ganglion neurons. Journal of Neuroscience Research 2011. 89(11):1707–1710.

[7] Cho, T. and V.V. Chaban, Interaction between P2X3 and ERalpha/ERbeta in ATP-mediated calcium signaling in mice sensory neurons. Journal of Neuroendocrinology 2012. 24(5): 789–97

[8] Srivastava DP et al. Rapid estrogen signaling in the brain: implications for the fine-tuning of neuronal circuitry. Journal of Neuroscience 2011. 31 (45): 16056–16063.

[9] Al-Chaer ED, Traub RJ. Biological basis of visceral pain: recent developments. Pain 2002. 96 (3): 221–225.

[10] Mayer EA. Gut feelings: the emerging biology of gut-brain communication. Nature Review Neuroscience 2011. 12 (8): 453–466.

[11] Malykhina AP. Neural mechanisms of pelvic organ cross-sensitization. Neuroscience 2007. 149(3): 660–672.

[12] Grover M, Herfarth H, Drossman DA. The functional-organic dichotomy: postinfectious irritable bowel syndrome and inflammatory bowel disease-irritable bowel syndrome. Clinical Gastroenterology and Hepatology 2009. 7(1): 48–53.

3

Inflammatory Bowel Disease: Epidemiology

Sumant S. Arora and Talha A. Malik

Abstract

Inflammatory bowel disease (IBD) is characterized by two partially distinct alimentary disease processes, namely Crohn's disease (CD) and ulcerative colitis (UC), affecting genetically predisposed individuals. CD and UC were first described in 1932 and 1859, respectively. It is estimated that 1.5 million in North America and 2.5 million persons in Europe have IBD. The peak incidence of CD and UC is between 20–30 years and 30–40 years of age, respectively. Both incidence and prevalence of CD and UC are similar across males and females. However, several studies suggest a female predominance in CD and a male predominance in UC. The pathogenesis of IBD is attributed to an uncontrolled immune-mediated inflammatory response to an unrecognized environmental trigger that interacts with the intestinal flora. Various determinants of IBD include the following: peculiar environmental triggers, intestinal immune mechanisms, heritable factors, gut flora, diet, mesenteric fat, medications, nicotine, infectious agents, immunization, hygiene, pregnancy, breastfeeding, stress and lifestyle. Predominant complications in IBD are surgery, malnutrition, disease exacerbations and cancer. Patients with CD have a higher mortality compared to general population. Epidemiological studies continue to expand our understanding of the distribution, determinants and mechanisms of IBD. This has enabled us to recognize safer and effective approaches to management.

Keywords: inflammatory bowel disease, Crohn's disease, ulcerative colitis, epidemiology, incidence, prevalence

1. Introduction

Inflammatory bowel disease (IBD) is an idiopathic chronic inflammatory disorder of the alimentary tract that encompasses two major closely related yet heterogeneously distinct disease entities—Crohn's disease (CD) and ulcerative colitis (UC). IBD is characterized by chronic or relapsing uncontrolled immune activation and inflammation in genetically predisposed individuals to a yet unknown environmental trigger that interacts with the gut flora and primarily affects the digestive tract [1–7]. Historically, Dr. Burrill Crohn, Dr. Leon Ginzburg and Dr. Gordon Oppenheimer first described CD in 1932 as regional or terminal ileitis—inflammation of terminal ileum [8–10]. In 1859, Dr. Samuel Wilks recognized UC as a discrete entity, but it was Sir Arthur Hurst, who described its endoscopic pattern and distinguished it from the more common bacillary dysentery [8, 9, 11]. Pathologically, CD usually consists of transmural inflammation (all layers from mucosa to serosa) and may discontinuously involve any part of the alimentary tract from mouth to anus, whereas UC is characterized by submucosal inflammation limited to the colon [6]. Approximately, one and a half million residents in the USA and two and a half million in Europe have IBD, with about half represented in each of the two discrete IBD subgroups [2, 12].

2. Incidence, prevalence and distribution

Though now recognized worldwide, traditionally IBD was considered a condition that primarily affected Caucasians across Europe, North America and Australia [1]. Hence, most of the available epidemiologic data on CD and UC have been derived from population-based studies conducted in these geographic regions [1]. The incidence and prevalence of CD and UC have stabilized in the aforementioned regions; however, it is still higher than in the rest of the world [1]. Further, the incidence and prevalence of IBD, predominantly CD, have increased in the developing world particularly in the Middle East, Southeast Asia and the Asia Pacific Region [7, 12, 13]. Meanwhile, South America and Africa have significantly low incidence and prevalence rates, albeit anecdotal reports have hinted an increase in incidence [14, 15].

Even in the West, IBD has become increasingly recognized among minority populations [1]. The most significant rise in incidence has occurred in second-generation immigrants from low-risk geographic regions to Western countries, that is, high-risk regions. This supports the concept of an equal if not higher contribution from environmental influences compared to genetic predisposition [1, 16]. Also, has been noted a higher incidence of IBD among immigrants and their families who migrated from socioeconomically backward regions [1]. Moreover, compared to minorities in the West, recent immigrants tend to have a milder disease course [1].

Globally, there remains a paucity of accurate epidemiologic data due to clinical overlap of the IBD entities with conditions such as infectious colitis and differences in the health care systems precluding reliable case estimation. The recognized IBD cases may further only represent a fraction of the actual disease burden due to diagnosis requiring invasive and expensive modalities. Moreover, at times, CD cannot be clearly distinguished from UC, especially early in the disease course before distinctive characteristics have manifested, often requiring reassignment of the IBD subgroup diagnosis [17]. Despite the aforementioned limitations, the incidence and prevalence of both CD and UC have demonstrated a distribution trend. The incidence and prevalence data vary across the globe depending upon geographic region, environment, immigration trends, ethnicity [1–3] and even differ within the same geographic region. Moreover, a north-south distribution gradient has been observed for IBD risk across the world [18]. This has been attributed to regional differences in sunlight and vitamin D exposure with high levels of exposure inversely correlated with risk of IBD [19, 20].

The annual incidence rates of CD are comparable across most of the developed world. It is estimated to be 20.2 per 100,000 person-years, 12.7 per 100,000 person-years, 29.3 per 100,000 person-years and 16.5 per 100,000 person-years in North America, Europe, Australia and New Zealand, respectively [21–23]. In contrast, Asia has a low incidence rate of approximately 0.54 per 100,000 person-years [24]. Similarly, the incidence rates for UC in North America, Europe and Asia range from 7.6 to 19.5 per 100,000 person-years, 1.7 to 13.6 per 100,000 person-years and 0.3 to 5.8 per 100,000 person-years, respectively [4]. In the past, UC was considered to be slightly more prevalent; however, an increased incidence of CD in the past few decades has resulted in a trend reversal. Most recent estimates of prevalence of CD in North America are 25–300 per 100,000 person-years and that for UC are 170–250 and 43–294 per 100,000 person-years, respectively, in North America and Europe [21, 25, 26]. Overall, both the incidence and prevalence of CD and UC are increasing with time. This can be attributed to a number of factors including improved sanitation, diet and medication exposures, increased IBD awareness among patients and clinicians, use of improved endoscopic and radiologic diagnostic modalities and widened health care access [21, 27].

2.1. Age and gender disparity

Although IBD can occur at any age, the peak age of onset for CD and UC is generally between 20–30 years and 30–40 years of age, respectively [1, 4, 6, 21]. However, some European cohorts have suggested a second peak between 60–70 years of age, especially for UC. The most plausible explanation for this additional peak is ascertainment bias due to increased health care access and more frequent evaluation of older patients. Majority of North American population-based study has shown that the median and mean age of diagnosis of CD and UC range between 30–45 years and 40–45 years, respectively [28, 29]. Additionally, these studies especially in adults have suggested a female predominance in CD and male predominance in UC [1, 30]. This gender-based disparity may be attributed to hormonal or life-style factors. However, the variation is inconsistent, particularly in low IBD incidence regions, where CD may be more prevalent among men [25, 31]. Men tend to be diagnosed with IBD, especially UC at a later age than their female counterparts [6]. On the other hand, in the pediatric population, the trend in gender distribution is reversed with more boys having CD than girls [32].

2.2. Racial and ethnic disparity

There appears to be a marked ethnic and racial variation in the incidence of IBD. Early studies from the 1960s reported a lower incidence of IBD, specifically UC among African-Americans [33]. However, these studies were conducted in regions with predominant white populations, and more recent studies from 1990s have challenged these findings with comparable incidence rates among Whites and non-Whites [34, 35]. Further, CD was proposed to be more aggressive with earlier age of onset in African-Americans. A recent systematic review, however, suggested that the variance in IBD severity extrapolates from socioeconomic inequalities such as health care affordability and accessibility, rather than inherent biologic or genetic dissimilarities [36, 37]. Ethnically, the Jews in particular are vulnerable to develop IBD, with incidence rates being several fold higher than in the general population across the globe. Further, IBD is more common among the Ashkenazi Jews than the Sephardic Jews in the Middle East, but this trend is reversed in the United States and northern Europe, indicating influence of environmental factors [38].

3. Pathogenesis and risk factors

Pathogenically, IBD is believed to be due to uncontrolled immune activation and inflammation of the alimentary tract in genetically predisposed individuals. It is triggered by the interaction of an unknown environmental agent with the autoantigens believed to reside on nonpathogenic commensal bacteria of the intestinal microbiota (**Figure 1**) [7]. The primary mechanism of inflammatory insult in IBD is immune mediated. Intestinal epithelial cells in active IBD express HLA class II molecules that activate macrophages to secrete pro-inflammatory cytokines (IL-1, IL-6, IL-8, and TNF-α) and suppress the downregulatory cytokines (IL-2, IL-10, and TGF-β) in the lamina propria, thereby fostering chronic inflammation [5, 7, 12].

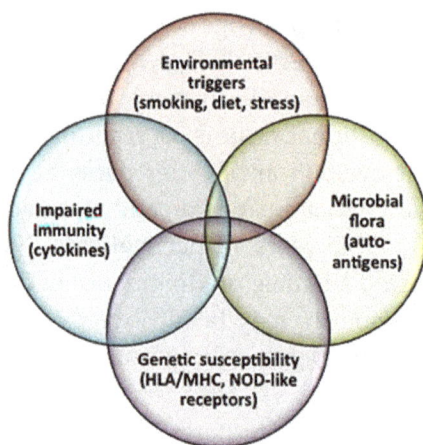

Figure 1. Factors implicated in the etiopathogenesis of IBD.

Various environmental triggers have been attributed to IBD causation. They include external antigens such as infectious pathogens (bacteria and viruses), dietary agents and autoantigens residing on the microbial gut flora [1, 6, 12]. In addition, both CD and UC tend to have genetic predisposition in about 15% cases. In regard to first-degree relative for CD and UC, the lifetime risk of developing IBD is approximately 5 and 2% among non-Jewish populations and 8 and 5% among Jewish populations, respectively [39]. The genetic predisposition is stronger for CD than UC based on higher concordance rates (50 and 10% vs. 16 and 4%) among monozygotic and dizygotic twins, respectively [40, 41].

Dietary factors more pronounced in typical western diet have been implicated in the pathogenesis of IBD. Comprehensive review of studies involving patients with CD has suggested possible association between increased consumption of refined sugars and animal meat and risk of development of IBD [42, 43]. The aforementioned dietary components are believed to interact with intestinal flora and produce pro-inflammatory agents [44]. Individuals who consume less dietary fiber, raw fruits and vegetables tend to have higher predilection for IBD [44]. Meanwhile, molecular studies have linked adipose tissue to intestinal inflammation [45, 46]. However, it remains unclear if this translates into a causal or clinically meaningful association between obesity and CD. Regardless, obese patients with CD tend to have a rapid disease progression compared to their underweight counterparts [47, 48]. Moreover, sedentary lifestyle is associated with overall higher IBD incidence [49].

Among environmental factors, smoking has a pivotal role in IBD with divergent effects in UC and CD [1]. Both current as well as former smoking, including exposure to passive smoking during childhood, is associated with twofold increase in the risk of CD [50, 51]. Smokers with CD tend to have an earlier age of onset, more aggressive (stricturing or penetrating) disease phenotype, heightened need for steroids and immunosuppressants and overall more surgical interventions as well as higher risk of postresection recurrence [52, 53]. In contrast to CD, smoking safeguards against UC and even indeterminate colitis, with an estimated 50% risk reduction in current smokers. However, this protective effect is less pronounced in females. Further, smokers with UC tend to have milder disease course, with less frequent proximal extension of disease and decreased need for immunosuppression and surgery [53, 54].

The precise mechanisms driving these contrasting effects of smoking on the two IBD subtypes remain unclear. It is hypothesized that smoking causes polymorphisms in genes regulating nicotine metabolism and decreases heat shock protein-70 resulting in reduced protection against cellular oxidative stress, which in turn impairs endothelial function in the intestinal mucosal barrier and promotes inflammation [55–58]. On the other hand, it is proposed that smoking alters the gut flora to reduce predisposition to UC [59].

Recent studies have suggested that infectious agents, such as *Salmonella* and *Campylobacter*, impart heightened risk for IBD development [60], while *Clostridium difficile* and cytomegalovirus have been linked with IBD exacerbations [61, 62]. However, no definite causal association has been identified.

Meanwhile, poor hygienic conditions, including large family size, lack of access to running water, consumption of unpasteurized milk, early exposure to farm animals and pets, have been suggested to protect against IBD development [1, 30, 63–65]. However, these associations are derived from studies conducted in the West and they failed to be replicated in the developing world [1, 66]. On the other hand, there is no definite association between immunization and risk of IBD. Early studies have linked attenuated live measles virus vaccine with IBD occurrence; however, recent studies support the contrary thereby suggesting a protective role [67].

Several pharmacologic agents have also been implicated as potential risk factors for IBD. They include NSAIDs, oral contraceptives, hormonal replacement therapy and antibiotics [68–73]. On the contrary, studies suggesting role of nutritional factors such as vitamin D in IBD development remain equivocal [1].

With regards to pregnancy, there is no definite association between the mode of childbirth (caesarian vs. vaginal delivery) and risk of IBD [74]. However, breastfeeding may play a protective role against IBD development later in life [1]. Meanwhile, depression and anxiety have not only been linked to higher risk of development of IBD but also to increased disease severity, need for surgical intervention, reduced quality of life and diminished response to immunosuppresants [75].

4. Classification

The heterogeneity of demographic, anatomic and disease behavior characteristics in IBD warranted a systematic grouping scheme to place its various phenotypes into simple categories. The first attempt was made by the Working Party of the World Congress of Gastroenterology that met in Vienna in 1998. Their report known as the "Vienna Classification" was published in the Journal of Inflammatory Bowel Diseases in 2000. This classification attempted to stratify CD into 24 disease clusters based on age at diagnosis, disease location and disease behavior (**Table 1**) [76]. Subsequently, the Vienna classification was critiqued owing to lack of universal clinical applicability [77].

	Vienna classification	Montreal classification
Age at diagnosis	A1: Below 40 years	A1 Below 16 years
	A2: Above 40 years	A2 Between 17 and 40 years
		A3 Above 40 years
Location	L1 Ileal	L1 Ileal
	L2 Colonic	L2 Colonic
	L3 Ileocolonic	L3 Ileocolonic
	L4 Upper	L4 Upper disease modifier or isolated upper disease
Behavior	B1 Nonstricturing, nonpenetrating	B1 Nonstricturing, Nonpenetrating
	B2 Stricturing	B2 Stricturing
	B3 Penetrating	B3 Penetrating
		p Perianal disease modifier

Table 1. Vienna and Montreal classification of Crohn's disease.

The Working Party of the Montreal World Congress of Gastroenterology then met in 2005 and put forth the Montreal classification of IBD (**Tables 1** and **2**) [78]. This new scheme grouped

CD primarily based on the same variables proposed by the experts at Vienna including patient's age at diagnosis (A1, 16 years and younger; A2, 17–40 years; A3, >40 years), disease location (L1, ileal: L2, colonic; L3, ileocolonic) and disease behavior (B1, nonstricturing, nonpenetrating; B2, stricturing; B3, penetrating). In addition, it introduced modifiers for upper tract disease location (L4) and for perianal disease (*p*). Further, it extended the classification to stratify UC based on the extent and severity of the disease (**Table 2**) [78].

Class	Extent	Description
E1	Ulcerative proctitis	Proximal extent of inflammation distal to rectosigmoid junction
E2	Left-sided UC (distal UC)	Involvement limited to proportion of colorectum distal to the splenic
E3	Extensive UC (pancolitis)	Involvement extending proximal to splenic flexure

Table 2. Montreal classification of ulcerative colitis.

5. Disease course

Based on phenotype by location, of all patients with CD at the time of diagnosis, one-third of patients have ileal involvement, one-third of patients have colonic involvement and the rest have ileocolonic disease. While with regard to disease behavior, 80% of all patients with CD at the time of diagnosis have nonpenetrating/nonstricturing disease with the remaining 20% having stricturing or penetrating disease [79]. As CD evolves, of all with nonpenetrating/ nonstricturing disease, up to one-third of patients progress to penetrating or stricturing complications at 5 years and about half at 20 years from diagnosis [79]. Further, in terms of disease activity, based on data from prebiologic era, about two-thirds of patients with CD tend to have a remitting and risk of CD relapsing course one-fifth remain active and about 13% enter long-term remission [80].

Meanwhile, for UC at the time of diagnosis, one-third of patients tend to have colonic involvement distal to rectosigmoid junction, one-third up to splenic flexure, while the remaining third have pancolitis, that is, contiguous involvement extending proximal to the splenic flexure [2]. The disease behavior is variable; 50% of UC patients with proctitis/proctosigmoiditis progress to extensive disease at 25 years [81]. While in regard to disease activity, based on data from prebiologic era, 57% of patients with UC tend to have a remitting and relapsing course, one quarter go into long-term remission, and about one-fifth remain active [39, 82].

6. IBD and morbidity

The key factors driving morbidity overlap between the two IBD subgroups—CD and UC. The predominant causes of morbidity in patients with CD are need for surgery, malnutrition followed by disease exacerbations and cancer [2, 4]. While among patients with UC, the major burden of morbidity is due to the development of cancer followed by requirement for surgery and disease exacerbations [2, 4]. Overall, surgery remains the most common cause of morbidity in CD and a significant cause of morbidity in UC. Recently, the cumulative risk of IBD, particularly patients with CD requiring surgery has significantly decreased with rates of surgery being approximately 10–14% and 18–35% after 1 and 5 years, respectively [83–88]. This is attributed to adoption of more aggressive medical therapy in recent times [1, 2, 83, 84, 89, 90]. Based on age, location and behavior of CD, the greatest need for surgery is with ileocecal location and stricturing or penetrating/fistulizing disease phenotype [2, 86, 87]. Similarly, in UC, the likelihood of need for colectomy has decreased recently with estimated rates of 6 and 10% after 1 and 5 years, respectively [83, 91–93]. The highest probability of colectomy is in those with relatively recent diagnosis and severe disease especially pancolitis [2].

An interesting association has been observed between appendectomy and IBD [1]. While appendectomy is found to protect against future occurrence of UC, it may lead to an increased incidence of CD [94–96].

With regard to cancer as one of the drivers of morbidity, the overall risk of colorectal cancer is significantly higher in patients with IBD compared to the general population. The primary factors influencing this risk include persistent active inflammation, immunosuppression, long-standing disease, extensive disease, young age at diagnosis, family history of colorectal cancer and coexisting primary sclerosing cholangitis [2, 97]. Overall, patients with IBD have heightened risk of extraintestinal cancers such as lymphoproliferative and skin cancers [2, 98–100].

7. IBD and mortality

Whether or not having IBD confers a higher mortality remains debated. Population-based studies from 1980s to 1990s suggested a moderate increase in mortality rate in CD [101, 102]. However, recent European studies have failed to replicate these findings and indicate a comparable mortality rate in CD to the general population [103–105]. Major causes of mortality in CD include direct, such as surgical complications and malnourishment, and indirect related to smoking [101, 106–107].

Similarly, there is lack of definitive evidence to support higher mortality rate in patients with UC [105, 107–110]. However, unlike CD, most deaths in UC are due to colorectal cancer than from surgical or other complications [106, 109].

8. Conclusion

In conclusion, IBD is a condition with a unique etiopathogenesis and significant epidemiologic burden. To the present day, epidemiological studies continue to expand our understanding of the distribution, determinants and mechanisms of IBD. This has enabled us to recognize safer and more effective approaches to management and therapeutics outside of mere immuno-suppression for IBD with emphasis on prevention, preemption and immunomodulation.

Author details

Sumant S. Arora[1*] and Talha A. Malik[2]

*Address all correspondence to: sumantarora@uabmc.edu

1 Department of Medicine, University of Alabama at Birmingham, Montgomery Residency Program, Montgomery, Alabama, USA

2 Department of Medicine-Gastroenterology and Department of Epidemiology, University of Alabama at Birmingham, Birmingham, Alabama, USA

References

[1] Ananthakrishnan AN. Epidemiology and risk factors for IBD. Nat Rev Gastroenterol Hepatol. 2015 Apr;12(4):205-17. doi: 10.1038/nrgastro.2015.34

[2] Burisch J, Munkholm P. The epidemiology of inflammatory bowel disease. Scand J Gastroenterol. 2015:1-10. doi: 10.3109/00365521.2015.1014407

[3] Malik TA. Inflammatory Bowel Disease: Historical Perspective, Epidemiology, and Risk Factors. Surg Clin North Am. 2015 Dec;95(6):1105-22. doi: 10.1016/j.suc.2015.07.006

[4] Cosnes J, Gower-Rousseau C, Seksik P, Cortot A. Epidemiology and natural history of inflammatory bowel diseases. Gastroenterology. 2011;140(6):1785-1794.

[5] Abraham C, Cho JH. Inflammatory bowel disease. The New England journal of medicine. 2009;361(21):2066-2078. doi: 10.1056/NEJMra0804647

[6] Podolsky DK. Inflammatory bowel disease. The New England journal of medicine. 2002;347(6):417-429. doi: 10.1056/NEJMra020831

[7] Loftus EV, Jr. Clinical epidemiology of inflammatory bowel disease: Incidence, prevalence, and environmental influences. Gastroenterology. 2004;126(6):1504-1517.

[8] Kirsner JB. Historical aspects of inflammatory bowel disease. Journal of clinical gastroenterology. 1988;10(3):286-297.

[9] Kirsner JB. Historical origins of current IBD concepts. World J Gastroenterol. 2001;7(2): 175-184. doi: 10.3748/wjg.v7.i2.175

[10] Crohn BB, Ginzburg L, Oppenheimer GD. Landmark article Oct 15, 1932. Regional ileitis. A pathological and clinical entity. By Burril B. Crohn, Leon Ginzburg, and Gordon D. Oppenheimer. JAMA : the journal of the American Medical Association. 1984;251(1):73-79.

[11] Hurst AF. Ulcerative colitis. Guy Hosp Rep 1909; 71:26.

[12] Kaplan GG. The global burden of IBD: from 2015 to 2025. Nat Rev Gastroenterol Hepatol. 2015 Dec;12(12):720-7. doi: 10.1038/nrgastro.2015.150

[13] Sood A, Midha V. Epidemiology of inflammatory bowel disease in Asia. Indian J Gastroenterol. 2007;26(6):285-289.

[14] Archampong TN, Nkrumah KN. Inflammatory bowel disease in Accra: what new trends. West Afr J Med. 2013;32(1):40-44.

[15] Ukwenya AY, Ahmed A, Odigie VI, Mohammed A. Inflammatory bowel disease in Nigerians: still a rare diagnosis? Annals of African medicine. 2011;10(2):175-179. doi: 10.4103/1596-3519.82067

[16] Kaplan GG. IBD: Global variations in environmental risk factors for IBD. Nat Rev Gastroenterol Hepatol. 2014 Dec;11(12):708-9. doi: 10.1038/nrgastro.2014.182

[17] Henriksen M, Jahnsen J, Lygren I, et al. Change of diagnosis during the first five years after onset of inflammatory bowel disease: Results of a prospective follow-up study (the IBSEN Study). Scand J Gastroenterol 2006; 41:1037-43. doi: 10.1080/00365520600554527

[18] Kappelman M, Rifas-Shiman S, Kleinman K, et al. The prevalence and geographic distribution of Crohn's disease and ulcerative colitis in the United States. Clin Gastroenterol Hepatol 2007; 5:1424-9. doi: 10.1016/j.cgh.2007.07.012

[19] Nerich V, Jantchou P, Boutron-Ruault MC, et al. Low exposure to sunlight is a risk factor for Crohn's disease. Aliment Pharmacol Ther 2011; 33:940-5. doi: 10.1111/j.1365-2036.2011.04601.x

[20] Ananthakrishnan AN, Khalili H, Higuchi LM, et al. Higher predicted vitamin D status is associated with reduced risk of Crohn's disease. Gastroenterology 2012; 142:482-9. doi: 10.1053/j.gastro.2011.11.040

[21] Molodecky NA, Soon IS, Rabi DM, et al. Increasing incidence and prevalence of the inflammatory bowel diseases with time, based on systematic review. Gastroenterology. 2012;142(1):46-54 e42; quiz e30. doi: 10.1053/j.gastro.2011.10.001

[22] Gearry RB, Richardson A, Frampton CM, et al. High incidence of Crohn's disease in Canterbury, New Zealand: Results of an epidemiologic study. Inflamm Bowel Dis 2006; 12:936-43. doi: 10.1097/01.mib.0000231572.88806.b9

[23] Wilson J, Hair C, Knight R, et al. High incidence of inflammatory bowel disease in Australia: A prospective population-based Australian incidence study. Inflamm Bowel Dis 2010; 16:1550-6. doi: 10.1002/ibd.21209

[24] Ng SC, Tang W, Ching J, et al. Incidence and phenotype of inflammatory bowel disease based on results from the Asia-Pacific Crohn's and Colitis Epidemiology Study. Gastroenterology 2013; 145:158-65. doi: 10.1053/j.gastro.2013.04.007

[25] Bernstein CN, Wajda A, Svenson LW, et al. The epidemiology of inflammatory bowel disease in Canada: a population-based study. The American journal of gastroenterology. 2006;101(7):1559-1568. doi: 10.1111/j.1572-0241.2006.00603.

[26] Pinchbeck BR, Kirdeikis J, Thomson AB. Inflammatory bowel disease in northern Alberta. An epidemiologic study. Journal of clinical gastroenterology. 1988;10(5): 505-515.

[27] Molodecky NA, Kaplan GG. Environmental risk factors for inflammatory bowel disease. Gastroenterol Hepatol 2010; 6:339-46.

[28] Loftus EV, Jr., Silverstein MD, Sandborn WJ, Tremaine WJ, Harmsen WS, Zinsmeister AR. Crohn's disease in Olmsted County, Minnesota, 1940-1993: incidence, prevalence, and survival. Gastroenterology. 1998;114(6):1161-1168.

[29] Loftus EV, Jr., Silverstein MD, Sandborn WJ, Tremaine WJ, Harmsen WS, Zinsmeister AR. Ulcerative colitis in Olmsted County, Minnesota, 1940-1993: incidence, prevalence, and survival. Gut. 2000;46(3):336-343. doi: 10.1136/gut.46.3.336

[30] Bernstein CN, Rawsthorne P, Cheang M, Blanchard JF. A population-based case control study of potential risk factors for IBD. The American journal of gastroenterology. 2006;101(5):993-1002. doi: 10.1111/j.1572-0241.2006.00381.x

[31] Devlin HB, Datta D, Dellipiani AW. The incidence and prevalence of inflammatory bowel disease in North Tees Health District. World journal of surgery. 1980;4(2):183-193.

[32] Auvin S, Molinie F, Gower-Rousseau C, et al. Incidence, clinical presentation and location at diagnosis of pediatric inflammatory bowel disease: a prospective population-based study in northern France (1988-1999). Journal of pediatric gastroenterology and nutrition. 2005;41(1):49-55.

[33] Mendeloff AI, Monk M, Siegel CI, Lilienfeld A. Some epidemiological features of ulcerative colitis and regional enteritis. A preliminary report. Gastroenterology. 1966;51(5):748-756.

[34] Kurata JH, Kantor-Fish S, Frankl H, Godby P, Vadheim CM. Crohn's disease among ethnic groups in a large health maintenance organization. Gastroenterology. 1992;102(6):1940-1948.

[35] Ogunbi SO, Ransom JA, Sullivan K, Schoen BT, Gold BD. Inflammatory bowel disease in African-American children living in Georgia. J Pediatr. 1998;133(1):103-107.

[36] Straus WL, Eisen GM, Sandler RS, Murray SC, Sessions JT. Crohn's disease: does race matter? The Mid-Atlantic Crohn's Disease Study Group. The American journal of gastroenterology. 2000;95(2):479-483. doi: 10.1111/j.1572-0241.2000.t01-1-01531.x

[37] Mahid SS, Mulhall AM, Gholson RD, Eichenberger MR, Galandiuk S. Inflammatory bowel disease and African Americans: a systematic review. Inflamm Bowel Dis. 2008;14(7):960-967. doi: 10.1002/ibd.20389.

[38] Yang H, McElree C, Roth MP, Shanahan F, Targan SR, Rotter JI. Familial empirical risks for inflammatory bowel disease: differences between Jews and non-Jews. Gut. 1993;34(4):517-524.

[39] Langholz E, Munkholm P, Davidsen M, Binder V. Course of ulcerative colitis: analysis of changes in disease activity over years. Gastroenterology. 1994;107(1):3-11.

[40] Sands BE. Inflammatory bowel disease: past, present, and future. J Gastroenterol. 2007;42(1):16-25. doi: 10.1007/s00535-006-1995-7

[41] Halme L, Paavola-Sakki P, Turunen U, Lappalainen M, Farkkila M, Kontula K. Family and twin studies in inflammatory bowel disease. World J Gastroenterol. 2006;12(23): 3668-3672. doi: 10.3748/wjg.v12.i23.3668

[42] Martini GA, Brandes JW. Increased consumption of refined carbohydrates in patients with Crohn's disease. Klinische Wochenschrift. 1976;54(8):367-371.

[43] Asakura H, Suzuki K, Kitahora T, Morizane T. Is there a link between food and intestinal microbes and the occurrence of Crohn's disease and ulcerative colitis? J Gastroenterol Hepatol. 2008;23(12):1794-1801. doi: 10.1111/j.1440-1746.2008.05681.x

[44] Thornton JR, Emmett PM, Heaton KW. Diet and Crohn's disease: characteristics of the pre-illness diet. Br Med J. 1979;2(6193):762-764.

[45] Bedford PA, Todorovic V, Westcott ED, et al. Adipose tissue of human omentum is a major source of dendritic cells, which lose MHC Class II and stimulatory function in Crohn's disease. Journal of leukocyte biology. 2006;80(3):546-554. doi: 10.1189/jlb. 0905501

[46] Karmiris K, Koutroubakis IE, Kouroumalis EA. Leptin, adiponectin, resistin, and ghrelin--implications for inflammatory bowel disease. Molecular nutrition & food research. 2008;52(8):855-866. doi: 10.1002/mnfr.200700050

[47] Blain A, Cattan S, Beaugerie L, Carbonnel F, Gendre JP, Cosnes J. Crohn's disease clinical course and severity in obese patients. Clinical nutrition. 2002;21(1):51-57. doi: 10.1054/ clnu.2001.0503

[48] Hass DJ, Brensinger CM, Lewis JD, Lichtenstein GR. The impact of increased body mass index on the clinical course of Crohn's disease. Clinical gastroenterology and hepatol- ogy : the official clinical practice journal of the American Gastroenterological Associa- tion. 2006;4(4):482-488. doi: 10.1016/j.cgh.2005.12.015

[49] Sonnenberg A. Occupational distribution of inflammatory bowel disease among German employees. Gut. 1990;31(9):1037-1040.

[50] Mahid SS, Minor KS, Stromberg AJ, Galandiuk S. Active and passive smoking in childhood is related to the development of inflammatory bowel disease. Inflamm Bowel Dis. 2007;13(4):431-438. doi: 10.1002/ibd.20070

[51] Higuchi LM, Khalili H, Chan AT, Richter JM, Bousvaros A, Fuchs CS. A prospective study of cigarette smoking and the risk of inflammatory bowel disease in women. The American journal of gastroenterology. 2012;107(9):1399-1406. doi: 10.1038/ajg.2012.196

[52] Cosnes J, Nion-Larmurier I, Afchain P, Beaugerie L, Gendre JP. Gender differences in the response of colitis to smoking. Clinical gastroenterology and hepatology : the official clinical practice journal of the American Gastroenterological Association. 2004;2(1):41-48.

[53] Lakatos PL, Szamosi T, Lakatos L. Smoking in inflammatory bowel diseases: good, bad or ugly? World J Gastroenterol. 2007;13(46):6134-6139. doi: 10.3748/wjg.v13.i46.6134

[54] Cosnes J, Carbonnel F, Carrat F, Beaugerie L, Cattan S, Gendre J. Effects of current and former cigarette smoking on the clinical course of Crohn's disease. Aliment Pharmacol Ther. 1999;13(11):1403-1411. doi: 10.1046/j.1365-2036.1999.00630.x

[55] McGilligan VE, Wallace JM, Heavey PM, Ridley DL, Rowland IR. Hypothesis about mechanisms through which nicotine might exert its effect on the interdependence of inflammation and gut barrier function in ulcerative colitis. Inflamm Bowel Dis. 2007;13(1):108-115. doi: 10.1002/ibd.20020

[56] Bergeron V, Grondin V, Rajca S, et al. Current smoking differentially affects blood mononuclear cells from patients with Crohn's disease and ulcerative colitis: relevance to its adverse role in the disease. Inflamm Bowel Dis. 2012;18(6):1101-1111. doi: 10.1002/ibd.21889

[57] Ananthakrishnan AN, Nguyen DD, Sauk J, Yajnik V, Xavier RJ. Genetic polymorphisms in metabolizing enzymes modifying the association between smoking and inflammatory bowel diseases. Inflamm Bowel Dis. 2014;20(5):783-789. doi: 10.1097/MIB.0000000000000014

[58] Hatoum OA, Heidemann J, Binion DG. The intestinal microvasculature as a therapeutic target in inflammatory bowel disease. Ann N Y Acad Sci. 2006;1072:78-97. doi: 10.1196/annals.1326.003

[59] Parkes GC, Whelan K, Lindsay JO. Smoking in inflammatory bowel disease: impact on disease course and insights into the aetiology of its effect. J Crohns Colitis. 2014;8(8):717-725. doi: 10.1016/j.crohns.2014.02.002

[60] Gradel KO, Nielsen HL, Schonheyder HC, Ejlertsen T, Kristensen B, Nielsen H. Increased short- and long-term risk of inflammatory bowel disease after salmonella or campylobacter gastroenteritis. Gastroenterology. 2009;137(2):495-501. doi: 10.1053/j.gastro.2009.04.001

[61] Ananthakrishnan AN, Issa M, Binion DG. Clostridium difficile and inflammatory bowel disease. Gastroenterology clinics of North America. 2009;38(4):711-728. doi: 10.1016/j.gtc.2009.07.003.

[62] Singh S, Graff LA, Bernstein CN. Do NSAIDs, antibiotics, infections, or stress trigger flares in IBD? The American journal of gastroenterology. 2009;104(5):1298-1313; quiz 1314. doi: 10.1038/ajg.2009.15

[63] Timm S, Svanes C, Janson C, et al. Place of upbringing in early childhood as related to inflammatory bowel diseases in adulthood: a population-based cohort study in Northern Europe. European journal of epidemiology. 2014;29(6):429-437. doi: 10.1007/s10654-014-9922-3

[64] Radon K, Windstetter D, Poluda AL, et al. Contact with farm animals in early life and juvenile inflammatory bowel disease: a case-control study. Pediatrics. 2007;120(2): 354-361. doi: 10.1542/peds.2006-3624

[65] Van Kruiningen HJ, Joossens M, Vermeire S, et al. Environmental factors in familial Crohn's disease in Belgium. Inflamm Bowel Dis. 2005;11(4):360-365. doi: 10.1097/01.MIB.0000158536.31557.90

[66] Sood A, Amre D, Midha V, et al. Low hygiene and exposure to infections may be associated with increased risk for ulcerative colitis in a North Indian population. Annals of gastroenterology : quarterly publication of the Hellenic Society of Gastroenterology. 2014;27(3):219-223.

[67] Davis RL, Kramarz P, Bohlke K, et al. Measles-mumps-rubella and other measles-containing vaccines do not increase the risk for inflammatory bowel disease: a case-control study from the Vaccine Safety Datalink project. Archives of pediatrics & adolescent medicine. 2001;155(3):354-359.

[68] Shaw SY, Blanchard JF, Bernstein CN. Association between the use of antibiotics in the first year of life and pediatric inflammatory bowel disease. The American journal of gastroenterology. 2010;105(12):2687-2692. doi: 10.1038/ajg.2010.398

[69] Chan SS, Luben R, Bergmann MM, et al. Aspirin in the aetiology of Crohn's disease and ulcerative colitis: a European prospective cohort study. Aliment Pharmacol Ther. 2011;34(6):649-655. doi: 10.1111/j.1365-2036.2011.04784.x

[70] Ananthakrishnan AN, Higuchi LM, Huang ES, et al. Aspirin, nonsteroidal anti-inflammatory drug use, and risk for Crohn disease and ulcerative colitis: a cohort study. Annals of internal medicine. 2012;156(5):350-359. doi: 10.7326/0003-4819-156-5-201203060-00007

[71] Cornish JA, Tan E, Simillis C, Clark SK, Teare J, Tekkis PP. The risk of oral contraceptives in the etiology of inflammatory bowel disease: a meta-analysis. The American journal of gastroenterology. 2008;103(9):2394-2400. doi: 10.1111/j.1572-0241.2008.02064.x

[72] Khalili H, Higuchi LM, Ananthakrishnan AN, et al. Hormone therapy increases risk of ulcerative colitis but not Crohn's disease. Gastroenterology. 2012;143(5):1199-1206. doi: 10.1053/j.gastro.2012.07.096

[73] Khalili H, Higuchi LM, Ananthakrishnan AN, et al. Oral contraceptives, reproductive factors and risk of inflammatory bowel disease. Gut. 2013;62(8):1153-1159. doi: 10.1136/gutjnl-2012-302362

[74] Bager P, Simonsen J, Nielsen NM, Frisch M. Cesarean section and offspring's risk of inflammatory bowel disease: a national cohort study. Inflamm Bowel Dis. 2012;18(5): 857-862. doi: 10.1002/ibd.21805

[75] Bernstein CN, Singh S, Graff LA, Walker JR, Miller N, Cheang M. A prospective population-based study of triggers of symptomatic flares in IBD. The American journal of gastroenterology. 2010;105(9):1994-2002. doi: 10.1038/ajg.2010.140

[76] Gasche C, Scholmerich J, Brynskov J, et al. A simple classification of Crohn's disease: report of the Working Party for the World Congresses of Gastroenterology, Vienna 1998. Inflamm Bowel Dis. 2000;6(1):8-15.

[77] Louis E, Collard A, Oger AF, Degroote E, Aboul Nasr El Yafi FA, Belaiche J. Behaviour of Crohn's disease according to the Vienna classification: changing pattern over the course of the disease. Gut. 2001;49(6):777-782. doi:10.1136/gut.49.6.777

[78] Silverberg MS, Satsangi J, Ahmad T, et al. Toward an integrated clinical, molecular and serological classification of inflammatory bowel disease: report of a Working Party of the 2005 Montreal World Congress of Gastroenterology. Canadian journal of gastroenterology. 2005;19 Suppl A:5A-36A.

[79] Thia KT, Sandborn WJ, Harmsen WS, Zinsmeister AR, Loftus EV, Jr. Risk factors associated with progression to intestinal complications of Crohn's disease in a population-based cohort. Gastroenterology. 2010;139(4):1147-1155. doi: 10.1053/j.gastro. 2010.06.070

[80] Munkholm P, Langholz E, Davidsen M, Binder V. Disease activity courses in a regional cohort of Crohn's disease patients. Scand J Gastroenterol. 1995;30(7):699-706.

[81] Solberg IC, Lygren I, Jahnsen J, et al. Clinical course during the first 10 years of ulcerative colitis: results from a population-based inception cohort (IBSEN Study). Scand J Gastroenterol. 2009;44(4):431-440. doi: 10.1080/00365520802600961

[82] Moum B, Vatn MH, Ekbom A, et al. Incidence of ulcerative colitis and indeterminate colitis in four counties of southeastern Norway, 1990-93. A prospective population-based study. The Inflammatory Bowel South-Eastern Norway (IBSEN) Study Group of Gastroenterologists. Scand J Gastroenterol. 1996;31(4):362-366.

[83] Vind I, Riis L, Jess T, et al. Increasing incidences of inflammatory bowel disease and decreasing surgery rates in Copenhagen City and County, 2003-2005: a population-based study from the Danish Crohn colitis database. The American journal of gastroenterology. 2006;101(6):1274-1282. doi: 10.1111/j. 1572-0241.2006.00552.x

[84] Nguyen GC, Nugent Z, Shaw S, Bernstein CN. Outcomes of patients with Crohn's disease improved from 1988 to 2008 and were associated with increased specialist care. Gastroenterology. 2011;141(1):90-97. doi: 10.1053/j.gastro.2011.03.050

[85] Lakatos L, Kiss LS, David G, et al. Incidence, disease phenotype at diagnosis, and early disease course in inflammatory bowel diseases in Western Hungary, 2002-2006. Inflamm Bowel Dis. 2011;17(12):2558-2565. doi: 10.1002/ibd.21607

[86] Burisch J, Pedersen N, Cukovic-Cavka S, et al. Initial disease course and treatment in an inflammatory bowel disease inception cohort in Europe: the ECCO-EpiCom cohort. Inflamm Bowel Dis. 2014;20(1):36-46. doi: 10.1097/01.MIB.0000436277.13917.c4

[87] Solberg IC, Vatn MH, Hoie O, et al. Clinical course in Crohn's disease: results of a Norwegian population-based ten-year follow-up study. Clinical gastroenterology and hepatology : the official clinical practice journal of the American Gastroenterological Association. 2007;5(12):1430-1438. doi: 10.1016/j.cgh.2007.09.002

[88] Sands BE, Arsenault JE, Rosen MJ, et al. Risk of early surgery for Crohn's disease: implications for early treatment strategies. The American journal of gastroenterology. 2003;98(12):2712-2718. doi: 10.1111/j.1572-0241.2003.08674.x

[89] Ramadas AV, Gunesh S, Thomas GA, Williams GT, Hawthorne AB. Natural history of Crohn's disease in a population-based cohort from Cardiff (1986-2003): a study of changes in medical treatment and surgical resection rates. Gut. 2010;59(9):1200-1206. doi: 10.1136/gut.2009.202101

[90] Lakatos PL, Golovics PA, David G, et al. Has there been a change in the natural history of Crohn's disease? Surgical rates and medical management in a population-based inception cohort from Western Hungary between 1977-2009. The American journal of gastroenterology. 2012;107(4):579-588. doi: 10.1038/ajg.2011.448

[91] Hoie O, Wolters F, Riis L, et al. Ulcerative colitis: patient characteristics may predict 10-yr disease recurrence in a European-wide population-based cohort. The American journal of gastroenterology. 2007;102(8):1692-1701. doi: 10.1111/j. 1572-0241.2007.01265.x

[92] Vester-Andersen MK, Prosberg MV, Jess T, et al. Disease course and surgery rates in inflammatory bowel disease: a population-based, 7-year follow-up study in the era of immunomodulating therapy. The American journal of gastroenterology. 2014;109(5): 705-714. doi: 10.1038/ajg.2014.45

[93] Vester-Andersen MK, Vind I, Prosberg MV, et al. Hospitalisation, surgical and medical recurrence rates in inflammatory bowel disease 2003-2011-a Danish population-based cohort study. J Crohns Colitis. 2014;8(12):1675-1683. doi: 10.1016/j.crohns.2014.07.010

[94] Andersson RE, Olaison G, Tysk C, Ekbom A. Appendectomy and protection against ulcerative colitis. The New England journal of medicine. 2001;344(11):808-814. doi: 10.1056/NEJM200103153441104

[95] Andersson P, Olaison G, Bodemar G, Nystrom PO, Sjodahl R. Surgery for Crohn colitis over a twenty-eight-year period: fewer stomas and the replacement of total colectomy by segmental resection. Scand J Gastroenterol. 2002;37(1):68-73. doi: 10.1080/003655202753387383

[96] Radford-Smith G, Pandeya N. Associations between NOD2/CARD15 genotype and phenotype in Crohn's disease--Are we there yet? World J Gastroenterol. 2006;12(44): 7097-7103. doi: 10.3748/wjg.v12.i44.7097

[97] Beaugerie L. Inflammatory bowel disease therapies and cancer risk: where are we and where are we going? Gut. 2012;61(4):476-483. doi: 10.1136/gutjnl-2011-301133

[98] Pedersen N, Duricova D, Elkjaer M, Gamborg M, Munkholm P, Jess T. Risk of extra-intestinal cancer in inflammatory bowel disease: meta-analysis of population-based cohort studies. The American journal of gastroenterology. 2010;105(7):1480-1487. doi: 10.1038/ajg.2009.760

[99] Kandiel A, Fraser AG, Korelitz BI, Brensinger C, Lewis JD. Increased risk of lymphoma among inflammatory bowel disease patients treated with azathioprine and 6-mercaptopurine. Gut. 2005;54(8):1121-1125. doi: 10.1136/gut.2004.049460

[100] Long MD, Herfarth HH, Pipkin CA, Porter CQ, Sandler RS, Kappelman MD. Increased risk for non-melanoma skin cancer in patients with inflammatory bowel disease. Clinical gastroenterology and hepatology : the official clinical practice journal of the American Gastroenterological Association. 2010;8(3):268-274. doi: 10.1016/j.cgh. 2009.11.024

[101] Jess T, Frisch M, Simonsen J. Trends in overall and cause-specific mortality among patients with inflammatory bowel disease from 1982 to 2010. Clinical gastroenterology and hepatology : the official clinical practice journal of the American Gastroenterological Association. 2013;11(1):43-48. doi: 10.1016/j.cgh.2012.09.026

[102] Wolters FL, Russel MG, Sijbrandij J, et al. Crohn's disease: increased mortality 10 years after diagnosis in a Europe-wide population based cohort. Gut. 2006;55(4):510-518. doi: 10.1136/gut.2005.072793

[103] Hovde O, Kempski-Monstad I, Smastuen MC, et al. Mortality and causes of death in Crohn's disease: results from 20 years of follow-up in the IBSEN study. Gut. 2014;63(5): 771-775. doi: 10.1136/gutjnl-2013-304766

[104] Romberg-Camps M, Kuiper E, Schouten L, et al. Mortality in inflammatory bowel disease in the Netherlands 1991-2002: results of a population-based study: the IBD South-Limburg cohort. Inflamm Bowel Dis. 2010;16(8):1397-1410. doi: 10.1002/ibd. 21189

[105] Manninen P, Karvonen AL, Huhtala H, et al. Mortality in ulcerative colitis and Crohn's disease. A population-based study in Finland. J Crohns Colitis. 2012;6(5):524-528. doi: 10.1016/j.crohns.2011.10.009

[106] Jess T, Gamborg M, Munkholm P, Sorensen TI. Overall and cause-specific mortality in ulcerative colitis: meta-analysis of population-based inception cohort studies. The American journal of gastroenterology. 2007;102(3):609-617. doi: 10.1111/j.1572-0241.2006.01000.x

[107] Bewtra M, Kaiser LM, TenHave T, Lewis JD. Crohn's disease and ulcerative colitis are associated with elevated standardized mortality ratios: a meta-analysis. Inflamm Bowel Dis. 2013;19(3):599-613. doi: 10.1097/MIB.0b013e31827f27ae

[108] Hoie O, Schouten LJ, Wolters FL, et al. Ulcerative colitis: no rise in mortality in a European-wide population based cohort 10 years after diagnosis. Gut. 2007;56(4): 497-503. doi: 10.1136/gut.2006.101519

[109] Winther KV, Jess T, Langholz E, Munkholm P, Binder V. Survival and cause-specific mortality in ulcerative colitis: follow-up of a population-based cohort in Copenhagen County. Gastroenterology. 2003;125(6):1576-1582.

[110] Kassam Z, Belga S, Roifman I, Hirota S, Jijon H, Kaplan GG, Ghosh S, Beck PL. Inflammatory bowel disease cause-specific mortality: a primer for clinicians. Inflamm Bowel Dis. 2014 Dec;20(12):2483-92. doi: 10.1097/MIB.0000000000000173

4

Non-Pharmacological Approach to Irritable Bowel Syndrome

Elsa M. Eriksson, Kristina I. Andrén and
Henry T. Eriksson

Abstract

Irritable bowel syndrome (IBS) is a commonly diagnosed gastrointestinal condition. It represents a significant healthcare burden and still remains a real challenge. Over the years, IBS has been described as a strict illness of the gastrointestinal tract (medical model) or as a more complex multi-symptomatic disorder of the brain-gut axis (biopsychosocial or psychosomatic model). The reason why IBS has been such a challenge and is so difficult to handle might be related to different approaches. These differences in the view of the syndrome have affected the assessment, treatment and handling of the IBS patient. Patients with IBS, where the symptoms from the gastrointestinal tract are one part of a multi-symptom palette sometimes hidden in the body or mind, need a more holistic outlook. The key to an effective treatment approach is a gastroenterological examination to exclude other diseases along with an assessment of the whole body and its awareness by a body-mind therapist. This chapter discusses the view of the patient together with patient evaluations and body-mind treatment from a practical point of view.

Keywords: irritable bowel syndrome, body awareness therapy, body-mind evaluation, treatment

1. Introduction

Irritable bowel syndrome (IBS) is one of the most commonly diagnosed gastrointestinal conditions and generates a significant healthcare burden with huge economic costs [1]. In Sweden, 10–20% of the inhabitants suffer from some kind of disturbed bowel function [2]. Many are on long-term sick leave and there are studies showing that about 46% of all sick leaves are due to these patient categories and thus generating high costs for the society [3]. About 30–40% of the patients, consulting healthcare for acute abdominal troubles, are not diagnosed, and hence there might be IBS patients hidden among this group of patients. Increased economic consequences are also incurred as a result of unnecessary surgery. IBS is a common disease with symptoms, including abdominal pain, cramping or bloating. It may also include alteration in bowel habits like faecal urgency or obstipation. Patients may find relief of pain and other discomfort upon defecation. The prevalence of IBS may vary with different definitions and more severe cases can be underestimated. IBS is more prevalent among women. IBS patients can be subdivided in relation to symptoms. The three subtypes are a constipation predominant group (C-IBS), a diarrhoea predominant group (D-IBS) and a group with alternating type (A-IBS) where stool fluctuates between diarrhoea and constipation. In some cases, the symptoms may be so severe that a risk for suicide might occur. A final diagnosis of IBS should be based on clinical symptoms together with exclusion of various somatic diseases [1].

IBS patients often have various other symptoms, beside their gastrointestinal problems. They may have pain in other parts of the body, they may score high psychological symptoms as well as low quality of life. We have also found that they show deviations in body parameters such as body tensions, bodily stress patterns, low body awareness and biochemical stress parameters. Many IBS patients have been subjected to traumatic events and may suffer from a low self-esteem, difficulties setting limits and hypersensitivity. They are often co-diagnosed with fibromyalgia, "burn-out" depression and/or panic disorder. Patients may consult a number of different specialists within gastroenterology (abdominal problems), psychiatry (panic attacks and depression), rheumatology (arthritis), dermatology (eczema and itch) or primary healthcare (chronic fatigue syndrome, fibromyalgia and myalgia). The diagnosis given to a patient with one of these conditions often depends on the characteristic symptoms and the expertise of the treating clinician [1, 2, 4–6].

IBS patients have been reported to have higher levels of stress and more traumatic experiences than patients without gastrointestinal disturbances. Rats, experimentally induced with chronic stress, showed gastrointestinal symptoms (GIS) comparable to IBS. Different parts of the autonomic nervous system (ANS) have been shown to vary in activity when patients display diarrhoea or constipation as pre-dominant symptom of their IBS. When the state of stress continues it may lead to dysfunction of the ANS, that is, an autonomic dysfunction, sometimes called a comprehensive health disturbance. The syndromes in patients with overlapping diagnoses and multi-symptoms have also been called functional somatic syndromes, medically unexplained symptoms, somatoform disorders, unexplained clinical conditions or bodily distress syndrome. It has been suggested that these conditions actually should be gathered under one common name [1–4, 7, 8].

1.1. IBS over the years

The year 1948, Collins defined the syndrome of irritable colon as a "hyperirritable, neuromuscular imbalance of the colon sufficiently severe to cause abdominal pain or distress." He continued that it was "due to functional as well as somatic causes and it is important to emphasise physiologic, local irritative and psychosomatic factors" [9]. In 1956, Bargen wrote "The so called irritable colon is primarily the result of an emotional disturbance, a tension state, abuse of laxative agents or a dietary indiscretion." Bargen continued "Measures should include particular attention to their emotional disturbances, their situation in respect to stress, and particularly their dietary problems" [10]. IBS was later on (during the 1960s), defined as a disease of the gastrointestinal region with mainly pharmacological treatment. Wessely et al. [11] wrote in 1999 an article entitled "Functional somatic syndromes: one or many?" leading to that several physicians expressed their frustration about the treatment of IBS. Enck and Martens [12] wrote in 2008, "The next consensus for the syndrome of the irritable bowel has to be interdisciplinary." In the late 1970s, the authors started to use the word "biopsychosocial" and up to now about 100 articles have been published according to PubMed using this term in relation to IBS. Throughout the literature, two views emerge, including the medical view of IBS as a strict disease of the gastrointestinal tract, as well as a psychosomatic/biopsychosocial view in which IBS is seen as a complex multi-symptomatic disorder [1].

2. Non-pharmacological treatments

Most research concludes that the management of the complex syndrome IBS should rely on a combination of non-pharmacological and pharmacological therapies with dietary and lifestyle modifications. Some authors claim that treatments involving body and mind are the most effective and powerful treatment strategies in IBS/body distress patients [13–15]. Different non-pharmacological regimens have been used for the treatment of IBS. Body-mind therapies such as gut-directed hypnotherapy, mindfulness therapy, functional relaxation and body awareness therapy have been used with promising results both during treatment and at follow-up. Over the years, treatments have progressed from mostly individual to more group sessions; and there is also a trend towards prolonged sessions. The treatment modalities have also gone from focusing either on the body or the mind to now focusing on both [1].

Hypnotherapy has been used to treat IBS patients with good results since Whorwell et al. introduced it in 1984 [16]. Hypnotherapy means to induce a state of relaxation or trance in response to verbal or other stimuli, with suggestions for improvement made. The patient is taught relaxation, ego strengthening and coping skills. Tailoring the therapy to the patient's symptomatology is essential and the importance of practice is vital and should ideally take place on a daily basis. Hypnotherapy is mostly used with individually tailored technique and 12 sessions of treatment are provided to gain maximum benefit. It has been mostly used with gut-directed therapy; however Carolusson [17] includes both gut-oriented hypnotherapy and hypnoanalysis either separately or in combination. She concludes that hypnosis treatment has to be designed depending on patients' personality and possible mental defence-functions in relation to the symptoms as well as the mental and social resources. This technique is exceptionally operator-dependent; and not suitable for everyone [18]. Whorwell suggests that "hypnotherapy incorporated into a programme with a contingency plan for dealing with individuals who do not respond to this particular form of treatment is the best form of treatment" [19].

To apply *mindfulness* is to practise awareness of internal sensations and to have a non-judgemental approach to all experiences, impressions, thoughts and feelings that comes into awareness and to be fully present in the activities. Gaylord et al. adapted this practice to an IBS population by encouraging the patients to apply this approach on IBS-related symptoms and perceptions. Participants were instructed to notice any sensations in the abdominal area and try to distinguish those sensations from thoughts about the sensations [1, 20].

Functional relaxation is assumed to be a treatment of autonomic dysfunction with proprioception and a part of body awareness. During relaxed expiration, very subtle movements of the small joints are performed, when at the same time, the patient, focus and explore the perceived body sensations which are triggered by the movements. This takes unconscious body-mind experiences into account and, due to rediscovery and development of basic motivational systems, previously forgotten forms of bodily self-awareness can be re-experienced [1, 21].

Body awareness therapy (BAT™) is structured movements based on human anatomical and physiological requirements to achieve optimal dynamics. The BAT™ alludes to help the body find its natural posture. Then the body systems (circular, muscular, nerves and breathing) facilitate to recover their natural function. By doing so, unconscious body and mind experiences can come into awareness. Practising body awareness includes presence, reflection and acceptance. BAT™ was developed in Sweden by physiotherapists in the early 1970s. Nowadays it is used for treatment of various stress and pain-related conditions in all Nordic countries, as well as in Estonia, Austria, Scotland, Switzerland, the Netherlands, Spain and Turkey [1, 22].

One common point of these methods is training on how to be in the here and now; to be aware of the present. Body-mind training affects the level of muscular tension, the posture, the breathing, together with the function and mobility of the inner organs. The bodily experiences always exist in the present, and the awareness of emotions is inseparable from the consciousness of their bodily expressions. Altogether, these express how a person feels mentally and physically. In this way, these therapies, embracing body and mind, are assumed to work through a physiological transformation accomplished via the ANS [21, 23]. Although the methods differ slightly in how they are addressed, either through the mind (hypnotherapy or mindfulness) or through the body (body awareness therapy or functional relaxation), the treatment results are similar [1].

3. The Studies of Functional Bowel Syndrome and Treatment (SOFT) project

A project was started in 2000 with the purpose of examining patients with functional bowel disorders and compare them with healthy volunteers (without bowel disorders), and further to evaluate the effects of body awareness therapy on the patients symptoms. Since 2004, the authors (KA, gestalt therapist/BSc in chemistry/biomedicine and EE, physiotherapist/PhD in biochemistry/physiology, both trained and certified in BAT) have worked together and treated approximately 340 patients. Patients are referred from both primary and special care units (medicine and surgery), about 30% from each. Due to IBS being such a complex syndrome and our diversified backgrounds, we were interested in evaluating as many symptoms as possible reported by the patients. In a smaller study of IBS patients, vitamins, fatty acids and minerals were followed. We have also tried to characterise the IBS subtypes according to the data measured. In an epidemiologic study including a random population sample from the general population in Gothenburg, Sweden, we studied the correlation of gastrointestinal symptoms to other symptomatology in the same population. The SOFT studies and their results are described on the following sections. For practical reasons, the IBS patient is referred to as a women (she) in the following text.

3.1. The examination procedure in the SOFT study

After a thorough interview including medical history and their narrated experience, the patients are examined with two physical examinations: a resource-oriented body examination (ROBE) and a moving test body awareness scale-health (BAS-H) (**Table 1**). The ROBE examination evaluates body posture, function, respiration, passive mobility, balance and muscular degree of palpation. BAS-H evaluates grounding, midline, respiration and ability to set limits. The BAS-H test is based upon observations made by a physiotherapist of defined items on basic movements (BASobs) as well as standardised questions concerning their body awareness (BASself). From these two examinations one can get a picture of, to what degree the patient herself is aware of her body and its tensions. Patients in the project complete self-assessment questionnaires concerning psychological and psychosocial symptoms, pain, bodily symptoms and also a questionnaire regarding gastrointestinal symp-

Anamnesis	
Psychosomatic physiotherapeutic examinations	
	Resource-oriented body examination (ROBE)
	Body awareness scale examination (BAS-H)
Blood and saliva samples	
	Cortisol, prolactin, C-peptide, TG (triglycerides), minerals
	Vitamins
Questionnaires	
	GIS (Gastro Intestinal Scale, gastrointestinal symptoms)
	SCL90 (Symptom Check List 90, general symptoms, rating how much)
	CS (Complaint scale, general symptoms, rating how often)
	SOC (sense of coherence, health concepts related to quality of life)
	PRS (psychosocial rating scale)
Pain body map	Women/man
Food diary	4 days (including Saturday and Sunday)

Table 1. Examinations of the patients in the SOFT project.

toms. The CS scale measures autonomic dysfunction and can be divided into a vegetative, muscular and psychological part. Stress parameters in blood and saliva are also measured [1, 4–6].

In our study, the patients are evaluated at the unit two to three times during a total time of approximately 3 h, before starting treatment. After these examinations and meetings, we can form an opinion of each patient and what she may need to reduce symptoms and improve quality of life. These procedures also give us a hint of to what extent the patient is able to comply with our group treatment, and if we need to strengthen and support her regarding this before the start of treatment. Individual dialogues are held and questionnaires are completed at four times, one before treatment, one after 12 and 24 weeks, respectively, and also 6 months after the end of treatment.

3.2. The subtype study

Eighty IBS patients (30 D-IBS, 16 C-IBS and 34 A-IBS) underwent physiotherapeutic examinations (for dysfunctions in body movements/awareness) and were compared to an apparently healthy control group. Both IBS patients and controls answered questionnaires regarding psychological (SCL90) and gastrointestinal symptoms. Biochemical variables were analysed in blood. The subtypes were compared with each other and the control group [6].

3.3. The mineral, vitamin and fatty acids study

In a sub-study, 30 IBS patients were analysed for whole blood or serum levels of vitamins (B6, B12, E, Q10 and folic acid), minerals (Na, K, Ca, Mg, Cu, Fe, P, PB, Li, Zn and Selenium) and fatty acids (saturated, mono-unsaturated, $\Omega 3$ and $\Omega 6$). Questionnaires for gastrointestinal symptoms (GIS) and psychological symptoms (SCL90) were completed and correlated. Results from questionnaires versus minerals were calculated. The patients were grouped according to reference ranges established by the laboratory (Lab. für spektralanalytische und biologische Untersuchungen, Stuttgart, Germany) [24].

3.4. The epidemiologic study

The study of "Men born 1913" started in Gothenburg in 1963. In 2003, women born 1953 were included for the first time and a total of 668 women of 50 years old were randomly selected from the general population. We focused on gastrointestinal symptoms such as "have you during the last three months suffered from diarrhoea and/or constipation." The women were extensively screened with examinations such as descriptive data (body weight, height, BMI, waist hip, circumference, smoking and alcohol), somatic data (blood pressure, cholesterol, triglycerides, glucose and diseases) and vegetative data such as (dizziness, perspiration, breathlessness, indisposition and chilliness). Additionally, questions regarding stress were included (experience of stress, burnout and absence from work due to stress), psychological expression (lack of sleep, nervous symptom and easily moved to tears), psychosocial symptoms (situation of work, home, economics, health, memory and energy), grade of occupation (work, sick list and early pension) and medication were registered [25, 26].

4. Results

4.1. Before treatment evaluation of IBS patients in the SOFT study

Before treatment, evaluations show that IBS patients have deviated movement patterns, for example, grounding, midline, centration, setting up limits and awareness of respiration (BAS-H). Further they may have an impact on posture, body function (flexibility, spontaneous movement and passive activity), respiration and the muscular system (ROBE). Stress-parameters in blood and saliva can be affected and some patients also have mineral and vitamin deficiencies. Furthermore, they often present a low quality of life, and in many cases have experienced traumatic events (such as bullying in school, parental premature death, sexual abuse, war experiences or violations by the healthcare). They may also have psychological symptoms and autonomic dysfunction. The IBS patient thus shows many signs of being in a chronic condition of strain. In other words – they have an internal stress. Patients may have difficulties with trusting healthcare providers. Several patients have been adversely affected by previous visits. Often they have been told: "This is stress you will have to live with"; "With positive thinking it will be better." They often feel wrecked and angry, and tell that they have lost their self-confidence and self-esteem [1, 3–6].

When assessed before treatment, the patients in our study showed mostly deviated patterns in the results from the gastrointestinal survey, the body-oriented examinations and the pain drawings, in contrast to the psychological and biochemical data which were within normal limits or deviated (**Table 2**). From our experience to date, none of the patient from more than 300 patients have expressed only gastrointestinal symptoms [1, 3].

4.2. Results subtype study

The IBS patients as a whole group, as well as divided into subtypes, show higher triglyceride values compared to controls. When the material is divided into subtypes, the D-IBS group differ from the other two subtypes with significantly higher C-peptide values and lower prolactin values. This group score an almost normal degree in the questionnaire of sense of coherence (SOC) and thus showed a good quality of life. This was also reflected from the

Parts	Comments
Body oriented (ROBE, BAS-H)	Deviating in most cases
Pain (bodymap)	Deviating in most cases
Psychological (questionnaires)	Deviating or normal
Biochemical (blood, saliva)	Deviating or normal

Table 2. General results from examinations of IBS-patients.

D-IBS patients in a less distorted psychosocial rating scale in comparison with the other two subtypes. However, they express a high pain score similar to the other subtypes. The D-IBS group shows a disturbed body movement pattern on BASobs of the same magnitude as that of the C-IBS and the A-IBS group. However, on self-estimation (BASself) they rate themselves as having less dysfunction (not in conformity with the rating of the physiotherapist) reflecting a lower sense of body awareness. Compared to C-IBS and A-IBS, the D-IBS has the same amount of gastrointestinal symptoms but less psychological symptoms.

The C-IBS patients have higher prolactin values both compared to the controls and the D-IBS subtype. To some extent, similar pattern is seen in the C-IBS and the A-IBS group. On BASself examination both C-IBS and A-IBS rate themselves at the same level as did the physiotherapist. Both these subtypes suffer from more psychological and gastrointestinal symptoms, than was seen among controls. And the C-IBS patients have more psychological symptoms than the A-IBS group. Both groups display a lower quality of life outlined in the psychosocial rating scale and in the sense of coherence scale. Besides, they are afflicted with higher pain scores compared to the controls.

4.3. Results mineral study

IBS patients show considerable deficiencies of predominant minerals in whole blood. The study shows that only a small number of the tested IBS patients have levels within reference ranges (**Figure 1**). Values, both above and below the reference range (outliers), correlate to both gastrointestinal and psychological symptoms. Mineral values within reference ranges correspond to less gastrointestinal symptoms, both totally (Mg**, Cu* and Ca*) and for the sub-items gastrointestinal pain (Mg**), nausea (Ca*) and motility (Mg* and Ca*), see example for Ca (**Figure 2**). Mineral values within reference ranges correspond to less psychological symptoms as seen for Zink (**Figure 3**). These mineral shortages can contribute to the symptom map of the IBS patient. For the other substances measured more individual patterns are seen.

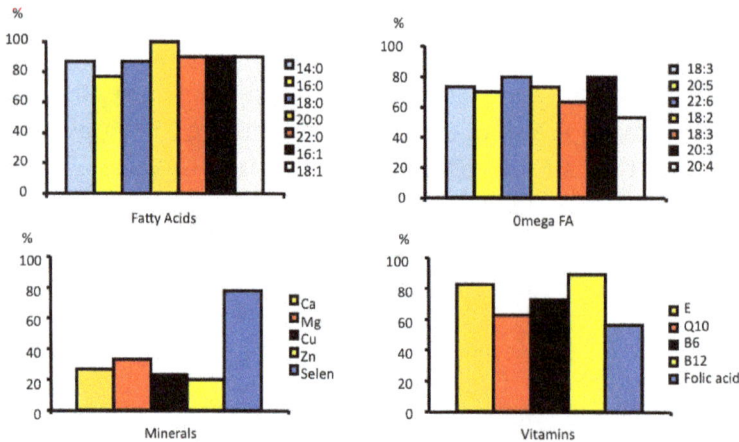

Figure 1. Percentage within reference ranges* for vitamins, minerals and fatty acids. *Lab. für spektralanalytische und biologische untersuchungen, Stuttgart, Germany.

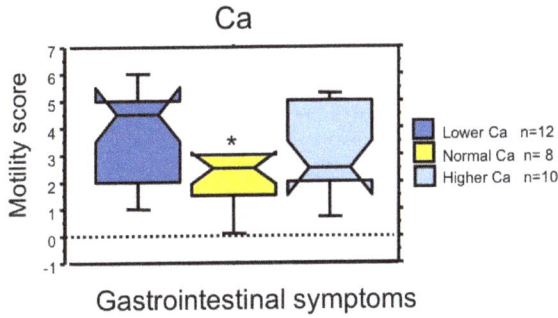

Figure 2. IBS patients with Ca levels within reference ranges express less gastro-intestinal symptoms, here illustrated as motility score. "Motility" = sensation of incomplete evacuation, sensation of urge to defecate. The higher score the more symptoms.

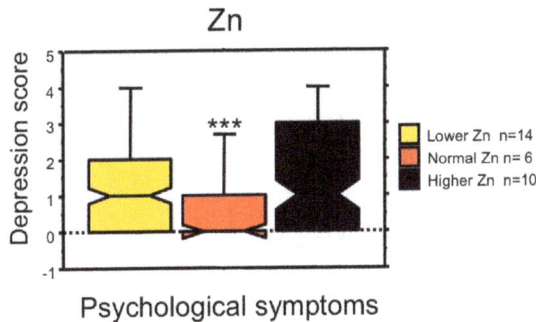

Figure 3. IBS patients with Zn levels within reference ranges express less psychological symptoms, here illustrated as depressive score. "Depression"—feelings of energy loss, suicidal ideation, easily crying and feeling—captured, lonely, depressed, anxious, hopeless or worthless. The higher score the more symptoms.

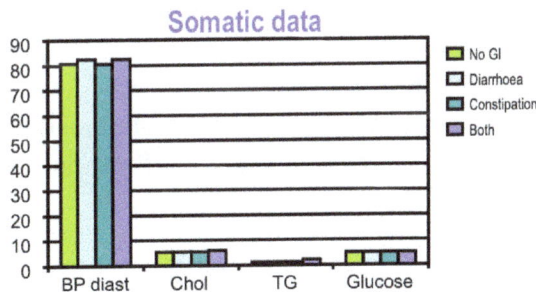

Figure 4. Score for some somatic data for the control group and the GI groups (diarrhoea, constipation and both).

4.4. Results epidemiologic study

Totally 668 of 994 invited 50-year-old women participated in the study. Of these 668 examined women, 492 (73.7%) had no gastrointestinal symptom. A total of 64 women (9.6%) reported diarrhoea, 85 (12.7%) stated constipation and 27 (4%) reported a mixture of diarrhoea and

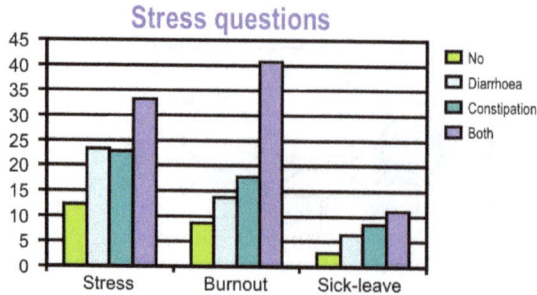

Figure 5. Score for stress, burnout and sick leave for the control group and the GI groups (diarrhoea, constipation and both).

constipation. No significant differences were seen between the controls (*no gastrointestinal problems*) and those women with gastrointestinal symptoms regarding *any of* the descriptive or somatic data (**Figure 4**). On the other hand, women reporting gastrointestinal symptoms showed significantly *more* vegetative and psychological symptoms, felt *more* stressed, had a *worse* psychosocial situation and were *more* on sick leave together with maintaining sickness pension in a *higher proportion* than did women without gastrointestinal symptoms (**Figure 5**). Our study shows that gastrointestinal symptoms are rather related to stress and psychosomatics, than to somatic parameters. The gastrointestinal symptoms contribute to an increased degree of sick leave and early retirement pension. These data underline the importance of considering *a more* psychosomatic attitude when treating patients with gastrointestinal symptoms.

5. The treatment procedure in the SOFT study

Process-oriented treatment is given in the form of body awareness practice in groups (8–12 individuals), 2 h per time on 24 occasions. Each occasion consists of bodily practice, theory and reflection. Psychosomatics, stress, anxiety, trauma, posture, allergy, IBS, food, body awareness, self-image, ANS and guilt and shame are theoretical themes that are addressed during each course. The structure of the treatment was inspired by Torrestad et al. [27], who developed a physiotherapeutic treatment model for awareness and relaxation. The bodily exercises derived mainly from basic body awareness (Institute for Basic Body awareness IBK™) [22].

5.1. The structure

Generally, the treatment is divided into three phases. The first phase is all about the body, its needs and body awareness. In the second phase, focus lies on changing the bodily behaviour. During the third part the training is aimed to integrate new insights and changes in everyday life. The same basic exercises are used each time; they are carried out easily from the beginning and are gradually expanded. Other exercises are included, if necessary. The focus lies on practicing body awareness, that is, to be aware of what is happening in the body. The order between lying, sitting, standing and walking exercises is varied in accordance with the group process. Most of the exercises can be performed in ways that are more stabilising or opening, and depending on the reaction of the patients, the exercises can be individually adjusted by the therapists. Every meeting begins and ends with a reflective discussion, in which each participant says her name and possibly something about how the past week has been, and how the body is feeling and at the end of the meeting, what has been noticed in the body during today's class.

5.2. The role of the leaders

Before each class the leaders outline a programme for the day which is adapted to the group process, focusing on the resources of the patients. Leaders keep diary on how the exercises are working and about themes that are expressed in the discussions. These notes created together with the leaders' own reflections, a basis for planning and the next training session. The purpose is to mediate the knowledge, both practical and theoretical, that each individual need in her process towards a better health. This purpose is reflected in the leaders' approach to the patients' questions and comments, as well as in planning the exercises and the theory.

6. The treatment results in the SOFT study

In conclusion, the studies in the SOFT project show that as the patients' gastrointestinal symptoms decrease, their pain decreases, they feel better and experience less anxiety and depression. They develop better relations to their own body and to the life around them. Patients change from having a feeling of being controlled by their gut and their symptoms to feeling safer and to be able to handle different situations in life, both physically and mentally. This treatment affects the patients' body, their feelings, thoughts and actions (**Table 3**).

6.1. Body examinations

ROBE shows that patients improve the variable function during treatment. They are also more relaxed and develop a higher degree of body awareness and a more normalised tension pattern at muscle palpation. In the BAS-H (the movement part of BAS-H), the IBS patients showed improvements. IBS patients also expressed awareness (the interview part of BAS-H) of their improvements, particularly in relation to the ground and in centring of the movements but also to breathing, and to the ability to set limits [3–5].

6.2. Surveys, SCL90, CS and SOC

Psychological symptoms at baseline scored with SCL90 were significantly more common in the IBS group than in the healthy control group. IBS patients score lower levels of psychological symptoms such as depression, obsession, paranoid ideation, anxiety, phobic anxiety and psychoticism after treatment, as measured by SCL90. The items of depression and somatisation were positively correlated. Patients show improvements in the vegetative part of the CS scale early in the treatment period (at the 12 weeks assessment) which then continued. The IBS patients showed a lower sense of coherence than the controls

I have noticed:	
"Body"	*how I am sitting, standing and walking, and if I am anxious or relaxed*
	that feelings quickly transmit to the stomach
"Mind"	*that I am better in expressing my needs, and how I want to do things without bullying others and when I am assertive, I get positive response and people listen to me*
I have started thinking about:	
"Body"	*to recognise when the stress in the body speeds up (to stop in time),*
	I respect more than previously how the body is feeling
	myself, I feel safe to listen to my body
"Mind"	*my past and how it has affected me*
	to take it easy, to cool down
	to not care so much about what other people think about me
I have started to change	
"Body"	*I have great use of the exercises that I learned at our meetings; I practice them daily and have now only minor phases of pain from the diverticulums*
	I feel more vitality and joy in my body.
"Mind"	*my ideas of achievement/performance, I don't have to do everything so much better than everyone else anymore*
	my way of interacting with others, I stand up for myself and my needs and I am, at the same time, more sensitive for the need of the other

Table 3. Patients' comments after 24 weeks of treatment.

before treatment. There were also differences in the items of comprehensibility, manageability and meaningfulness. Their sense of coherence or coping ability shows improvement during the treatment period in total and for each subtype. Before treatment, some patients scored themselves very low, comparable to levels reported from patients who had tried to commit suicide.

6.3. Pain drawings

At baseline, pain drawing gives higher scores for IBS patients than for healthy controls. In addition to pain in the stomach, IBS patients also have other bodily pain of different qualities, for example, in shoulders, arms, back, breast, head, leg and foot. No difference is seen between the subtypes (D-IBS, C-IBS and A-IBS) in this respect and the pain gradually decreased with treatment [3–5].

6.4. Saliva cortisol

Measurements of saliva cortisol indicate that IBS patients can be classified into two groups according to how cortisol levels are reflected in the saliva during the day (diurnal cortisol). One group showed increased diurnal slope and another group lower diurnal slope, which may be interpreted as "overstressed" and "burnt out," respectively. Diurnal cortisol went towards normalisation after treatment with BAT, irrespective of the starting levels. Somatic symptoms correlated with biochemical symptoms. There was a correlation between the most normal score of muscle palpation and a more optimal slope of saliva cortisol [6].

6.5. Observations during treatment

In our study, we as leaders have recurrently noted indications that patients become more grounded and more relaxed during treatment. We observe, for example, better balance in movements and decreased facial tension. The patients develop a better relationship with their own bodies, which, for example, is noticeable when they find it easier to relate to their own body and express more positive opinions about it. They also score lower levels of psychological symptoms after treatment. As the patients become more aware of their symptoms, they improve their body awareness and their symptoms decrease. In the group situation, the changes are also reflected. For example, patients who are very silent when treatment starts will gradually become more confident and start talking more in the group, and those who early on, do not take part in pair exercises will later on join these exercises. Other patients reported that they no longer are dwelling on injustices in the past, and now could let them go and move on forward in their lives [3–5].

7. Working relationship between patient and therapist

Many authors emphasise the importance of a good working treatment relationship between the patient and the therapist/clinician. In order to get an optimal treatment, the therapists need to explore how to create practicable channels of contact. A person with a cognitive orientation wants to obtain a theoretically plausible explanation of her problems in order to feel safe and secure. A person with alexithymia, who cannot express and do not have words for her emotions, needs to increase her body awareness, in order to become comfortable with her body. A person with a vivid and colourful imagination is probably receptive to exercises that include mental visualisation. An optimal treatment plan should comprise all of these components [1].

7.1. Aspects of performing body-mind therapies

When treating IBS patients, who has tendency to dissociate, the therapist must be careful not to re-victimise the patient and thus risk the patient dropping out. By noticing early warning signs for dissociation and with careful guidance, the patients can learn how to build a trusting relationship with themselves and others, in order to maintain both a psychological and a physical integrity (setting up limits) and also to facilitate for the patients to find words to describe the body-signals and sensations. With increasing body awareness, the patients will learn how to stabilise themselves when emotional systems are aroused. In order to first perceive the body and then to connect the sensations in the body with a certain sense or emotion is crucial for the treatment to be effective. The patient may express after several treatment sessions: "Before I just had a stomach ache, but now it is like that just before I get pain, I feel angry" [1, 3].

7.2. Duration of body-mind treatment

The length of treatment can be crucial [1]. Short treatment duration is not always sufficient for all patients; some can be left behind as they display more symptoms. In our studies we have found different patient treatment processes. IBS patients grade themselves on different symptom questionnaires, and both body and biochemical parameters are evaluated; the process can be determined by such parameters. For example, one patient can estimate high levels of symptoms before treatment that are reduced after treatment. Another patient might start by estimating low levels before treatment and score higher at 12 weeks and then lower again after 24 weeks. Such a patient probably need more time to become aware of her bodily sensations, and thus "underestimated" the levels of her symptoms/sensations before the treatment start. A third patient can score increasing symptoms throughout the entire treatment period. This example shows a patient who started out with having a substantially low body awareness, whose experiences have been out of reach/hidden in the body and then slowly arouse into awareness during the treatment process. Hence, treatment of this patient should not be concluded until the patient's symptoms decrease [1, 3–6].

8. Discussion

Many authors, including Collins et al. [9], Bargen [10] and Enck et al. [12], have stressed that IBS is a complicated condition with both physiological and psychological factors involved in the pathogenesis [1]. Moser points out that in practice, functional gastrointestinal disorders are the most frequent disorder seen and suggest that integrated psychosomatic care should be provided [28]. This is in line with the results from our SOFT project with physical, psychological and biochemical examinations and treatment of the "whole person" using body awareness therapy.

The SOFT study has shown that as the patients' gastrointestinal symptoms decreases, the pain decreases, they feel better and experience less depression and anxiety. The patients express a greater awareness of their own potential to affect their symptoms and are more able to control their lives. They change from feeling controlled by their gut and their symptoms to feel safer and able to handle different situations in life, both physically and mentally. Other studies confirm that patients' gastrointestinal symptoms and the extra-intestinal manifestations improve along with increased body awareness [1, 3].

Levels of anxiety and depression are significantly higher among patients with IBS in comparison with apparently healthy persons without IBS [7, 9, 10]. Something that may contribute to the reduction in health-related quality of life in patients with IBS is the ability to cope with stressful circumstances in life. Antonovsky [29] says that a person needs a strong sense of coherence (SOC) to be able to cope with significant life stressor. Patients having alternating constipation and diarrhoea may be a great problem of daily life that could be considered highly stressful. Thus, a strong SOC might lessen the impact of various stressors on well-being or the stressors themselves can weaken SOC. Motzer et al. [30] have searched for therapeutic ways to increase SOC and quality of life and thus ease the psychological distress associated with IBS. Sperber et al. [31] questioned whether SOC represent a predictor of treatment success or is an outcome variable (which is changeable). We believe that SOC can act both as a predictor and an outcome variable. A low SOC may be a predictor at baseline reflecting the severity of IBS, and thus could prolong the duration of treatment (predictor). However, in the end of the study patients altered their sense of coherence (outcome variable) towards normality values as a result of the therapy [5].

Saliva cortisol in healthy persons has straight downward slopes during daytime. A more negative stress response is reflected by a lower saliva cortisol slope and is an indicator of accumulated physiological and psychosocial stress [32]. A lower slope associated with too high or too low muscle palpation grade was seen in our study. An increased slope of saliva cortisol belonged for the most part to the group with a somewhat increased muscle palpation grade. An increased slope may represent the first phase of the body trying to compensate for stress while a lower slope represents chronic stress and/or exhaustion [33]. Saliva cortisol in the IBS patients changed during treatment; both the lower and the increased slope approached the slope of the controls.

From the SOFT subtype study, it seems the D-IBS patients differ from the other subtypes. D-IBS patients, with a higher proportion of men, scored less psychological symptoms, less body awareness, but scored a better sense of coherence and showed higher C-peptide values in blood. They were not aware of their lack of body awareness and did not realise entirely their depreciated state of health. Overall, they showed themselves to be ambitious persons, and there were more men compared to the other subtypes. Also, many of them were in the middle of their professional careers. The higher C-peptide and triglyceride levels may be parts of a metabolic syndrome, which is known to correlate with psychosocial stress possibly indicating an adrenergic onset that could represent an unconscious mental stress. When studying predominant symptoms in IBS and correlation with autonomic nervous system deviations it was found that the D-IBS subgroup was associated with adrenergic nervous system malfunctions. Prolactin may be important in the process of coping with stress and traumatic experience and it has been reported that active soldiers have lower prolactin values. A strong correlation has been shown between prolactin and alexithymia especially the item "difficulty to identifying feelings." The D-IBS group in our study had both lower prolactin values and lower body awareness [6].

The C-IBS and A-IBS patients are characterised by their psychological symptoms, with more depression and anxiety and with impaired sense of coherence. They express higher degree of body awareness compared to the D-IBS group. Emotional strain and an increased vagal tone are correlated to increased levels of prolactin which could be one reason for the measured prolactin increase in the C-IBS group [6]. Although the sample size of the present study of subtypes is fairly modest, all subjects were recruited from patients with rather advanced IBS disease with several years' history of symptoms. Since they were referred from various doctors from different clinics they could represent a general population of IBS patients.

According to Gonsalkorale et al. [34], IBS has gained the reputation of being somewhat unrewarding to treat. As a consequence, many physicians although performing thorough examinations ensure their patients that there are nothing seriously wrong but offer no remedy to treat the condition. Many patients, especially those who have had their troublesome symptoms for a long time have lost their confidence and feel like "failures" with no hope when they enter our study [1]. Dysregulation of the autonomic nervous system and the emotional system can involve reactions in which the distress inside the body is not recognised because of location or due to low body awareness. This may be one explanation why patients have difficulty identifying their symptoms and can contribute to the fact that there might be misunderstandings between the IBS patients and healthcare providers [1, 3–6]. Another possible explanation could be the two different views of IBS, as mentioned earlier; when the treating doctor views IBS as a strict gastrointestinal disease he will be more apt to a reassuring approach. On the other hand, the doctor who embraces the view that IBS is a more complex disorder will refer the patient to a competent body-mind therapist or a multi-professional team offering a more psychosomatic therapy.

As IBS patients express a great deal of symptoms, they often find themselves somewhat lost within the normal healthcare system with its specialisation. For example, within the field of gastroenterology, some hospitals have various departments for the upper and lower gastrointestinal tract. This involves a great risk that the patients with multiple symptoms and multiple diagnoses are inadequately treated since their cases fall in between different categories [1, 3]. When practising a team approach to management with a graduated treatment programme, extremely high levels of satisfaction in patients and in staff can be achieved [34]. As we saw in the epidemiologic study of 50-year-old women, gastrointestinal symptoms were common in that population and showed a strong correlation to psychosomatic symptoms. Therefore, a more psychosomatic attitude in diagnosis and treatment of these women might have great impact on their well-being.

Many authors stress the importance of a thorough examination of IBS patients with their many symptoms after having excluded important somatic diseases. In the SOFT project, the comprehensive body examination gave us a hint about the treatment duration needed for the patient to improve. When IBS patients are receiving too short treatment duration, the patient may experience relief from some symptoms, but with the underlying distress still present, they will remain untreated and symptoms can be replaced by other symptoms (known as a symptom shift). In these cases, there is a risk that the patients will continue to seek treatment elsewhere and thus get caught between specialities and might never come to understand their internal body mind communication [17]. Patients who need longer treatment periods could be patients that can be defined as non-responders, males with D-IBS, fibromyalgia patients or those who have severe social stress; all factors are likely to cause detraction from the efficacy of the treatment.

Hypnotherapy, mindfulness treatment and body awareness therapy will almost certainly improve the patients' coping skills in various life situations. These methods involve the body by normalising tension, and they also emphasise the importance of being present in the moment. It is only in the present time that you can access and influence the experience and behaviour patterns, which are established in the nervous system [35]. A plausible consequence of this is that consciousness of the "here and now" is very substantial for changing the processes and should be the focus of therapy from the beginning. The habits of non-optimal movement and tension patterns, whether due to chronic stress or other mechanisms, can become so established in the body that you are incapable of changing them on your own. These habits are integrated as part of the self-perception and can be unconsciously hidden together with other suppressed feelings and tensions. To deal with ingrained muscular pattern, the patients must be re-educated and trained until the new patterns feel at least equally familiar as the old ones [36]. Paradoxically, patients need body awareness training to be aware of their tensed bodies before they can start to change and in a deeper sense learn to apply the body awareness therapy [1, 3]. The body awareness technique can thus be used to take control of unwanted symptoms and to reduce psychological distress and improve coping skills [1, 3].

9. Conclusion

From the SOFT project it can be concluded that IBS patients, in comparison with healthy controls have higher degree of body tension and gastrointestinal and psychological symptoms and also biochemical stress markers compared to healthy controls. Our treatment with body awareness therapy reduced these parameters and helped these multi-symptomatic patients feel better. This treatment can be practised for all types of IBS, and since it is performed in groups it is therefore suitable for treating quite a large number of patients at the same time. Our structure of treatment in the SOFT study, combining bodily exercises with theoretical reflections and including time for reflexions in the group, has proven to be beneficial for our patients.

The future health problems are generally considered to be of psychosomatic or psychosocial nature. This should cause us great concern, and we need a new approach for these multi-symptomatic patients and not least the IBS patients. Good teamwork is important during this new approach to treat multi-symptom patients. Therapists/physicians should talk to each other about IBS cases and/or work in a team to ensure that any real or potential problem that may arise can be promptly resolved. When planning effective treatment strategies it is of utmost importance to understand the diversity of this syndrome. Thus, treatment should be aimed at body-mind intervention after having performed a good evaluation survey of each patient both by a gastroenterologist and a body-mind therapist. The duration of treatment should be individually adjusted. Following the same patients systematically, before, during and after treatment seems to be the best method of choice at present. These patients need a psychosomatic approach which is emphasised from our epidemiologic study. Applying a more psychosomatic attitude when diagnosing and treating these patients will give a more optimal caring and in the long run lowered medical healthcare costs.

Author details

Elsa M. Eriksson*, Kristina I. Andrén and Henry T. Eriksson

*Address all correspondence to: elsa.eriksson@surgery.gu.se

Department of Functional Gastroenterology, Sahlgrenska University Hospital, Göteborg, Sweden

References

[1] Eriksson EM, Andrén KI, Kurlberg GK, Eriksson HT. Aspects of the non-pharmacological treatment of irritable bowel syndrome. *World J Gastroenterol* 2015; **21**: 11439–11449. DOI:10.3748/wjg.v21.i40.11439. Review.

[2] Ålander T, Svärdsudd K, Agréus L. Functional gastrointestinal disorder is associated with increased non-gastrointestinal healthcare consumption in the general population. *Int J Clin Pract* 2008; **62**: 234–240. DOI:10.1111/j.1742-1241.2007.01549.x

[3] Biguet G, Keskinen-Rosenqvist R, Levy-Berg A. Understanding the body's message – approaches from the physiotherapists' point of view. 1st ed. Lund: Studentlitteratur, 2012. ISBN:9789144073217

[4] Eriksson E, Nordwall V, Kurlberg G, Rydholm H. Effects of body awareness therapy in patients with irritable bowel syndrome. *Adv Physiol Educ* 2002; **4**: 125–135. DOI:10.1080/140381902320387540

[5] Eriksson EM, Möller IE, Söderberg RH, Eriksson HT, Kurlberg GK. Body awareness therapy: a new strategy for relief of symptoms in irritable bowel syndrome patients. *World J Gastroenterol* 2007; **13**: 3206–3214. PMID: 17589899 DOI:10.3748/WJG.v13.i23.3206

[6] Eriksson EM, Andrén KI, Eriksson HT, Kurlberg GK. Irritable bowel syndrome subtypes differ in body awareness, psychological symptoms and biochemical stress markers. *World J Gastroenterol* 2008; **14**: 4889–4896. PMID: 18756596 DOI:10.3748/wjg.14.4889

[7] White DL, Savas LS, Daci K, Elserag R, Graham DP, Fitzgerald SJ, Smith SL, Tan G, El-Serag HB. Trauma history and risk of irritable bowel syndrome in women veterans. *Aliment Pharmacol Ther* 2010; **32**: 551–561. DOI:10.1111/j.1365-2036.2010.04387.x

[8] Vicario M, Guilarte M, Alonso C, Yang P, Martínez C, Ramos L, Lobo B, González A, Guilà M, Pigrau M, Saperas E, Azpiroz F, Santos J. Chronological assessment of mast cell-mediated gut dysfunction and mucosal inflammation in a rat model of chronic psychological stress. *Brain Behav Immun* 2010; **24**: 1166–1175. DOI:10.1016/j.bbi.2010.06.002

[9] Collins EN. The diagnosis and treatment of irritable colon; physiologic, local irritative and psychosomatic factors. *Med Clin North Am* 1948; **32**: 398–407. PMID:18902879

[10] Bargen JA. The problem of the syndrome of irritable bowel. *Gastroenterology* 1956; **30**: 703–706. PMID:13318254

[11] Wessely S, Nimnuan C, Sharpe M. Functional somatic syndromes: one or many? *Lancet* 1999; **354**: 936–939. DOI:10.1016/S0140-6736(98)08320-2

[12] Enck P, Martens U. The next consensus for the irritable bowel syndrome has to be interdisciplinary. *Z Gastroenterol* 2008; **46**: 211–215. DOI:10.1055/s-2007-963341

[13] Fink P, Schröder A. One single diagnosis, bodily distress syndrome, succeeded to capture 10 diagnostic categories of functional somatic syndromes and somatoform disorders. *J Psychosom Res* 2010; **68**: 415–426. DOI:10.1016/j.jpsychores.2010.02.004

[14] Grundmann O, Yoon SL. Complementary and alternative medicines in irritable bowel syndrome: an integrative view. *World J Gastroenterol* 2014; **20**: 346–362. DOI:10.3748/wjg.v20.i2.346. Review.

[15] Schenström O. Introduction to mindfulness, CD. On the CD he says "It is the most powerful tool that I have come in contact with during my 30 years as a physician" 2006. Available from: http://www.mindfulnesscenter.se

[16] Whorwell PJ, Prior A, Faragher EB. Controlled trial of hypnotherapy in the treatment of severe refractory irritable-bowel syndrome. *Lancet* 1984; **2**: 1232–1234. DOI:10.1016/S0140-6736(84)92793-4

[17] Carolusson S. Dynamic hypnosis, IBS, and the value of individualizing treatment: a clinical perspective. *Int J Clin Exp Hypn* 2014; **62**: 145–163. DOI:10.1080/00207144.2014.869127

[18] Whorwell PJ. Effective management of irritable bowel syndrome – the Manchester Model. *Int J Clin Exp Hypn* 2006; **54**: 21–26. DOI:10.1080/00207140500323006

[19] Whorwell PJ. The history of hypnotherapy and its role in the irritable bowel syndrome. *Aliment Pharmacol Ther* 2005; **22**: 1061–1067. DOI:10.1111/j.1365-2036.2005.02697.x. Review.

[20] Gaylord SA, Palsson OS, Garland EL, Faurot KR, Coble RS, Mann JD, Frey W, Leniek K, Whitehead WE. Mindfulness training reduces the severity of irritable bowel syndrome in women: results of a randomized controlled trial. *Am J Gastroenterol* 2011; **106**:1678–1688. DOI:10.1038/ajg.2011.184

[21] Lahmann C, Röhricht F, Sauer N, Noll-Hussong M, Ronel J, Henrich G, von Arnim A, Loew T. Functional relaxation as complementary therapy in irritable bowel syndrome: a randomized, controlled clinical trial. *J Altern Complement Med* 2010; **16**: 47–52. DOI:10.1089/acm.2009.0084

[22] BAT™, The Institute for Body Awareness Therapy™. Available from: http://www.ibk.nu

[23] Landsman-Dijkstra JJ, van Wijck R, Groothoff JW. The long-term lasting effectiveness on self-efficacy, attribution style, expression of emotions and quality of life of a body

awareness program for chronic a-specific psychosomatic symptoms. *Patient Educ Couns* 2006; **60**: 66–79. PMID:16332472

[24] Eriksson E, Holmquist Å, Wolfgang Bayer W, Bergman B. Blood levels of vitamins, minerals and fatty acids in patients with irritable bowel syndrome (IBS). In proceedings of the European Conference on Psychosomatic Research (ECPR); 27–30 September 2006; Cavtat, Croatia. *J Psychosom Res* 2006; **61**: 422 DOI:10.1016/j.jpsychores.2006.06.004

[25] Welin C, Wilhelmsen L, Welin L, Johansson S, Rosengren A. Perceived health in 50-year-old women and men and the correlation with risk factors, diseases, and symptoms. Gend Med 2011; **8**: 139–149. DOI:10.1016/j.genm.2011.03.005

[26] Eriksson E, Johansson S, Wallander MA, Welin C, Kurlberg G, Eriksson H. Gastrointestinal symptoms in 50 year old women shows a strong correlation to psychosomatics. Continuation of the epidemiological study "Men born 1913". In proceedings of the European Conference on Psychosomatic Research (ECPR); 27–30 September 2006; Cavtat, Croatia. *J Psychosom Res* 2006; **61**: 405–406. DOI:10.1016/j.jpsychores.2006.06.004

[27] Torrestad A, Håkansson M, Axelli T. Development of a program for the treatment of chronic pain and anxiety. A learning process leading from unsound to sound assessment. *Int J Technol Assess Health Care* 1992; **8**: 85–92. PMID:1601597

[28] Moser G. Psychosomatic aspects of bowel diseases. *Z Psychosom Med Psychother* 2006; **52**: 112–126. PMID:16790162

[29] Antonovsky A. The structure and properties of the sense of coherence scale. *Soc Sci Med* 1993; **36**: 725–733. PMID:8480217

[30] Motzer SA, Hertig V, Jarrett M, Heitkemper MM. Sense of coherence and quality of life in women with and without irritable bowel syndrome. *Nurs Res* 2003; **52**: 329–337. PMID:14501547

[31] Sperber AD, Carmel S, Atzmon Y, Weisberg I, Shalit Y, Neumann L, Fich A, Buskila D. The sense of coherence index and the irritable bowel syndrome. A cross-sectional comparison among irritable bowel syndrome patients, with and without coexisting fibromyalgia, irritable bowel syndrome non patients, and controls. *Scand J Gastroenterol* 1999; **34**: 259–263. PMID:10232869

[32] Sephton SE, Sapolsky RM, Kraemer HC, Spiegel D. Diurnal cortisol rhythm as a predictor of breast cancer survival. *J Natl Cancer Inst* 2000; **92**: 994–1000. PMID:10861311

[33] Rosmond R, Bjorntorp P. Low cortisol production in chronic stress. The connection stress-somatic disease is a challenge for future research. *Lakartidningen* 2000; **97**: 4120–4124. PMID:11068377

[34] Gonsalkorale WM, Houghton LA, Whorwell PJ. Hypnotherapy in irritable bowel syndrome: a large-scale audit of a clinical service with examination of factors influencing responsiveness. *Am J Gastroenterol* 2002; **97**: 954–961. PMID:12003432

[35] Gottwald C. Awareness and mindfulness in consciousness-centred body psychotherapy. *Int Body Psychother J* 2014; **13**:67–79. Available from: Academic Search Index, Ipswich, MA.

[36] Lundvik Gyllensten A, Hansson L, Ekdahl C. Patient experiences of basic body awareness therapy and the relationship with the physiotherapist. *J Bodywork Mov Ther* 2003; **7**: 173–183. DOI:10.1111/j.1471-6712.2004.00272.x

5

Intestinal Fibroblast/Myofibroblast TRP Channels in Inflammatory Bowel Disease

Lin Hai Kurahara, Keizo Hiraishi, Kunihiko Aoyagi,
Yaopeng Hu, Miho Sumiyoshi and Ryuji Inoue

Abstract

Inflammatory bowel disease (IBD) is characterized by the repeated cycles of inflammation and healing of the gut, which ultimately progress into intestinal fibrosis. Colonic fibroblast/myofibroblast's functions such as transformation, proliferation, invasion, migration, stress fiber formation, collagen synthesis, and cytokine/chemokine secretion are well estimated. However, the detailed mechanism can rarely be found so far. Thus, we focused on transient receptor potential (TRP) protein super family activated by various physical/chemical stimulations based on the above-described recognitions and also conducted the following examinations for the potential roles in Ca^{2+} signal transduction in fibroblast/myofibroblasts cells, which play an important role in intestinal inflammation and tissue remodeling. This chapter not only facilitates the understanding about the new role of intestinal fibroblast/myofibroblasts TRP channel for regulating inflammation, fibrotic processes but also suggests a novel molecular target of IBD treatment in future.

Keywords: inflammatory bowel disease (IBD), myofibroblast, TRP channels

1. Introduction

The prevalence of inflammatory bowel disease (IBD), a group of idiopathic disorders such as Crohn's disease (CD) and ulcerative colitis (UC) that cause chronic inflammation or ulcers in large- and small-intestinal mucosa, has been rapidly increasing since the Second World War. Because IBD follows a course of repeated severe diarrhea and constipation from a young age, it deteriorates an individual's quality of life for a long period of time as a refractory disorder.

Currently, most IBD treatments are limited to symptomatic relief. With increasing incidence, there is an escalating need to clarify a cause and establish definitive treatments [1, 2].

Located at the interface between the epithelium and lamina propria in most mucosal tissues, intestinal fibroblast/myofibroblast cells have ultrastructural features reminiscent of both smooth muscle cells and fibroblasts. Accumulating evidence suggests that myofibroblasts play crucial roles in intestinal homeostasis, inflammation, and neoplasia. In addition, these cells are known to play an essential role in modulating wound healing and fibrosis processes at the time of tissue damage or inflammation [3–5]. For instance, during skin-wound healing, fibroblast cells differentiate into myofibroblasts that secrete cytokines and growth factors to reduce wound size by contracting granulation tissue. Similarly, fibroblast-derived hepatic stellate cells (also known as Ito cells) located in the sinusoidal space of the liver support sinusoidal structure. Fibroblasts with similar transformation ability are also distributed in renal tubular epithelia, where they can be transformed in response to tissue damage, inflammatory substances, or growth factors to promote collagen production and stress fiber formation for tissue fibrosis [6–8]. Furthermore, fibroblast/myofibroblast cells produce cytokines, chemokines, growth factors, and inflammatory mediators involved in immune and inflammatory responses. The activation of myofibroblasts can induce excessive fibrosis, causing pathological tissue modifications (remodeling) such as wound closure, keloid formations, hepatic fibrosis (cirrhosis), and digestive tract obstructions [9]. However, mechanisms underlying myofibroblast transformation and cytokine secretion remain almost completely unknown, despite their importance in inflammatory tissue modifications.

Fibroblasts/myofibroblasts play important roles during the processes of intestinal inflammation and tissue remodeling [10, 11]; however, detailed mechanisms have rarely been identified. Based on previously described recognitions, we therefore focused on the transient receptor potential (TRP) superfamily as a new Ca^{2+} channel gene group activated by various physical and chemical stimuli. Mammalian TRP proteins form a non-selective cation channel superfamily that includes approximately 30 isoforms categorized into six subfamilies [12], including TRPC (canonical or classical: TRPC1–7), TRPV (vanilloid: TRPV1–6), TRPM (melastatin: TRPM1–8), TRPP (polycystin: TRPP1–4), TRPML (mucolipin: TRPML1–3), and TRPA (ankyrin: TRPA1). Implicated in a variety of cellular functions, TRP proteins form large non-voltage-gated cation channels constitutively activated by various physicochemical stimuli. Known activators for TRP channels include chemical stimuli (such as receptor stimulation, change in pH, and spicy or cooling agents), as well as temperature changes and various forms of mechanical stimuli including osmotic stress, membrane stretching, and shear forces. Proposed mechanisms are primarily associated with lipid bilayer mechanics, specialized force-transducing structures, biochemical reactions, membrane trafficking, and transcriptional regulation. TRP channels are assumed to form a tetrameric structure with four homologous subunits consisting of a six transmembrane segments, S1–S6, which are flanked by N- and C-terminal cytosolic regions. Although the six-time membrane-spanning configuration and a short helical pore loop between S5 and S6 segments are the hallmarks of voltage-gated cation channels, in TRP channels, periodically arranged, positively charged amino acid residues in the S4, which are essential for voltage-sensing, are missing [13]. Further, many additional protein-to-protein interaction domains and phosphorylation motifs exist within the N- and C-terminals of TRP channels. It is believed that, within specific membrane domains (e.g., caveola), a variety of signaling complexes are formed through these interaction sites, wherefrom diverse intracellular signal transductions are initiated. Owing to ubiquitous expression over the whole body including the central/peripheral nerve, cardiovascular, respiratory, digestive, renal urogenital, and erythroid/immune systems, TRP channels are thought to contribute to diverse biological functions, which are not restricted to innocuous and noxious multimodal sensory transduction (heat, cold, touch, proprioception, pain, taste, etc.) but also involve cardiac function, gut motility, psychomotor activity, and cell survival, proliferation, and death. In addition, several specific mutations have been identified in the *trp* genes for some hereditary disorders [12, 14–17].

The expression of TRP proteins in the alimentary tract is not confined to sensory neurons. The repertoire includes the other major classes of cells constituting the tract such as epithelial, endothelial, and smooth muscle cells and has recently been extended to fibroblasts/myofibroblasts [13], which belong to a special category of cells tightly associated with colonal/intestinal remodeling with the ability to transform and replicate to produce various cytokines under inflammatory circumstances. For instance, calcitonin gene-related peptide and substance P are known to be released by increased intracellular Ca^{2+} concentration through TRPV1 channel activation in sensory neurons [18, 19]. It has been proposed that excessive expression of this channel may be causally related with the occurrence and/or progression of IBD [20, 21]. Moreover, a nonselective cation channel TRPC4, which can be activated by muscarinic G-protein-coupled receptor stimulation, may be important for the excitatory control of intestinal smooth muscle cells [22–24]. Subsequent reports have implicated Ca^{2+} influx through TRPC4 channels in the initiation of spontaneous excitations in interstitial cells of Cajal, which regulate the gut automaticity [25]. More recently, we explored the potential roles of TRP channels in myofibroblastic Ca^{2+} signaling during intestinal inflammation and fibrosis. By using myofibroblast cell lines (CCD-18Co and InMyoFib) established from human colon epithelial and murine neonatal intestinal tissues, respectively, we could gain some key insights into the mechanisms underlying intestinal inflammatory and fibrotic remodeling processes [26].

In this chapter, we first describe the expression and function of TRPC channels in fibroblasts/myofibroblasts and then briefly discuss their potential roles in gastrointestinal disorders. Since the tumor-transforming factor (tumor necrosis factor (TNF))-α has been shown to affect the expression level of TRPC1 protein and its associated Ca^{2+}-transporting activity, the first part will be dedicated mainly to elucidating how TNF-α stimulates cyclooxygenase-2 (COX-2)-dependent prostaglandin E2 (PGE2) production through the activation of TRPC1 channels and enhances Ca^{2+} dynamics in CCD-18Co myofibroblasts. We next clarify the impact of PGE2 production on myofibroblastic function, with particular interest in Ca^{2+}-dependent regulation of transcription factors, that is, the nuclear factor of activated T-cell (NFAT) and the nuclear factor kB (NF-kB). The results suggest that negative feedback regulation of PGE2 production in intestinal myofibroblasts through TRPC1-associated Ca^{2+} influx may be of significant clinical importance to protect the gut from exacerbation of inflammatory process and, thus, progression of IBD [27].

In the second part, we describe the functional implications of transforming growth factor β1 (TGF-β1)-induced TRP channel activation in InMyoFib cells. Our studies so far suggest that TRP channels effectively regulate the expression of fibrosis-associated molecules and TGF-β signaling in InMyoFib cells. Consistent with this, expressions of TRP channels and fibrosis-associated factors were found to be increased in the stenotic but not in non-stenotic regions of biopsy samples from CD patients' intestines, implying a therapeutic potential of targeting the channels [28]. From these advances, we further anticipate gaining a good clue to elucidating the complex interplay among commensal microbiota, intestinal cells, and the immune system of the gut, and how such interactions, with genetic susceptibility and modification by environmental factors, contribute to the pathogenesis of IBD.

2. Roles of TRP proteins for the occurrence/progression of inflammatory bowel disease

Consultation with the literature indicates that there is close correlation between IBD initiation/progression and autoimmune abnormalities, which is characterized by aberrances in inflammatory responses of intestinal bacteria within the digestive tract. CD14-positive macrophages are markedly increased in the intestinal tract with CD pathology, where inflammatory cytokines including interleukin-6 and interleukin-23 (IL-6/IL-23) and TNF-α are excessively produced. The production of these cytokines, which can in turn activate adaptive immune reactions along with the production of IL-12 and IL-23, occurs at lower levels in the normal intestinal tract. However, suppressed immune responses of intestinal bacteria are inducible with higher production of IL-10, an anti-inflammatory cytokine involved in immune tolerance [29]. However, when chronic intestinal inflammation occurs, TNF-α or IL-6 can be excessively produced, initiating an excessive inflammatory response. Originally, adaptive immune responses were considered to play the dominant role in the pathogenesis of IBD; however, novel immunological and genetic studies have demonstrated that innate immune responses are of comparable significance in inducing gut inflammation. Recent progress in understanding IBD pathogenesis sheds light on related disease mechanisms, including innate and adaptive immunities, and interactions between genetic influences and microbial or environmental factors [2].

TNF-α is central to inflammatory processes and acts as an endogenous tumor promoter [30]. Therapeutic antibodies against TNF-α exert dramatic ameliorating effects on inflammatory bowel syndrome; myofibroblasts have been found to play a key role in this disorder [31]. TNF-α activates PGE2 production in myofibroblasts, fulfilling both protective and destructive roles in the gut. Although genetic deletion of the PGE2 receptor EP4 is detrimental to the gut, high concentrations of PGE2 analogs have also been shown to worsen clinical colitis (eventually leading to tumorigenesis), likely through the induction of pro-inflammatory reactions [32–34]. The formation of PGE2 in myofibroblasts is primarily catalyzed by COX-2, which is expressed at low levels in unstimulated conditions before being rapidly induced in response to inflammatory cytokines, growth factors, and tumor promoters [35].

The myofibroblast cell line CCD-18Co expresses both COX forms and secretes PGE2, a feature that is significantly enhanced by TNF-α or IL-1β [30]. Evidence suggests that COX-2 expression and PGE2 production in myofibroblasts are controlled by intracellular Ca^{2+} concentration [36, 37]. However, the exact sources of Ca^{2+}, which contribute to this process, remain entirely unclear. In general, there are two distinct sources of Ca^{2+} for elevating intracellular Ca^{2+} levels: Ca^{2+} influx across the plasma membrane and Ca^{2+} release from the endoplasmic reticulum (ER). Ca^{2+} influx can occur through voltage-gated Ca^{2+} channels, receptor-operated Ca^{2+}-permeable channels (ROCs), and store-operated Ca^{2+} channels (SOCs). Recent studies have demonstrated that the canonical members of the TRP superfamily of proteins (TRPC) may contribute to SOC and ROC. The TRPC family consists of seven distinct isoforms designated as TRPC1-TRPC7 [12, 14, 38, 39]. Presently, TRPC1 is regarded as one of the most plausible candidate molecules for SOC in many cell types [38, 39] and plays a critical role in intestinal epithelial restitution [40]. In some cell types, TRPC1 dynamically assembles with both stromal-interacting molecule 1 (STIM1) and Orai1 to generate a greater complexity in store-dependent Ca^{2+} influx mechanisms [41], although whether TRPC1 serves as a pore-forming SOC subunit still remains unclear.

In CCD-18Co cells, treatment with TNF-α greatly enhanced both Ca^{2+} influx induced by store depletion and cell-surface expression of TRPC1 protein and induced a cationic conductance. Selective inhibition of TRPC1 expression occurs by small interfering RNA or functionally effective TRPC1 antibody targeting the near-pore region of TRPC1 antagonized enhancement of store-dependent Ca^{2+} influx by TNF-α, whereas TNF-α potentiated the induction of PGE2 production. Overexpression of TRPC1 in CCD-18Co produced opposite consequences [27]. We further elucidated that NF-kB and NFAT serve as important positive and negative transcriptional regulators, respectively, of TNF-α-induced COX-2-dependent PGE2 production in colonic myofibroblasts, at the downstream of TRPC1-associated Ca^{2+} influx [27]. NFAT and NF-kB are widely distributed Ca^{2+}-dependent transcription factors capable of regulating a multitude of physiological and pathophysiological processes [42–44]. NFAT is activated through dephosphorylation by calcineurin, which is activated upon binding of Ca^{2+}/calmodulin. NFAT is reported to regulate COX-2 expression in colon carcinoma cells [45], and its activation can occur through Ca^{2+} influx associated with TRPC1-, TRPC3-, or TRPC6-associated SOC or ROC activities [46, 47]. The NF-kB transcription factor family plays a key role in several cellular functions (inflammation, apoptosis, cell survival, proliferation, angiogenesis, and innate and acquired immunity) as well as in regulating the expression of more than 500 different genes involved in inflammatory and immune responses [48, 49]. The anti-inflammatory natural compound curcumin acts as a principal mechanism to suppress the NF-kB-mediated signaling, thereby modulating immune responses [50–52].

The fact that high doses of exogenous PGE2 analogs exacerbate clinical colitis in the TNBS model might be relevant to the use of misoprostol to prevent ulcers in patients who take antiarthritis medication. The side effects listed for misoprostol include a variety of gastrointestinal tract problems, and these deleterious actions of PGE2 are likely associated with the stimulation of the release of interleukin-23 from activated dendritic cells, which in turn facilitate the differentiation of helper T lymphocytes to the pro-inflammatory phenotype Th17. These opposing actions of PGE2 may imply that the extent of its production is crucial to determine the fate of intestinal mucosa, that is, the maintenance of integrity or disintegration. In this regard, the negative feedback regulation of PGE2 production in intestinal myofibroblasts through TRPC1-associated Ca^{2+} influx may be of significant clinical importance to protect the gut from exacerbation of inflammatory process and thus the progression of inflammatory bowel syndrome.

3. Intestinal fibroblast/myofibroblast TRP channel and fibrosis

Repeated cycles of inflammation and healing of the gut ultimately progress into intestinal fibrosis (**Figure 1**). Innate immune-signaling pathways are also important drivers of myofibroblast transdifferentiation, as they cause cellular activation and fibrosis. Numerous mediators, including PDGF, EGF, IGF-1 and -2, CTGF, IL-1, IL-13, stem cell factor, endothelins, angiotensin II, TGF-α, TGF-β, bFGF, and peroxisome proliferator activator receptor-γ, promote myofibroblast proliferation and extracellular matrix (ECM) production. These activated myofibroblasts are central to fibrogenesis [53, 54].

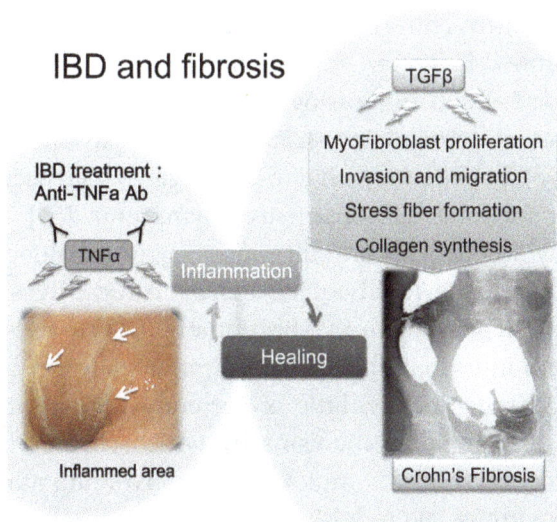

Figure 1. Inflammatory bowel disease and fibrosis. Repeated cycles of inflammation and healing of the gut ultimately progress into intestinal fibrosis. Endoscopic view of the inflamed area and a lower gastrointestinal series from a CD patient with fibrosis are shown. Colonoscopy and biopsy sampling showed a fibrotic lesion responsible for a colon stenosis.

TGF-β is principal to the development of fibrotic stenosis in CD and in numerous cell types. TGF-β secretion augments myofibroblast transformation. Canonical TGF-β signaling commences with its binding to a TGF-β type 2 receptor, which subsequently heterodimerizes with a TGF-β type 1 receptor to form an active TGF-βR1 receptor complex. Activated TGF-β type 1 receptor complex phosphorylates proteins against decapentaplegic homologs 2 and 3 (SMAD-2 and SMAD-3); activation of these transcription factors promotes collagen synthesis

[55]. TGF-β can also signal through noncanonical pathways involving extracellular signal-regulated kinases (ERKs), c-Jun N-terminal kinase, and p38-mitogen-activated protein kinase (p38-MAPK). Both canonical and noncanonical TGF-β-signaling pathways are implicated in myofibroblast cytokine production and fibrosis in the gut [5, 53]. TGF-β levels are elevated in the inflamed intestines of CD and ulcerative colitis patients, and abnormal TGF-β signaling impairs intestinal immune tolerance and tissue repair [56]. In addition, TGF-β receptor-triggered-signaling cascades can be enhanced by calcineurin inhibitors cyclosporin A and FK506 [57, 58]. However, neutralizing TGF-β1 *in vivo* as an anti-fibrotic approach in CD may be highly problematic, as this may actually lead to disease exacerbation, despite the potent anti-inflammatory and immunoregulatory properties of this cytokine. In addition to TGF-β1, emerging evidence has shown that IL-13 and IL-17 are involved in intestinal fibrosis. IL-13 signaling via IL-13 receptor type 2 (IL-13R2) and subsequent TGF-β1 production comprises the main fibrotic pathway in a model of chronic colitis [59]. IL-17A expression was found to be increased in the inflamed areas of patients with inflammatory bowel disease [60].

In response to tissue injury and profibrotic mediators including TGF-β and PDGF, fibroblasts differentiate into myofibroblasts, and the activation and/or recruitment of fibroblasts with resistance to apoptosis result in fibrogenesis and subsequent fibrosis [61, 62]. It has been estimated that about 45% of human deaths are associated with fibroproliferative disorders including fibrosis [63]. Recently, anti-TNF-α antibodies were successfully introduced as anti-inflammatory IBD therapies. However, for patients with fibrotic stenosis, there are only surgical treatments such as balloon dilation [64]. Approximately one-third of CD patients have severe intestinal strictures and obstructions (caused by excessive fibrosis) that are eventually fatal. In addition, treating CD patients with anti-TNF agents increases the risk of developing recurrent intestinal stenosis and sub-obstructive symptoms [65], necessitating repeated surgery [66]. In fact, many IBD patients are still suffering from re-stenosis of surgically treated regions, which greatly impairs the quality of life and can risk the lives of patients. Thus, there is an urgent need to establish alternative anti-fibrotic strategies to treat CD patients and other individuals suffering from intestinal fibrotic complications beyond currently available anti-inflammatory therapies. Unfortunately, little is currently known about intestinal wound-healing processes and pathogenic mechanisms by which chronic intestinal inflammation causes detrimental fibrosis, although a complex scenario involving numerous humoral factors has been suggested in experimental models [6–8].

Fibroblasts (vimentin+, α-SMA−), located in the submucosal area of normal tissues, are central in maintaining structural formation, healing, and regeneration. Increased resident fibroblast populations are pivotal to fibrosis development. Fibroblasts isolated from IBD mucosa proliferate faster than normal, and this increase occurs after exposure to growth factors and pro-inflammatory cytokines, and after direct cell-to-cell contact with inflammatory cells. Fibroblast-to-myofibroblast (vimentin+, α-SMA+) transformation plays a critical role in wound healing and tissue remodeling after injury [8, 67]. Myofibroblasts synthesize ECM components and generate high contractile forces for wound retraction or tissue remodeling in develop-mental processes. However, persistent myofibroblast activity can underlie hypertrophic scarring, loss of tissue compliance, and even rampant fibrosis that is the basis for fibrotic disorders of the heart, skin, lung, kidney, skeletal muscle, and liver [6, 68, 69]. The myofibroblast is considered a hybrid cell type with both smooth muscle and fibroblast properties [8]. A defining feature of myofibroblast differentiation is the formation of α-SMA stress fibers that provides a structural network for generating contractile forces [70]. Furthermore, intestinal stricture formation in CD is driven by the local excessive production of TGF-β [5, 71]. It is well known that fibrosis is associated with excessive accumulation of ECM components, such as collagens, matrix metalloproteinases (MMPs), and tissue inhibitors of metalloproteinases (TIMPs) [63, 72, 73]. In addition, other ECM proteins, such as fibronectins, elastins, and fibrillins, are upregulated during the development of fibrosis. This is due mainly to increased synthesis and decreased degradation of ECM components. Notably, during this process, MMPs that degrade the ECM are upregulated, whereas TIMPs are downregulated [74].

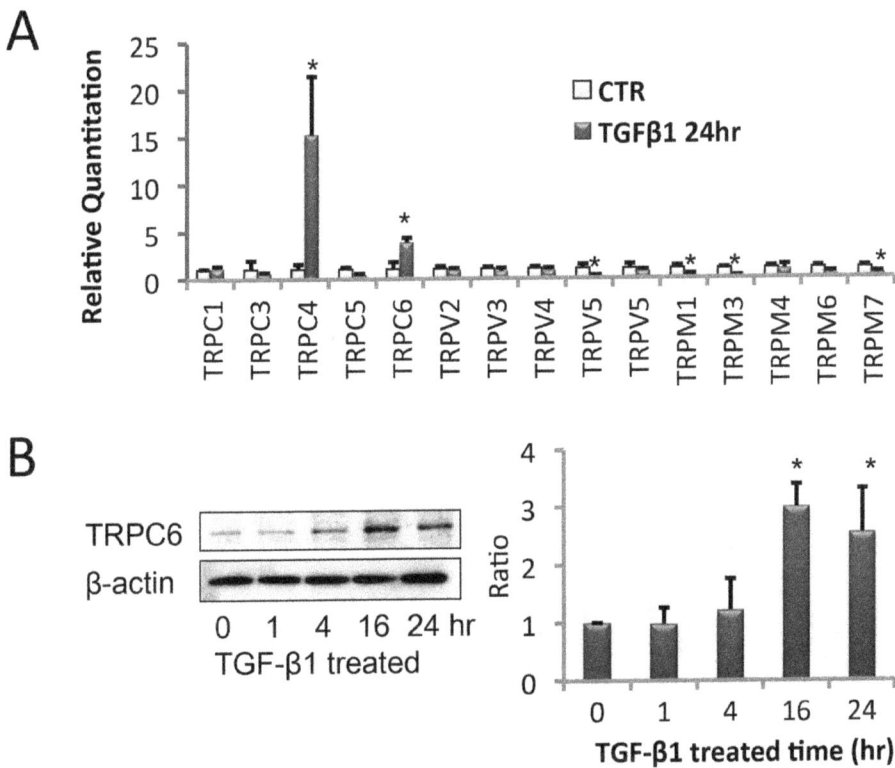

Figure 2. (A) *TRP* isoforms' mRNA in InMyoFibs. Results of real-time PCR analysis of the mRNA expression levels of *TRPC1, -C3, -C4, -C5, -C6, -V2, -V3, -V4, -V5, -V6, -M1, -M3, -M4, -M6,* and *-M7* after treatment with TGF-β1 (5 ng/mL, 24 h) are shown. (B) Immunoblot data of time-dependent changes in TRPC6 protein expression (left panel). Data were normalized to an internal control (β-actin) and are an average of four independent experiments (right panel). *$P < 0.05$ compared with untreated cells ($n = 4$). This figure was modified from a figure in Ref. [28].

TRP channels are cellular sensors for a wide variety of physical and chemical stimuli [75–77]. For example, they are involved in the sensation of touch, smell, taste, temperature, and pain [75, 78–80]. Recent studies have revealed that TRP channels also play essential roles in cell signaling and responses to innocuous or harmful environmental changes [15, 16, 81]. In addition, the activation of TRP channels changes the membrane potential, passes important signaling ions across the cell membrane, changes enzymatic activity, and initiates endocytosis or exocytosis [12, 75, 82]. Ca^{2+} is an essential signaling molecule implicated in various long-term cellular consequences, such as differentiation, gene expression, and cell proliferation, growth, and death, and it plays a significant role in regulating fibroblast functions [83–85]. TRPC channels are non-voltage-gated nonselective Ca^{2+}-permeable channels. Enhanced Ca^{2+} influx has been implicated in both differentiation and cytoskeletal rearrangements of various cell types. Accumulating evidence suggests that fibrosis-associated events in myofibroblasts are controlled by intracellular Ca^{2+} concentration, which is mediated by some members of the TRP channel superfamily [14, 86–88]. For example, TRPC1-mediated Ca^{2+} influx is essential for intestinal homeostasis/inflammation and progesterone-induced endometrial decidualization [27, 89]. Ca^{2+} signaling through TRPM7 channels likely plays a key role in TGF-β1-elicited fibrogenesis in human atrial fibroblasts [88]. Similarly, TRPC6/calcineurin-mediated signaling is essential for dermal and cardiac myofibroblast transformation, which occurs through complex interwoven pathways involving TGF-β, p38 mitogen-activated protein kinase, and serum response factor [70]. The formation of cell-to-cell contact is governed by Ca^{2+} signaling through TRPC4, which co-immunoprecipitates with junction proteins β-catenin and cadherin in vascular endothelial cells [90]. However, whether TRP channels play a role in intestinal fibrosis is not clearly understood.

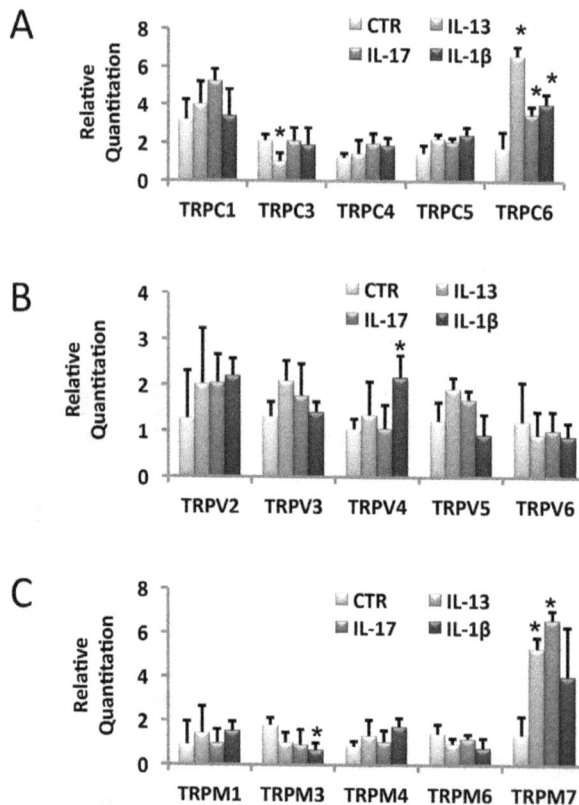

Figure 3. Real-time PCR analysis of *TRPC1, -C3, -C4, -C5, -C6, -V2, -V3, -V4, -V5, -V6, -M1, -M3, -M4, -M6,* and *-M7* after a 24-h treatment with IL-13 (10 ng/mL), IL-17 (10 ng/mL), and IL-1β (10 ng/mL). This figure was modified from a supplementary figure in Ref. [28].

In intestinal myofibroblasts, not only TGF-β1 but also IL-13 and IL-17 significantly upregulated TRPC6 expression (**Figures 2** and **3**). Myofibroblast TRPC6 is a key factor to modulate fibrosis through TGF signaling, and thus targeting TRPC6 may be a useful therapeutic regimen for CD patients with intestinal fibrosis [28]. The results showed that while increased TRPC6 activity promoted the TGF-β1-mediated expression of α-SMA and N-cadherin and strengthened interactions between the three molecules, it also negatively regulated collagen synthesis and secretion of anti-fibrotic factors, such as IL-10 and IL-11 (ERK and p38-MAPK dependent) [91–93]. Upregulated TRPC6 expression is essential for the formation of α-SMA stress fibers and N-cadherin-mediated adherens junctions, which, respectively, enable myofibroblasts to gain contractility and reinforce mutual intercellular connections [6, 94, 95]. Interestingly, adherens junctions appear in fibrotic tissues but are absent in normal tissues where fibroblasts do not develop the stress fibers [10]. These findings are consistent in part with a previous study that TRPC6-mediated Ca^{2+} influx was obligatory for myofibroblast differentiation in dermal and cardiac wound healing, although greater complexity appears to exist in the relationship between TRPC6-mediated signaling and intestinal fibrosis.

Furthermore, in our biopsy study, we examined samples from CD patients for the expression of TRPC4, TRPC6, α-SMA, N-cadherin, cytokines, and ECM, and found that these molecules were all increased in TGF-β1-treated InMyoFibs. The mRNA levels of *TRPC6, ACTA2, CDH2, IL-10, IL-11,* and *COL1A1* were significantly higher in stenotic areas than in non-stenotic mucosal areas of CD patients, whereas that of *TRPC4* was not significantly changed in 12 paired biopsy samples obtained from six patients (**Figure 4**). Stenotic lesions can be either inflammatory, fibrogenic, or neoplastic, or possess all of these characteristics. This means that therapeutic strategies distinguishing between these processes would yield improved outcomes compared with the currently available approaches. In this regard, more direct evidence that TRPC6 vitally contributes to the progression of excessive fibrosis in both an experimental model and in human tissues should help to elucidate the mechanism underlying the fibrotic process. This may be relevant not only to intestinal fibrosis but also to other fibrotic lesions of the skin, lung, and liver, where these channels are expressed at significant levels.

In addition to aforementioned mechanisms, the imbalance between MMP and TIMP, which maintain the state of remodeling and restitution, can accelerate structural changes of the bowel wall [1]. Microarray experiments showed that InMyoFib cells primarily express *MMP-1, MMP-2, TIMP-1,* and *TIMP-2*. When we next measured transcript expression of these molecules in stenotic areas from biopsy samples and TGF-β1-treated cells, we found that their mRNA levels were significantly unregulated; however, *TRPC6* siRNA pretreatment did not affect expression in TGF-β1-treated cells.

The studies with intestinal fibroblast/myofibroblast propose a new proof of concept that TRPC6 may act as an anti-fibrotic mediator. The upregulation of this channel appears to inhibit the signaling cascades associated with intestinal fibrosis including SMAD-2 phosphorylation and myocardin expression, which in turn modulate collagen synthesis, actin fiber formation, and expression of N-cadherin. Further evidence from biopsy samples suggests that the same mechanism may also operate in stenotic lesions of IBD. These results not only facilitate our understanding about this new role for TRPC6 in regulating fibrotic processes but also provide a novel molecular target for anti-fibrotic therapies to treat IBD in the future.

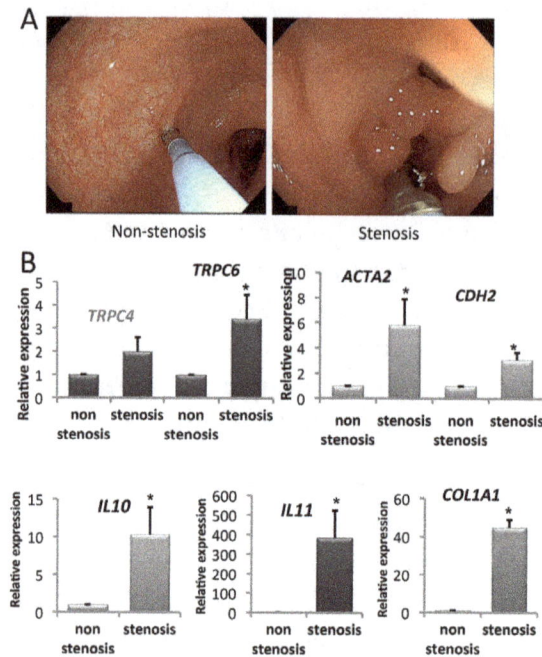

Figure 4. (A) Fibrosis in the colon: a clinical problem. Ulcerations and tissue damage are caused by chronic inflammation. This is followed by bowel wall fibrosis, leading to pseudopolyps or strictures reducing the colon. (B) Crohn's disease (CD) patient biopsies from non-stenotic and stenotic intestinal areas. The mRNA levels of TRPC4, TRPC6, ACTA2 (α-SMA), CDH2 (N-cadherin), IL-10, IL-11, and COL1A1 in biopsies were examined by real-time RT-PCR in non-stenotic and stenotic-inflamed mucosal tissues of CD patients. $*P < 0.05$ versus non-stenotic samples (12 paired biopsy samples obtained from six patients). **Figure 4B** was modified from a figure in Ref. [28].

4. Summary

Several studies including our study have underscored the importance of intestinal fibroblast/ myofibroblast cells in IBD pathophysiology and epithelial barrier integrity, and accumulating evidence from preclinical and clinical studies has started to note an important contribution of TRP channels to many gastrointestinal remodeling processes. In this chapter, we summarized recent advances in this field, with particular emphasis on TNF-α-activated TRPC1 and TGF-β-activated TRPC6 expression and function in primary-cultured fibroblasts/myofibroblasts in the gastrointestinal tract, in conjunction with limited but interesting results from biopsy samples from CD patients. A noteworthy possibility from it is that the functionality of TRP channels may have unexpectedly tight correlation with inflammation- and fibrosis-associated processes in myofibroblasts *in vitro* and *in vivo*. Further investigation will be warranted to substantiate our yet-premature knowledge about this newly emerging field, which would hopefully lead to the exploitation of an unprecedentedly unique treatment for highly intractable inflammatory/fibrotic disorders with greatly compromised quality of life, such as IBD.

Acknowledgements

This study was supported by the grants in aid to L.-H.K. from the Ministry of Education, Culture, Sports, Science, and Technology (Nos. 15K08978, 22790677, 25860571), a MEXT-Supported Program funding research activities of female researchers, the Clinical Research Foundation, and the Central Research Institute of Fukuoka University.

Author details

Lin Hai Kurahara[1*], Keizo Hiraishi[1], Kunihiko Aoyagi[2], Yaopeng Hu[1], Miho Sumiyoshi[1] and Ryuji Inoue[1]

*Address all correspondence to: hailin@fukuoka-u.ac.jp

1 Department of Physiology, Fukuoka University School of Medicine, Fukuoka University, Fukuoka, Japan

2 Department of Gastroenterology, Fukuoka University School of Medicine, Fukuoka University, Fukuoka, Japan

References

[1] Karantanos, T. and Gazouli M., Inflammatory bowel disease: recent advances on genetics and innate immunity. Ann Gastroenterol, 2011. 24(3): p. 164–72.

[2] Zhang, Y.Z. and Li, Y.Y., Inflammatory bowel disease: pathogenesis. World J Gastroenterol, 2014. 20(1): p. 91–9.

[3] Meier, J.K., et al., Specific differences in migratory function of myofibroblasts isolated from Crohn's disease fistulae and strictures. Inflamm Bowel Dis, 2011. 17(1): p. 202–12.

[4] Valentich, J.D., et al., Phenotypic characterization of an intestinal subepithelial myofibroblast cell line. Am J Physiol, 1997. 272(5 Pt 1): p. C1513–24.

[5] Biancheri, P., et al., The role of transforming growth factor (TGF)-beta in modulating the immune response and fibrogenesis in the gut. Cytokine Growth Factor Rev, 2014. 25(1): p. 45–55.

[6] Hinz, B. and Gabbiani, G., Fibrosis: recent advances in myofibroblast biology and new therapeutic perspectives. F1000 Biol Rep, 2010. 2: p. 78.

[7] Latella, G., et al., Can we prevent, reduce or reverse intestinal fibrosis in IBD? Eur Rev Med Pharmacol Sci, 2013. 17(10): p. 1283–304.

[8]   Hinz, B., Formation and function of the myofibroblast during tissue repair. J Invest Dermatol, 2007. 127(3): p. 526–37.

[9]   Hourigan, L.F., et al., Fibrosis in chronic hepatitis C correlates significantly with body mass index and steatosis. Hepatology, 1999. 29(4): p. 1215–9.

[10] Hinz, B., et al., Myofibroblast development is characterized by specific cell-cell adherens junctions. Mol Biol Cell, 2004. 15(9): p. 4310–20.

[11] Hinz, B., et al., The myofibroblast: one function, multiple origins. Am J Pathol, 2007. 170(6): p. 1807–16.

[12] Flockerzi, V., An introduction on TRP channels. Handb Exp Pharmacol, 2007. 179: p. 1–19.

[13] Phillips, A.M., Bull, A., and Kelly, L.E., Identification of a Drosophila gene encoding a calmodulin-binding protein with homology to the trp phototransduction gene. Neuron, 1992. 8(4): p. 631–42.

[14] Inoue, R., et al., Transient receptor potential channels in cardiovascular function and disease. Circ Res, 2006. 99(2): p. 119–31.

[15] Inoue, R., Jian, Z., and Kawarabayashi, Y., Mechanosensitive TRP channels in cardio-vascular pathophysiology. Pharmacol Ther, 2009. 123(3): p. 371–85.

[16] Inoue, R., et al., Regulation of cardiovascular TRP channel functions along the NO-cGMP-PKG axis. Expert Rev Clin Pharmacol, 2010. 3(3): p. 347–60.

[17] Nilius, B., TRP channels in disease. Biochim Biophys Acta, 2007. 1772(8): p. 805–12.

[18] Szallasi, A. and Blumberg, P.M., Complex regulation of TRPV1 by vanilloids, in TRP Ion Channel Function in Sensory Transduction and Cellular Signaling Cascades, Liedtke, W.B. and Heller, S., Editors. Boca Raton, FL; CRC Press/Taylor & Francis 2007.

[19] Szallasi, A., et al., The vanilloid receptor TRPV1: 10 years from channel cloning to antagonist proof-of-concept. Nat Rev Drug Discov, 2007. 6(5): p. 357–72.

[20] Yiangou, Y., et al., ATP-gated ion channel P2X(3) is increased in human inflammatory bowel disease. Neurogastroenterol Motil, 2001. 13(4): p. 365–9.

[21] Yiangou, Y., et al., Increased acid-sensing ion channel ASIC-3 in inflamed human intestine. Eur J Gastroenterol Hepatol, 2001. 13(8): p. 891–6.

[22] Inoue, R., TRP channels as a newly emerging non-voltage-gated CA2+ entry channel superfamily. Curr Pharm Des, 2005. 11(15): p. 1899–914.

[23] Kuriyama, H., et al., Physiological features of visceral smooth muscle cells, with special reference to receptors and ion channels. Physiol Rev, 1998. 78(3): p. 811–920.

[24] Insuk, S.O., et al., Molecular basis and characteristics of KATP channel in human corporal smooth muscle cells. Int J Impot Res, 2003. 15(4): p. 258–66.

[25] Torihashi, S., et al., Calcium oscillation linked to pacemaking of interstitial cells of Cajal: requirement of calcium influx and localization of TRP4 in caveolae. J Biol Chem, 2002. 277(21): p. 19191–7.

[26] Yu, X., et al., TRP channel functions in the gastrointestinal tract. Semin Immunopathol, 2016 May;38(3):385–96.

[27] Hai, L., et al., Counteracting effect of TRPC1-associated Ca2+ influx on TNF-alpha-induced COX-2-dependent prostaglandin E2 production in human colonic myofibroblasts. Am J Physiol Gastrointest Liver Physiol, 2011. 301(2): p. G356–67.

[28] Kurahara, L.H., et al., Intestinal myofibroblast TRPC6 channel may contribute to stenotic fibrosis in Crohn's disease. Inflamm Bowel Dis, 2015. 21(3): p. 496–506.

[29] Neurath, M.F., Cytokines in inflammatory bowel disease. Nat Rev Immunol, 2014. 14(5): p. 329–42.

[30] Kim, E.C., et al., Cytokine-mediated PGE2 expression in human colonic fibroblasts. Am J Physiol, 1998. 275(4 Pt 1): p. C988–94.

[31] Di Sabatino, A., et al., Functional modulation of Crohn's disease myofibroblasts by anti-tumor necrosis factor antibodies. Gastroenterology, 2007. 133(1): p. 137–49.

[32] Kabashima, K., et al., The prostaglandin receptor EP4 suppresses colitis, mucosal damage and CD4 cell activation in the gut. J Clin Invest, 2002. 109(7): p. 883–93.

[33] Sheibanie, A.F., et al., The proinflammatory effect of prostaglandin E2 in experimental inflammatory bowel disease is mediated through the IL-23-->IL-17 axis. J Immunol, 2007. 178(12): p. 8138–47.

[34] Sugimoto, Y. and Narumiya, S., Prostaglandin E receptors. J Biol Chem, 2007. 282(16): p. 11613–7.

[35] Smith, W.L., DeWitt, D.L., and Garavito, R.M., Cyclooxygenases: structural, cellular, and molecular biology. Annu Rev Biochem, 2000. 69: p. 145–82.

[36] Ogata, S., et al., Ca2+ stimulates COX-2 expression through calcium-sensing receptor in fibroblasts. Biochem Biophys Res Commun, 2006. 351(4): p. 808–14.

[37] Zhu, Y., et al., Ca2+- and PKC-dependent stimulation of PGE2 synthesis by deoxycholic acid in human colonic fibroblasts. Am J Physiol Gastrointest Liver Physiol, 2002. 283(3): p. G503–10.

[38] Ambudkar, I.S., et al., TRPC1: the link between functionally distinct store-operated calcium channels. Cell Calcium, 2007. 42(2): p. 213–23.

[39] Putney, J.W., Physiological mechanisms of TRPC activation. Pflugers Arch, 2005. 451(1): p. 29–34.

[40] Rao, J.N., et al., TRPC1 functions as a store-operated Ca2+ channel in intestinal epithelial cells and regulates early mucosal restitution after wounding. Am J Physiol Gastrointest Liver Physiol, 2006. 290(4): p. G782–92.

[41] Ong, H.L., et al., Dynamic assembly of TRPC1-STIM1-Orai1 ternary complex is involved in store-operated calcium influx. Evidence for similarities in store-operated and calcium release-activated calcium channel components. J Biol Chem, 2007. 282(12): p. 9105–16.

[42] Crabtree, G.R. and Olson, E.N., NFAT signaling: choreographing the social lives of cells. Cell, 2002. 109(Suppl.): p. S67–79.

[43] Timmerman, L.A., et al., Rapid shuttling of NF-AT in discrimination of Ca2+ signals and immunosuppression. Nature, 1996. 383(6603): p. 837–40.

[44] Yates, L.L. and Gorecki, D.C., The nuclear factor-kappaB (NF-kappaB): from a versatile transcription factor to a ubiquitous therapeutic target. Acta Biochim Pol, 2006. 53(4): p. 651–62.

[45] Duque, J., Fresno, M., and Iniguez, M.A., Expression and function of the nuclear factor of activated T cells in colon carcinoma cells: involvement in the regulation of cyclooxygenase-2. J Biol Chem, 2005. 280(10): p. 8686–93.

[46] Ohba, T., et al., Upregulation of TRPC1 in the development of cardiac hypertrophy. J Mol Cell Cardiol, 2007. 42(3): p. 498–507.

[47] Thebault, S., et al., Differential role of transient receptor potential channels in Ca2+ entry and proliferation of prostate cancer epithelial cells. Cancer Res, 2006. 66(4): p. 2038–47.

[48] Basak, S., et al., A fourth IkappaB protein within the NF-kappaB signaling module. Cell, 2007. 128(2): p. 369–81.

[49] Karin, M. and Greten, F.R., NF-kappaB: linking inflammation and immunity to cancer development and progression. Nat Rev Immunol, 2005. 5(10): p. 749–59.

[50] Vecchi Brumatti, L., et al., Curcumin and inflammatory bowel disease: potential and limits of innovative treatments. Molecules, 2014. 19(12): p. 21127–53.

[51] Holt, P.R., Katz, S., and Kirshoff, R., Curcumin therapy in inflammatory bowel disease: a pilot study. Dig Dis Sci, 2005. 50(11): p. 2191–3.

[52] Holt, P.R., Curcumin for inflammatory bowel disease: a caution. Clin Gastroenterol Hepatol, 2016. 14(1): p. 168.

[53] Leask, A., Potential therapeutic targets for cardiac fibrosis: TGFbeta, angiotensin, endothelin, CCN2, and PDGF, partners in fibroblast activation. Circ Res, 2010. 106(11): p. 1675–80.

[54] Derynck, R. and Zhang, Y.E., Smad-dependent and Smad-independent pathways in TGF-beta family signalling. Nature, 2003. 425(6958): p. 577–84.

[55] Medina, C., et al., Transforming growth factor-beta type 1 receptor (ALK5) and Smad proteins mediate TIMP-1 and collagen synthesis in experimental intestinal fibrosis. J Pathol, 2011. 224(4): p. 461–72.

[56] Babyatsky, M.W., Rossiter, G., and Podolsky, D.K., Expression of transforming growth factors alpha and beta in colonic mucosa in inflammatory bowel disease. Gastroenterology, 1996. 110(4): p. 975–84.

[57] Akool el, S., et al., Molecular mechanisms of TGF beta receptor-triggered signaling cascades rapidly induced by the calcineurin inhibitors cyclosporin A and FK506. J Immunol, 2008. 181(4): p. 2831–45.

[58] Chiasson, V.L., et al., Endothelial cell transforming growth factor-beta receptor activation causes tacrolimus-induced renal arteriolar hyalinosis. Kidney Int, 2012. 82(8): p. 857–66.

[59] Fichtner-Feigl, S., et al., IL-13 signaling via IL-13R alpha2 induces major downstream fibrogenic factors mediating fibrosis in chronic TNBS colitis. Gastroenterology, 2008. 135(6): p. 2003–13.

[60] Biancheri, P., et al., The role of interleukin 17 in Crohn's disease-associated intestinal fibrosis. Fibrogenesis Tissue Repair, 2013. 6(1): p. 13.

[61] Arribillaga, L., et al., Therapeutic effect of a peptide inhibitor of TGF-beta on pulmonary fibrosis. Cytokine, 2011. 53(3): p. 327–33.

[62] Biernacka, A., Dobaczewski, M., and Frangogiannis, N.G., TGF-beta signaling in fibrosis. Growth Factors, 2011. 29(5): p. 196–202.

[63] Ghosh, A.K. and Vaughan, D.E., Fibrosis: is it a coactivator disease? Front Biosci (Elite Ed), 2012. 4: p. 1556–70.

[64] Bettenworth, D. and Rieder, F., Medical therapy of stricturing Crohn's disease: what the gut can learn from other organs—a systematic review. Fibrogenesis Tissue Repair, 2014. 7(1): p. 5.

[65] Condino, G., et al., Anti-TNF-alpha treatments and obstructive symptoms in Crohn's disease: a prospective study. Dig Liver Dis, 2013. 45(3): p. 258–62.

[66] Rieder, F., et al., Wound healing and fibrosis in intestinal disease. Gut, 2007. 56(1): p. 130–9.

[67] Tomasek, J.J., et al., Myofibroblasts and mechano-regulation of connective tissue remodelling. Nat Rev Mol Cell Biol, 2002. 3(5): p. 349–63.

[68] Wynn, T.A., Cellular and molecular mechanisms of fibrosis. J Pathol, 2008. 214(2): p. 199–210.

[69] Wang, Y.S., et al., Role of miR-145 in cardiac myofibroblast differentiation. J Mol Cell Cardiol, 2014. 66: p. 94–105.

[70] Davis, J., et al., A TRPC6-dependent pathway for myofibroblast transdifferentiation and wound healing in vivo. Dev Cell, 2012. 23(4): p. 705–15.

[71] Di Sabatino, A., et al., Transforming growth factor beta signalling and matrix metallo-proteinases in the mucosa overlying Crohn's disease strictures. Gut, 2009. 58(6): p. 777–89.

[72] Muro, A.F., et al., An essential role for fibronectin extra type III domain A in pulmonary fibrosis. Am J Respir Crit Care Med, 2008. 177(6): p. 638–45.

[73] Zeisberg, M. and Kalluri, R., Cellular mechanisms of tissue fibrosis. 1. Common and organ-specific mechanisms associated with tissue fibrosis. Am J Physiol Cell Physiol, 2013. 304(3): p. C216–25.

[74] Hemmann, S., et al., Expression of MMPs and TIMPs in liver fibrosis - a systematic review with special emphasis on anti-fibrotic strategies. J Hepatol, 2007. 46(5): p. 955–75.

[75] Zheng, J., Molecular mechanism of TRP channels. Compr Physiol, 2013. 3(1): p. 221–42.

[76] Inoue, R., Ito, Y., and Mori, Y., TRP-related proteins as new target molecules: their correspondence to native receptor-operated cation channels. Tanpakushitsu Kakusan Koso, 2000. 45(6 Suppl): p. 1038–46.

[77] Inoue, R., Ito, Y., and Mori, Y., The TRP proteins, a rapidly expanding Ca2+ entry channel family and a new molecular target for drug development. Nihon Rinsho, 2002. 60(1): p. 18–24.

[78] Clapham, D.E., Runnels, L.W., and Strubing, C., The TRP ion channel family. Nat Rev Neurosci, 2001. 2(6): p. 387–96.

[79] Clapham, D.E., TRP channels as cellular sensors. Nature, 2003. 426(6966): p. 517–24.

[80] Ramsey, I.S., Delling, M., and Clapham, D.E., An introduction to TRP channels. Annu Rev Physiol, 2006. 68: p. 619–47.

[81] Cheng, Y. and Nash, H.A., Drosophila TRP channels require a protein with a distinctive motif encoded by the inaF locus. Proc Natl Acad Sci USA, 2007. 104(45): p. 17730–4.

[82] Xu, T., et al., Novel insights into TRPM7 function in fibrotic diseases: a potential therapeutic target. J Cell Physiol, 2015. 230(6): p. 1163–9.

[83] Berridge, M.J., Calcium signalling remodelling and disease. Biochem Soc Trans, 2012. 40: p. 297–309.

[84] Yue, L.X., Xie, J., and Nattel, S., Molecular determinants of cardiac fibroblast electrical function and therapeutic implications for atrial fibrillation. Cardiovas Res, 2011. 89(4): p. 744–753.

[85] Saliba, Y., et al., Evidence of a role for fibroblast transient receptor potential canonical 3 Ca2+ channel in renal fibrosis. J Am Soc Nephrol, 2015. 26(8): p. 1855–1876.

[86] Nishida, M., et al., Galpha12/13-mediated up-regulation of TRPC6 negatively regulates endothelin-1-induced cardiac myofibroblast formation and collagen synthesis through nuclear factor of activated T cells activation. J Biol Chem, 2007. 282(32): p. 23117–28.

[87] Onohara, N., et al., TRPC3 and TRPC6 are essential for angiotensin II-induced cardiac hypertrophy. EMBO J, 2006. 25(22): p. 5305–16.

[88] Du, J., et al., TRPM7-mediated Ca2+ signals confer fibrogenesis in human atrial fibrillation. Circ Res, 2010. 106(5): p. 992–1003.

[89] Kawarabayashi, Y., et al., Critical role of TRPC1-mediated Ca(2)(+) entry in decidualization of human endometrial stromal cells. Mol Endocrinol, 2012. 26(5): p. 846–58.

[90] Graziani, A., et al., Cell-cell contact formation governs Ca2+ signaling by TRPC4 in the vascular endothelium: evidence for a regulatory TRPC4-beta-catenin interaction. J Biol Chem, 2010. 285(6): p. 4213–23.

[91] Aoki, H., et al., Autocrine loop between TGF-beta1 and IL-1beta through Smad3- and ERK-dependent pathways in rat pancreatic stellate cells. Am J Physiol Cell Physiol, 2006. 290(4): p. C1100–8.

[92] Saraiva, M. and O'Garra, A., The regulation of IL-10 production by immune cells. Nat Rev Immunol, 2010. 10(3): p. 170–81.

[93] Kido, S., et al., Mechanical stress activates Smad pathway through PKCdelta to enhance interleukin-11 gene transcription in osteoblasts. PLoS One, 5(9): e744–e744 (2010).

[94] Ina, K., et al., Significance of alpha-SMA in myofibroblasts emerging in renal tubulointerstitial fibrosis. Histol Histopathol, 2011. 26(7): p. 855–66.

[95] Speca, S., et al., Cellular and molecular mechanisms of intestinal fibrosis. World J Gastroenterol, 2012. 18(28): p. 3635–61.

6

Psychiatric Comorbidities in Irritable Bowel Syndrome (IBS)

Mihaela Fadgyas Stanculete

Abstract

FA lot of research has pointed out that irritable bowel syndrome (IBS) is a multifactorial illness involving visceral hypersensitivity, alteration of communication between the enteric nervous system (ENS) and central nervous system (CNS), increased intestinal permeability, minimal intestinal inflammation, and altered intestinal microflora. Psychological, social, and genetic factors appear to be important in the development of IBS symptomatology through several mechanisms. This chapter addresses the relationships between irritable bowel syndrome (IBS) and psychiatric comorbidities. The aim of this chapter is to provide an overview of explanatory hypothesis and to describe a variety of approaches which integrate the vast research data about IBS and psychiatric comorbidities, including genetic, brain imaging, and neuropsychological findings. The section of this chapter which overlooks the psychotropic treatment reviews the comparative efficacy of various drugs.

Keywords: irritable bowel syndrome, neuroimaging, psychiatric comorbidities, psychosocial factors

1. Introduction

Irritable bowel syndrome (IBS) is a chronic functional gastrointestinal (GI) disorder that has been reported to be associated with increased use of health-care resources and impaired quality of life.

Over the last two decades, it is becoming increasingly clear that many factors are involved in IBS, and they interact in very complex ways, which have not been yet elucidated.

The biopsychosocial model has been developed to explain the IBS pathogenesis better. According to this model, the gastrointestinal function is modulated via brain-gut axis by psychosocial factors. Particular attention is given to stress, emotion, and psychological factors in the IBS pathogenesis.

Emerging data reveals the interaction between psychiatric disorders and IBS, which suggests that this association should not be ignored when developing strategies for screening and treatment. The simultaneous presence of a mental disorder and IBS worsen the prognosis of both diseases involved to a significantly greater extent.

It is very important to understand better how social and psychological factors influence biological processes both in IBS and psychiatric conditions. Several mechanisms have been proposed to explain this association. In this chapter, we highlight data from a wide range of research including genetic, neurotransmitter, and brain imaging studies.

Stressful life events can lead to the activation of hypothalamic-pituitary-adrenal (HPA) axis. Neurotransmitters including serotonin, norepinephrine, and corticotropin-releasing factor change the motility and the perception in the gut. Brain regions necessary for pain processing and pain and emotional regulation may be involved. The psychological burden of a chronic relapsing illness can increase the maladaptive behaviors and negative emotions and decrease the coping abilities. A better understanding of these processes will be crucial for developing more useful treatments.

Although pharmacological treatments have proven efficacy in IBS, the illness remains chronic with the symptomatic and functional problems only partially influenced for most patients.

A lot of papers have documented improved clinical prognosis in IBS through psychological and pharmacologic interventions. Despite these promising data, the evidence is still limited by underpowered sample sizes.

With this growing awareness of the importance of psychosocial factors in IBS care, medical professionals experience an increased need for accessible background information and practical guidelines for diagnosis and management of psychiatric comorbidities.

Over the last two decades, it is becoming increasingly clear that many factors are involved in IBS and they interact in very complex ways, which have not been yet elucidated.

2. Psychosocial factors linked to IBS

The biopsychosocial model aims to integrate the multidimensional mechanisms to understand how IBS can be developed under such multiple interactions. The most important characteristic of this model is the bidirectional causality: the psychosocial factors influence the brain and the gut, and the gut interacts with the brain via the autonomic nervous system and the hypo-thalamic-pituitary-adrenal (HPA) axis [1]. The principal psychological and social factors that have been reported to contribute to the onset, the severity, and the evolution of IBS are presented in **Table 1**.

Sociological factors	– Parental beliefs and behaviors
	– Illness behavior
	– Learning through positive reinforcement or reward and modeling
	– Adverse life events (sexual, emotional, physical abuse)
	– Chronic life stress
	– Social support
	– Culture (cultural beliefs, norms)
Psychological factors	– Anxiety, depression
	– Anger
	– Cognitive-affective processes: gastrointestinal anxiety, hypervigilance, and attentional bias, catastrophizing, alexithymia
	– Coping mechanisms

Table 1. Psychological and sociological factors involved in IBS.

• Parental beliefs and behaviors. It is accepted that there is a familial aggregation of IBS. Studies demonstrated that not only the genetic factors could explain why IBS tends to cluster in families, but the development of gastrointestinal symptoms could also be explained by reinforcement and modeling of gastrointestinal illness behavior by parents [2].

• Positive reinforcement of illness behavior. Children whose parents reinforce sickness behavior (through parental protective behaviors) report more severe pain and more school absences than other children. Studies of childhood learning have also suggested that social learning through modeling processes (children observing and learning to exhibit the behaviors they witness) may also contribute to the intergenerational transmission of GI illness behavior and play a significant role in development and maintenance of IBS symptoms [3–5].

• Various types of early adverse life events (EALs) are associated with the development of IBS, in particular sexual, emotional, and physical abuse [6]. The relationship between abuse and severity of gastrointestinal symptoms and poorer health-related quality of life (HRQOL) seems to be partially mediated by concomitant mood disturbances [7]. Studies have shown that other types of EALs have been associated with an increased vulnerability toward developing IBS (parental death, divorce, or separation) [8]. A substantial body of evidence suggests that epigenetic mechanisms play a major role in the causal link between EALs and IBS. Findings from animal models and human studies highlighted the long-term effects of exposure to stress in early life through changes in gene expression [9]. Furthermore, prospective studies have demonstrated that chronic life stress is the most significant predictor of IBS symptom severity over 16 months. Stress has a marked impact on mucosal immune activation, intestinal sensitivity, permeability, secretion, and motility and through various mechanisms can affect the IBS treatment outcomes [10–12].

- Social support is related to many aspects of IBS. It was shown that social support is reduced in chronic illnesses. The association between the quality of social support and the severity of IBS symptoms was mostly investigated. Perceived adequacy of social support appears to have a positive influence on pain possibly through a reduction in stress levels [13]. In contrast, negative social relationship correlates with increased symptom severity.

- Culture. The impact of culture on the perception and description of IBS symptoms is already known. It was emphasized that cultural beliefs, norms, and behaviors should be taken into account when evaluating the IBS presentation and management of the symptoms. Cultural norms could shape the acceptability of expressing symptomatology and the willingness to seek health-care assistance.

- Gastrointestinal-specific anxiety (GSA) represents "the cognitive, affective, and behavioral response stemming from fear of gastrointestinal symptoms, and the context in which these visceral symptoms occur" indicating awareness of and concern about gastrointestinal sensations. It has been suggested that GSA may be more relevant than general anxiety for symptom severity and health outcome and represents a key predictor of IBS diagnosis. Moreover, GSA was found to be associated with the mental component of quality of life, suggesting that GSA is an important endpoint for different interventions [14].

- Hypervigilance. IBS patients selectively attend to gastrointestinal sensations compared to healthy individuals. Some researchers indicated that visceral hypersensitivity is linked with the hypervigilance toward visceral sensations and a tendency to label them negatively [15]. Hypervigilance may reflect poor coping with gastrointestinal-specific anxiety.

- Attentional bias. Studies indicate that attentional bias toward gastrointestinal sensations is exaggerated and could represent a potential factor in IBS development and maintenance. Researchers reported that focusing attention on bodily sensations leads to increased physical symptom complaints and illness behavior.

- Catastrophizing has been defined as a psychological construct characterized by the tendency to have a distorted negative view of health problems and amplify the threat of symptoms. Cross-sectional studies have found that catastrophizing in IBS is associated with increased pain, increased health-care utilization, and increased disability [16].

- Alexithymia is a multidimensional construct defined as an inability in experiencing, expressing, and describing emotions in a verbal manner. Alexithymia can be conceptualized as a deficit in cognitive processing and emotional regulations. IBS patients present higher levels of alexithymia than general population. Also, studies suggest that alexithymia, a stable trait, could be a stronger predictor of IBS severity than GSA, thus implying that impaired affective awareness may weigh in the clinical presentation of IBS [17].

- Anger represents a negative emotional state that has several dimensions: anger experience, anger expression, and anger control. Inhibited anger expression is associated with depression, pain interference, and the frequency of pain behaviors. There are results that higher levels of trait anger characterize IBS patients when compared to healthy population, and this may be associated with clinical manifestations [18]. Other studies demonstrated that IBS patients appear to have higher levels of anger than a group of patients with organic bowel diseases.

• Coping mechanisms. Studies have begun to focus on the coping mechanisms because these factors influence treatment options, patients' expectations, and treatment outcome. Coping represents the cognitive and behavioral efforts to deal (reduce or tolerate) with a perceived stressful situation. As mentioned above, the coping can influence the outcome of the illness. Therefore the quality of a coping strategy should be evaluated according to with its effect on the outcome. Lazarus has defined two categories of coping from the cognitive perspective: problem focused and emotion focused [19].

Problem-focused strategies strive for resolving the stressful situation or event or altering the source of the stress. It includes strategies such as:

– Problem solving (managing external aspects of the stressor)

– Seeking information or support in handling the situation (instrumental support)

– Accepting responsibility

– Removing oneself from a stressful situation

Emotion-focused coping represents the efforts to regulate the emotions associated with the situation. It involves strategies as:

– Positive reappraisal

– Distancing

– Escape-avoidance

– Seeking social support

Studies showed that in cases of chronic illnesses, the effects of coping are not influenced by the type of problem, or emotion-focus strategies are used but rather if active or avoidant methods are employed. Moreover, in IBS patients, it seems that the presence or absence of depression and/or anxiety influences how they cope with illness. Maladaptive coping and visceral sensitivity appear to be significantly associated with psychological distress, illness perception directly affecting the maladaptive coping.

Phillips et al. evaluated the role of psychosocial factors in predicting the belonging to IBS group and severity of IBS symptoms [20]. They found that four coping strategies (active coping, instrumental support, self-blame, and positive reframing) were best predictors of IBS.

Coping seems to be a relevant factor in mediating the adverse impact of IBS symptomatology on daily activities. Patients' quality of life could be impaired by the lack of adequate social support and by lower coping abilities acquired through social learning during childhood. Also, the impact of IBS symptoms on HRQOL impairment is mediated by dysfunctional attitudes and avoidant-oriented coping. Inefficient coping strategies represent important treatment targets for cognitive-behavioral therapy (CBT) because coping styles are modulated by the use of cognitive abilities [21].

3. Genes and IBS

As discussed before, IBS is a chronic disease characterized by familial clustering. In the recent years, the hypothesis of a genetic contribution to the development of IBS has gained some support [22].

It was postulated that IBS is a multifactorial, polygenic complex disorder. A candidate gene study evaluates a specific polymorphism or set of polymorphisms. Until now, approximately 60 candidate genes were investigated to determine whether specific genetic variants may be associated with IBS. Until now the data sustaining the genetic hypothesis are scarce, and some results have not been replicated.

Many epidemiological studies reported psychiatric comorbidities, and also reported higher rates of these comorbidities than in the general population. Different pathways could be affected in the subgroup of IBS patients with psychiatric comorbidities. Recent studies tried to evaluate if the IBS and mental disorders share common genetic pathways (primary cortico-tropin-releasing system and serotoninergic pathway).

Data are sustaining that HPA axis and serotoninergic system are likely to be involved in the genetic susceptibility to major depressive disorder, but currently, there is no clinical evidence for a common gene in IBS and major depression.

Eight genes involved in psychiatric disorders were investigated with mixed results:

1. FKBP5 gene (the gene encoding FK506-binding protein 51) is located on the short arm of chromosome 5; some variants were associated with stress reactivity and post-traumatic stress disorder (PTSD) risk.

2. Catechol-O-methyltransferase (COMT) gene: COMT Val158Met was related to IBS with constipation. The same variant was associated with obsessive-compulsive disorder (OCD), panic disorder (PD), and cognitive performance.

3. Opioid receptor Mu 1 (OPRM1) gene: diseases related to this gene include opioid dependence, pain sensitivity, and social sensitivity. OPRM1 118AG variant was associated with IBS-mixed and IBS-diarrhea (IBS-D).

4. Brain-derived neurotrophic factor (BDNF) gene: psychiatric diseases related to this gene include schizophrenia, anorexia and bulimia nervosa, PTSD, and mood disorders. BDNF Val166Met was associated with IBS with psychiatric comorbidities.

5. Neuropeptide Y (NPY) gene is implicated in stress response

6. Ankyrin repeat and kinase domain containing 1 (ANKK1) gene: it was associated with impulse control disorders and alexithymia.

7.   Dopamine receptor D2 (DRD2) gene: it seems to have a role in cocaine dependence.

8.   Fatty acid amide hydrolase (FAAH) gene also has a role in substance dependence.

A recent study found preliminary evidence that IBS patients with comorbid anxiety or depression are more likely to present functional variant alleles of serotonin transporters than IBS patients without psychiatric comorbidities.

Maybe the new technological advances in genomic studies will make it possible to identify common and rare variants on genomic deoxyribonucleic acid (DNA) [23]. Until now, based on candidate gene studies, it appears that there may be a different molecular basis for IBS with comorbid anxiety versus IBS without comorbid anxiety. Thus the role of environmental factor contributors to IBS development should not be underestimated.

4. Psychiatric comorbidity in IBS

Many studies reported an increased frequency of psychiatric comorbidities (diagnosis and symptoms) among patients with IBS. It has been estimated that IBS patients have high rates of psychiatric comorbidities (50 %–90 %). There are multiple factors involved in the determination of this comorbidity. The latest disease models of IBS encompass the overlap of brain circuits involved in emotion regulation, autonomic responses, and pain modulation as the most important features.

Clinical reports indicate that the relationship between IBS and psychiatric illnesses is bidirectional between the gastrointestinal tract and the brain, through various pathways (neural, neuroimmune, and neuroendocrine). Among mental disorders, mood disorders, anxiety disorders, and somatoform disorders have been the most frequently diagnosed conditions [24]. The complexity of the underlying pathophysiological processes is not completely understood. The hypothesis linking cognitive and emotional areas in the central nervous system (CNS) with the autonomic nervous system (ANS) and the enteric system (ENS) had a significant contribution to the understanding of the pathogenesis of IBS.

The increased comorbidity among IBS and psychiatric disorders is well established. Even though data refers to patients seen in tertiary gastroenterology centers, recent data pointed out that psychiatric comorbidity is also present in primary care.

Another important aspect that should be emphasized is that the majority of the study results are based on the administration of self-report screening instruments rather than a psychiatric interview. The screening tools only assess the probability of a psychiatric diagnosis, but further investigations are necessary. Moreover, studies of a causal relationship between IBS and psychiatric comorbidities are still limited in number and provide contradictory data.

Some authors argued that the data are applying only to those patients who have sought treatment and are not applicable to the non-consulters. Others suggested that could be a subset of patients with IBS characterized by high psychiatric comorbidity. Nevertheless, there is some evidence supporting the biological association between IBS and mental disorders.

Approximately 50 % of patients with a psychiatric disorder develop the disease before the GI symptoms became manifest, and psychiatric symptoms appear to develop at the same time in a majority of the remaining 50 %.

Many studies pointed out that worry-rumination can influence the brain-gut axis. Moreover, it has been identified as one fundamental factor that mediates the high co-occurrence of the two most frequent psychiatric comorbidities in IBS patients (anxiety and depression) [25].

It is noteworthy that the patients with severe IBS and comorbid psychiatric disorders have been found to have a higher impairment in HRQOL, elevated symptom burden, increased functional disability, and increased health-care costs.

4.1. Mood disorders and IBS

Many studies have investigated the prevalence of depression among IBS patients, but the results are vastly variable, ranging from high to much lower rates. There are also studies showing that patients with major depressive disorders present gastrointestinal symptoms.

Relevant findings from a large-scale population-based study suggest that depression and stress are independent risk factors for IBS. In this study, the incidence rate of IBS was higher in the patients with mild depression than in those with severe depression.

Several authors reported that IBS is associated with suicidality. The findings of one study indicate that 4 % of IBS patients who sought help from primary care, 16 % from secondary care, and 38 % from tertiary care endorsed suicidal ideation determined primary by the gastrointestinal symptoms. A systematic review indicated that IBS patients were two to four times more likely to recognize a history of suicidal behavior, even in the absence of depression.

A study conducted by Guthrie et al. revealed three definite groups of IBS patients [26]:

– Distressed high utilizers: characterized by multiple psychosocial comorbidities, increase levels of health-care utilization, high frequency of sexual abuse, and low pain thresholds to rectal balloon distension; the patients from this group reported suicidal ideation and self-harm history.

– Distressed low utilizers: marked by high psychiatric comorbidity, low physician consultations, low frequency of sexual abuse, and low pain threshold.

– Tolerant low utilizers: characterized by low rates of psychiatric comorbidities, low levels of consultations, and high pain thresholds.

It should be taken into account that an increase in suicidal ideation is not entirely explained by the symptom intensity and the presence of anxiety or depressive comorbidity. Therefore, IBS patients, especially distressed high utilizers, should be assessed for suicidality [27].

4.2. Anxiety disorders and IBS

As mentioned earlier, there is a higher prevalence of anxiety disorders among IBS patients than in the general population (47 % versus 26 %). According to the available literature, the most prevalent anxiety disorders among patients with IBS are generalized anxiety disorder (GAD) and panic disorder (PD). Some studies suggest that mixed IBS (IBS-M) patients are more likely to present higher scores for anxiety, especially in comparison with IBS with constipation (IBS-C) [25].

It must be noted that recent studies suggest that the strong association between GAD morbidity and IBS observed in tertiary centers was not a consequence of increased help-seeking behavior.

PD and IBS share common characteristics such as gastrointestinal symptoms, anticipatory anxiety, and avoidant behavior because of fear of symptoms. Based on results of different studies, it appears that the presence of IBS is associated with greater severity of agoraphobia, anticipatory anxiety, and panic attacks in PD patients. Moreover, patients with IBS reported having high scores of anxiety sensitivity, as the PD patients. Further information on IBS and PD came from a review emphasizing that the experience of feeling uncontrollable somatic symptoms, very common in IBS, could be a stimulating component for PD in patients with subclinical PD symptoms [28].

4.3. Somatoform disorders and IBS

IBS is considered a functional disorder, and it is congruent with the definition of somatoform disorders. The Diagnostic and Statistical Manual for Mental Disorders (DSM-4-TR) and the International Classification of Diseases (ICD) classify physical symptoms that cannot be medically explained together with persistent requests for medical investigations in a separate somatoform category. In the DSM-5 this category was renamed as "somatic symptoms disorder" (SSD) and redefined; there is no longer a demand for lack of "medical" explanation of symptoms. It means that this diagnosis could be a primary diagnosis (somatic symptoms may be medically unexplained) or could be a secondary diagnosis in patients who have an organic illness. The documented prevalence rates of somatoform disorders among IBS patients vary from 15 % to 48 % [29].

5. Neuroimaging in IBS

Studies using structural and functional techniques in IBS patients showed abnormalities that were associated with:

- Visceral hypersensitivity

- Impairment of affective processes involved in visceral pain modulation

- Alteration of descending pain inhibitory pathways

Data obtained from brain imaging studies in IBS demonstrated physiological differences that distinguish patients with IBS from a healthy population. The results obtained have varied maybe because of different study designs or due to the heterogeneity of study populations [30, 31].

5.1. Structural neuroimaging

Nowadays, structural approaches are provided mainly by diffusion tensor imaging (DTI) and by structural magnetic resonance imaging (sMRI). The studies focus on structural connectivity.

IBS patients with chronic pain have regional cortical thickness (CT) alterations in comparison with healthy controls. CT represents the results of neural reorganization of pain circuits and regions associated with sensorial processing.

IBS patients present decreased gray matter density in prefrontal and parietal regions and in emotional circuits. Ellingson et al. demonstrated in a study using DTI that IBS patients have microstructural changes in areas involved in the cortical pain modulatory areas and cortico-thalamic modulation. The anterior insula and basal ganglia (BS) have a prominent role in the integration of sensory and non-sensory information.

Another study demonstrated that IBS patients showed lower cortical thickness (CT) in the interoceptive association cortex (aINS) in the right hemisphere than in healthy controls.

The anterior insular subregion has multiple roles:

- Integration of food-related (olfaction and taste), interoceptive, emotional, and cognitive functions

- Provides output to autonomic and pain modulation systems

- Plays a key role in prediction, error processing, and self-awareness of sensations

In the relationship with these roles, insular regions seem to be involved in psychopathology. As already highlighted, patients with IBS have an abnormal processing of visceral pain in this area as a result of the dysfunctional inhibition of the pain in cortical areas. Patients reporting higher levels of pain intensity associated with their IBS symptoms presented an important CT in the bilateral orbitofrontal cortex (OFC). Also, it was observed that disease duration and pain intensity were correlated with CT in the dorsolateral prefrontal cortex (DLPFC) and OFC, bilaterally.

Other studies reported CT in the anterior midcingulate cortex (aMCC), ventrolateral prefrontal cortex (vlPFC), and thalamus. The structural changes of gray matter density in the periaqueductal gray (PAG) region may be a reflection of the compromised descending modulation of pain.

Blankstein evidenced increased gray matter density in the hypothalamus of the IBS patients.

Depression and anxiety have a well-established role in the modulation of pain. It was suggested that the decreased gray matter density in the anterior/medial thalamus in patients with IBS could be related to the clinical levels of anxiety or depression.

Interestingly, some authors suggested that structural changes in the primary interoceptive cortex, as well as in the attentional and emotional network, could represent endophenotypes of IBS.

5.2. Functional neuroimaging

Functional approaches are provided by single-positron emission computerized tomography (SPECT), positron emission tomography (PET), resting-state magnetic resonance (MRI) and functional magnetic resonance (fMRI), magnetic resonance spectroscopy (MRS), near-infrared spectroscopic imaging (NIRSI), and magnetoencephalography (MEG).

A recent meta-analysis of research on cortical responses to rectal distension suggests the conclusion that brain responses to rectal distension are different in IBS patients and healthy controls. IBS patients showed greater activation in brain regions involved in emotional processing, cognitive modulation, and interoceptive analysis.

Using the functional neuroimaging techniques in IBS patients, it was identified the hyperactivity of the amygdala (an essential component in the emotional arousal network). The amygdala network is involved in processing visceral input in relation to emotional stimuli, modulation of sensorial information, and emotional regulation.

Another area that exhibited functional alteration during experimental pain in IBS patients is represented by the basal ganglia (BG). The data obtained are consistent with the reduction of the dendritic density in cortico-basal ganglia-thalamic-cortical circuits involved in modulation of pain. Moreover, hypersensitive IBS patients present more DLPFC activation than normosensitive patients.

The results obtained in studies using neuroimaging techniques sustain the hypothesis that IBS have a biological substrate, but the same changes could be noticed in other chronic disorders. Furthermore, psychosocial factors (early-life trauma, catastrophizing, anxiety, and depression) have had a substantial impact on the neuroimaging correlations of IBS. An association was noticed (either positive or negative) between the level of psychopathology and neuroimaging findings, thus emphasizing the relevance of psychological factors in IBS determinism [32–34].

6. Neuropsychological findings in IBS

Stress induces changes in HPA axis functioning with neurobiological and cognitive consequences. The brain-gut axis appears to have a major importance of cognitive performance. The psychiatric comorbidity has also impact in the neurocognitive functioning [15, 35].

In general, normal cognitive functioning was reported in IBS, but some researchers demonstrated subtle cognitive deficits that remained after the correction for psychiatric comorbidity.

6.1. Attention and IBS

Attention is a behavioral and cognitive process involving the selection of sensory information to optimize current behavioral responses to specific stimuli relevant for the organism.

Researchers suggest that IBS patients have specific abnormalities in attentional network functioning. IBS patients present attentional biases for pain words. Attentional alterations are associated with increased pain report and illness behavior.

6.2. Memory and IBS

Currently, there are data suggesting impairment in visuospatial memory in patients with IBS. The researchers found that IBS patients displayed poorer performance in hippocampal-mediated visuospatial tasks than non-IBS controls. They made twice to three times as many errors on the visuospatial test as the healthy control group. It was suggested that visuospatial memory dysfunction could represent a common component of IBS [36].

6.3. Executive function and IBS

Cognitive flexibility in IBS patients was evaluated with Wisconsin Card Sorting Test (WCST). Recent researches have shown that IBS patients present latent impairments in the cognitive flexibility. The biological substrate for those findings seems to be the modified activity of the DLPFC, hippocampus, and insula. Also, the altered connectivity between the DLPFC and pre-supplementary motor area appears to be involved [37].

7. Psychopharmacology of IBS

Treatment of IBS could be classified in pharmacologic and non-pharmacological strategies. The choice of therapy depends on types of symptoms and their severity and frequency. It is clear that many aspects of IBS may be linked to psychosocial stressors and psychiatric comorbidities. More recent research emphasized that the psychotropic drugs can play a major role in the treatment of IBS patients [38].

7.1. Antidepressants

IBS is characterized by abnormalities in visceral sensations and dysregulation of central pain perception. Thus, the antidepressants represent a treatment option in patients with moderate and severe symptoms. The antidepressants were found to be efficacious for abdominal pain but have no effect on bowel habit. Moreover, their tolerance may represent a problem. Currently, antidepressants are used as a second-line therapy. The beneficial effects of antide-pressants could be the results of influence in central pain threshold (an increase of threshold). Other mechanisms of action are represented by the anticholinergic effects (influence on gastrointestinal motility and secretion) and by reducing the pain sensitivity of peripheral nerves [39].

7.1.1. Tricyclics antidepressants (TCA)

Most recent research supports the use of TCAs in IBS treatment. The effects of several TCAs including clomipramine, nortriptyline, and imipramine were investigated in IBS patients. The results showed that the required dose of TCAs is lower than that used to treat patients with depression. TCAs are effective in IBS-D due to the prolongment of whole-gut transit times. A systematic review of 11 randomized controlled trials RCTs comparing TCAs and placebo revealed that the benefit attributable to TCA therapy relative to placebo was 12.5 %. The numbers needed to treat (NNT) were four, equal or superior to other pharmacological agents (like motility agents and probiotics). The TCAs slow gut-transit time and could be used in diarrhea-predominant IBS.

7.1.2. Selective serotonin reuptake inhibitors (SSRIs)

Efficacy of SSRIs in the treatment of IBS was evaluated in seven randomized trials comparing SSRIs with placebo. The SSRIs studied were fluoxetine, paroxetine, and citalopram. One small open trial demonstrated the efficacy of paroxetine on abdominal pain. A common limitation of all the studies is represented by the short duration of the study (12 weeks) and the small sample size. The relative risks (RR) in the treatment of IBS symptoms were 0.62, but significant heterogeneity characterized the studies. The SSRIs decrease orocecal transit and would be of greater benefit in constipation-predominant IBS. According to Cochrane database of systematic reviews, SSRIs are prescribed at dosages standard for treating psychiatric disorders and should be used as a third-line treatment.

7.1.3. Serotonin-noradrenaline reuptake inhibitors (SNRIs)

Both serotonin and norepinephrine have a role in visceral motility and visceral sensation. It was noticed that low-dose SNRIs (duloxetine and venlafaxine) seem to be more efficacious than SSRIs. One study performed on healthy volunteers showed that venlafaxine reduced pain sensation ratings in response to grade distensions but did not have a significant impact on the colonic transit. SNRIs are promising, but more studies need to be done.

7.2. Atypical antipsychotics

Quetiapine may help patients with IBS by decreasing the anxiety and ameliorating sleep disturbances. It also augments the effect of antidepressants and provides an independent analgesic effect [40].

7.3. Anticonvulsants

Preliminary data from animal models provides evidence suggesting that the γ-aminobutyric acidergic (GABA) agents (gabapentin) and $\alpha2\delta$ ligand (pregabalin) may also be efficient in reducing central sensitization in hyperalgesia [41]. Gabapentin has more recently been used in the treatment of chronic pain. Pregabalin has been shown to be more potent than gabapentin. In patients with IBS, both gabapentin and pregabalin have been shown to reduce rectal sensitivity to balloon distension, but currently, there are no results published from clinical trials examining the efficacy of $\alpha2\delta$ ligands on symptoms in IBS patients.

7.4. Anxiolytic agents

The rationale for the use of anxiolytic drugs for the treatment of IBS likely came from the observation that the majority of patients also present of comorbid anxiety. Buspirone, an azapirone, is an anti-anxiolytic nonbenzodiazepine drug. It is a partial serotonin 1A (5-HT1A) receptor agonist used to augment the effects of antidepressants. The effects on gastrointestinal motility are represented by the reduction of funding tone and the delay of emptying. Also, a relaxation effect on the rectal tone was observed [42].

8. Conclusions

There is a general agreement that a global assessment of IBS patient should be done. The significant overlap between IBS and mental disorders should encourage the clinicians to evaluate for comorbid psychiatric disorders routinely. It is very important to recognize the linkage between psychiatric diagnoses and IBS because these comorbid conditions are characterized by increased symptom burden and additive functional impairment. Thus, successful management of patients with IBS requires careful attention to all psychosocial factors involved.

Author details

Mihaela Fadgyas Stanculete[1,2*]

Address all correspondence to: mihaelastanculete@yahoo.com

1 Department of Neurosciences, Discipline of Psychiatry and Pediatric Psychiatry, University of Medicine and Pharmacy "Iuliu Hațieganu", Cluj-Napoca, Romania

2 Second Psychiatric Clinic, Emergency County Hospital Cluj, Cluj-Napoca, Romania

References

[1] Tanaka Y, Kanazawa M, Fukudo S, Drossman DA. Biopsychosocial model of irritable bowel syndrome. J Neurogastroenterol Motil. 2011;2:131–9. DOI: 10.5056/jnm. 2011.17.2.131

[2] Levy RL, Whitehead WE, Walker LS, Von Korff M, Feld AD, et al. Increased somatic complaints and health-care utilization in children: effects of parent IBS status and parent response to gastrointestinal symptoms. Am J Gastroenterol. 2004;99(12):2442–51. DOI: 10.1111/j.1572-0241.2004.40478.x

[3] Van Oudenhove L, Levy RL, Crowell MD, Drossman DA, Halpert AD, Keefer L, Lackner JM, Murphy TB, Naliboff BD. Biopsychosocial aspects of functional gastrointestinal disorders: how central and environmental processes contribute to the development and expression of functional gastrointestinal disorders. Gastroenterology. 2016;150(6):1355–67. DOI: http://dx.doi.org/10.1053/j.gastro.2016.02.027

[4] Vervoort T, Huguet A, Verhoeven K, Goubert L. Mothers' and fathers' responses to their child's pain moderate the relationship between the child's pain catastrophizing and disability. PAIN®. 2011;152(4):786–93. DOI: 10.1016/j.pain.2010.12.010

[5] Van Tilburg MA, Levy RL, Walker LS, Von Korff M, Feld LD, Garner M, Feld AD, Whitehead WE. Psychosocial mechanisms for the transmission of somatic symptoms from parents to children. WJG. 2015;21(18):5532. DOI: 10.3748/wjg.v21.i18.5532.

[6] Bradford K, Shih W, Videlock EJ, Presson AP, Naliboff BD, Mayer EA, Chang L. Association between early adverse life events and irritable bowel syndrome. Clin Gastroenterol Hepatol. 2012;10(4):385–90. DOI: 10.1016/j.cgh.2011.12.018

[7] Drossman DA. Abuse, trauma, and GI illness: is there a link?. Am J Gastroenterol. 2011;106(1):14–25. DOI: 10.1038/ajg.2010.453

[8] Chitkara DK, van Tilburg MA, Blois-Martin N, Whitehead WE. Early life risk factors that contribute to irritable bowel syndrome in adults: a systematic review. Am J Gastroenterol. 2008;103(3):765–74. DOI: 10.1111/j.1572-0241.2007.01722.x

[9] O'Mahony SM, Hyland NP, Dinan TG, Cryan JF. Maternal separation as a model of brain–gut axis dysfunction. Psychopharmacology. 2011;214(1):71–88. DOI: 10.1007/s00213-010-2010-9

[10] Moloney RD, Johnson AC, O'Mahony SM, Dinan TG, Meerveld GV, Cryan JF. Stress and the microbiota–gut–brain axis in visceral pain: relevance to irritable bowel syndrome. CNS Neurosci Ther. 2016;22(2):102–17. DOI: 10.1111/cns.12490

[11] Vanuytsel T, van Wanrooy S, Vanheel H, Vanormelingen C, Verschueren S, Houben E, Rasoel SS, Tóth J, Holvoet L, Farré R, Van Oudenhove L. Psychological stress and corticotropin-releasing hormone increase intestinal permeability in humans by a mast cell-dependent mechanism. Gut. 2014;63(8):1293–9. DOI: 10.1136/gutjnl-2013-305690

[12] Van Oudenhove L, Aziz Q. Recent insights on central processing and psychological processes in functional gastrointestinal disorders. Dig Liv Dis. 2009;41(11):781–7. DOI: 10.1016/j.dld.2009.07.004

[13] Lackner JM, Brasel AM, Quigley BM, Keefer L, Krasner SS, Powell C, Katz LA, Sitrin MD. The ties that bind: perceived social support, stress, and IBS in severely affected patients. Neurogastroenterol Motil. 2010;22(8):893–900. DOI: 10.1111/j.1365-2982.2010.01516.x

[14] Jerndal P, Ringström G, Agerforz P, Karpefors M, Akkermans LM, Bayati A, Simrén M. Gastrointestinal-specific anxiety: an important factor for severity of GI symptoms and

quality of life in IBS. Neurogastroenterol Motil. 2010;22(6):646-e179. DOI: 10.1111/j.
1365-2982.2010.01493

[15] Kennedy PJ, Clarke G, Quigley EM, Groeger JA, Dinan TG, Cryan JF. Gut memories:
towards a cognitive neurobiology of irritable bowel syndrome. Neurosci Biobehav Rev.
2012;36(1):310–40. DOI: 10.1016/j.neubiorev.2011.07.001

[16] Hunt MG, Milonova M, Moshier S. Catastrophizing the consequences of gastrointestinal symptoms in irritable bowel syndrome. J Cogn Psychother. 2009;23(2):160–73. DOI:
10.1891/0889-8391.23.2.160

[17] Porcelli P, De Carne M, Leandro G. Alexithymia and gastrointestinal-specific anxiety
in moderate to severe irritable bowel syndrome. Compr Psych. 2014;55(7):1647–53.
DOI: 10.1016/j.comppsych.2014.05.022

[18] Fadgyas Stănculete M, Pojoga C, Dumitrascu DL. Experience of anger in patients with
irritable bowel syndrome in Romania. Clujul Medical. 2014;87(2):98. DOI: 10.15386/
cjmed-290

[19] Lazarus RS. Coping theory and research: past, present, and future. Psychosom Med.
1993;55(3):234–47.

[20] Phillips K, Wright BJ, Kent S. Psychosocial predictors of irritable bowel syndrome
diagnosis and symptom severity. J Psychosom Res. 2013;75(5):467–74. DOI: 10.1016/
j.jpsychores.2013.08.002.

[21] Grodzinsky E, Walter S, Viktorsson L, Carlsson AK, Jones MP, Faresjö Å. More negative
self-esteem and inferior coping strategies among patients diagnosed with IBS compared with patients without IBS-a case–control study in primary care. BMC Fam Pract.
2015;16(1):1. DOI: 10.1186/s12875-015-0225-x

[22] Saito YA. The role of genetics in IBS. Gastroenterol Clin North Am. 2011;40(1):45–67.
DOI: 10.1016/j.gtc.2010.12.011

[23] Henström M, D'Amato M. Genetics of irritable bowel syndrome. Mol Cell Pediatr.
2016;3(1):1. DOI: 10.1186/s40348-016-0038-6

[24] Garakani A, Win T, Virk S, Gupta S, Kaplan D, Masand PS. Comorbidity of irritable
bowel syndrome in psychiatric patients: a review. Am J Ther. 2003;10(1):61–7. DOI:
10.1097/00045391-200301000-00014

[25] Fond G, Loundou A, Hamdani N, Boukouaci W, Dargel A, Oliveira J, Roger M,
Tamouza R, Leboyer M, Boyer L. Anxiety and depression comorbidities in irritable
bowel syndrome (IBS): a systematic review and meta-analysis. Eur Arch Psychiatry
Clin Neurosci. 2014;264(8):651–60. DOI: 10.1007/s00406-014-0502-z

[26] Guthrie E, Barlow J, Fernandes L, Ratcliffe J, Read N, Thompson DG, Tomenson
B, Creed F, North of England IBS Research Group. Changes in tolerance to rectal
distension correlate with changes in psychological state in patients with severe

irritable bowel syndrome. Psychosom Med. 2004;66(4):578–82. DOI: 10.1097/01.psy.0000128899.22514.c0

[27] Spiegel BM. The burden of IBS: looking at metrics. Curr Gastroenterol Rep. 2009;11(4):265–9. DOI: 10.1007/s11894-009-0039-x

[28] Hausteiner-Wiehle C, Henningsen P. Irritable bowel syndrome: relations with functional, mental, and somatoform disorders. World J Gastroenterol WJG. 2014;20(20):6024–30. DOI: 10.3748/wjg.v20.i20.60240.6024

[29] Wouters MM, Boeckxstaens GE. Is there a causal link between psychological disorders and functional gastrointestinal disorders?. Expert Rev Gastroenterol Hepatol. 2016;10(1):5–8. DOI: 10.1586/17474124.2016.1109446

[30] Weaver KR, Sherwin LB, Walitt B, Melkus GD, Henderson WA. Neuroimaging the brain-gut axis in patients with irritable bowel syndrome. WJGPT. 2016;7(2):320–33. DOI: 10.4292/WJGPT.v7.i2.320

[31] Beauregard M. Mind does really matter: evidence from neuroimaging studies of emotional self-regulation, psychotherapy, and placebo effect. Prog Neurobiol. 2007;81(4):218–36.DOI: 10.1016/j.pneurobio.2007.01.005

[32] Mayer EA, Labus JS, Tillisch K, Cole SW, Baldi P. Towards a systems view of IBS. Nat Rev Gastroenterol Hepatol. 2015;12(10):592–605. DOI: 10.1038/nrgastro.2015.121

[33] Ma X, Li S, Tian J, Jiang G, Wen H, Wang T, Fang J, Zhan W, Xu Y. Altered brain spontaneous activity and connectivity network in irritable bowel syndrome patients: a resting-state fMRI study. Clin Neurophysiol. 2015;126(6):1190–7. DOI: 10.1016/j.clinph.2014.10.004

[34] Blankstein U, Chen J, Diamant NE, Davis KD. Altered brain structure in irritable bowel syndrome: potential contributions of pre-existing and disease-driven factors. Gastroenterology. 2010;138(5):1783–9. DOI: 10.1053/j.gastro.2009.12.043

[35] Attree EA, Dancey CP, Keeling D, Wilson C. Cognitive function in people with chronic illness: inflammatory bowel disease and irritable bowel syndrome. Appl Neuropsychol. 2003;10(2):96–104. DOI: 10.1207/S15324826AN1002_05

[36] Kennedy PJ, Clarke G, O'Neill A, Groeger JA, Quigley EM, Shanahan F, Cryan JF, Dinan TG. Cognitive performance in irritable bowel syndrome: evidence of a stress-related impairment in visuospatial memory. Psychol Med. 2014;44(07):1553–66. DOI: 10.1017/S0033291713002171

[37] Aizawa E, Sato Y, Kochiyama T, Saito N, Izumiyama M, Morishita J, Kanazawa M, Shima K, Mushiake H, Hongo M, Fukudo S. Altered cognitive function of prefrontal cortex during error feedback in patients with irritable bowel syndrome, based on FMRI

and dynamic causal modeling. Gastroenterology. 2012;143(5):1188–98. DOI: 10.1053/j.gastro.2012.07.104

[38]   Sinagra E, Romano C, Cottone M. Psychopharmacological treatment and psychological interventions in irritable bowel syndrome. Gastroenterol Res Pract. 2012;2012:486067. DOI: 10.1155/2012/486067

[39]   Ruepert L, Quartero AO, de Wit NJ, van der Heijden GJ, Rubin G, Muris JW. Bulking agents, antispasmodics and antidepressants for the treatment of irritable bowel syndrome. Cochrane Datbase Syst Rev. 2011. DOI: 10.1002/14651858.CD003460.pub3

[40]   Halland M, Talley NJ. New treatments for IBS. Nat Rev Gastroenterol Hepatol. 2013;10(1):13–23. DOI: 10.1038/nrgastro.2012.207

[41]   Lee KJ, Kim JH, Cho SW. Gabapentin reduces rectal mechanosensitivity and increases rectal compliance in patients with diarrhoea-predominant irritable bowel syndrome. Aliment Pharmacol Ther. 2005;22(10):981–8. DOI: 10.1111/j.1365-2036.2005.02685.x

[42]   O'Mahony S, Chua AS, Quigley EM, Clarke G, Shanahan F, Keeling PW, Dinan TG. Evidence of an enhanced central 5HT response in irritable bowel syndrome and in the rat maternal separation model. Neurogastroenterol Motil. 2008;20(6):680–8. DOI: 10.1111/j.1365-2982.2007.01065.x

7

Microbial Neuro-Immune Interactions and the Pathophysiology of IBD

Mònica Aguilera and Silvia Melgar

Abstract

Inflammatory bowel disease (IBD), encompassing Crohn's disease (CD) and ulcerative colitis (UC), is a group of debilitating disorders affecting patient's quality of life and with unknown aetiology. The collected evidence indicates that individuals can develop IBD as a result of genetic susceptibility, a dysregulated immune response and the influence of certain environmental factors. Common symptomatology includes abdominal pain, fever and bowel diarrhoea with blood and/or mucus excretion. The location and extent of disease differ between UC and CD, affecting the mucosal layer in the colon in UC patients, whereas in CD patients, a transmural inflammation is found anywhere in the gastrointestinal tract. Factors associated with IBD pathophysiology include alterations in immune responses, characterized by an atypically T helper (Th)-2 profile in UC, and a Th1/Th17 profile in CD, modifications in epithelial barrier function and alterations in the commensal microbiota composition with blooming of specific pathobionts, for example, adherent-invasive *Escherichia coli* (AIEC), and with diet. Recent research has uncovered that inflammation, *per se*, can activate the enteric nervous system inducing neurogenic inflammation and increasing visceral sensitivity, leading to pain. Similarly, alterations in the commensal microbiota composition/ligands have also led to modifications in intestinal nociceptive markers and in visceral pain. In this chapter, we aim to review the mechanisms implicated in microbial neuro-immune axis and its potential contribution to IBD pathophysiology and symptomatology. We focus on the findings identified in animal models and in IBD patients and on the prospective translation of targeting the microbial neuro-immune axis as future therapeutic treatment for intestinal inflammatory conditions.

Keywords: IBD, microbiota, intestinal neuro-immune interaction, visceral pain, microbiota–gut–brain axis

1. Introduction IBD

Inflammatory bowel disease (IBD) is a group of diseases comprising mainly two entities, ulcerative colitis (UC) and Crohn's disease (CD), of unknown aetiology. Ulcerative colitis was described in the late nineteenth century by Wilks and Moxon [1] and CD was described by Crohn et al. in the early 1930s as terminal ileitis [2]. Since the beginning of the twenty-first century, the incidence of IBD is increasing worldwide, especially in Westernized areas such as the United States, Europe, Australia and New Zealand as well as in South America, Asia and the Middle East and in specific populations, for example, paediatric-onset IBD. The prevalence in the Western World is currently up to 0.5% of the population [3].

IBD affects the patients' quality of life and is characterized by unpredictable flares of re-mission and relapses with symptoms of bloody diarrhoea, abdominal pain and rectal bleeding. The onset of IBD is at a young age ranging initially from 20 to 39 years and with a second onset in patients over 60 years of age [4]. IBD affects both males and fe-males, with a higher prevalence of CD in females and no major differences in UC patients [5]. The inflammation in UC is localized to the colonic superficial mucosa while the in-flammation in CD is transmural and can be found anywhere along the gastrointestinal (GI) tract, although the inflammation is predominantly located to the ileo-caecal area and the proximal colon [6, 7]. Ulcerative colitis is characterized by the formation of crypt ab-scesses, formed by extravasation of neutrophils through the intestinal epithelium while CD is characterized by the presence of skip lesions, granulomas, fibrosis and strictures. Extra-intestinal features in CD can result in major complications, for example, fibrotic strictures, and a subsequently need for surgery [8, 9]. To date, there is no cure for IBD, with most treatments primarily aiming to suppress disease severity and to keep the pa-tient in remission by using biologics, anti-suppressants and steroids.

The cause of IBD is unknown but the collected evidence suggest that IBD can be manifested in genetically susceptible individuals who mount inappropriate local immune responses against microbial antigens after exposure to environmental factors [7, 10].

To date, genomewide association studies (GWAS) have identified at least 163 susceptible genes for IBD, with loci associated to bacterial recognition (NOD2) and autophagy (ATG16L1, IRGM) conferring a higher risk for CD. In contrast, genes involved in mucosal barrier function (e.g. HNF4a, CDH1, LAMB1, ECM1), IL-10 signalling and HLA haplotype DRB1*0103 have been associated with UC. Interestingly, genes linked with adaptive immune responses such as IL-23R, IL-12B and STAT3 confer a higher risk for both CD and UC. Despite the large number of loci identified, only approximately 20–25% of patients are linked to at least one of these loci suggesting that there are most likely other factors potentiating its development [11–13].

Alterations in barrier function, dysregulation in tight junction proteins and increased bacterial uptake has been reported in experimental models of colitis and in patients with UC and CD supporting the GWAS identified genes on barrier function [14, 15]. Others have also suggested that Peyer's patches are the sites of initial lesions in CD with M cells playing an important role in sampling microbes from the gut lumen and presenting to immune cells to mount inflammatory responses [16, 17]. Furthermore, unaffected relatives of CD patients have shown increased intestinal permeability [14, 15].

2. Intestinal immune mechanisms and IBD

The main function of the intestinal immune system is to protect the host from harmful signals, for example, pathogens, by mounting specific responses as well as to keep a tolerance against A myriad of food and microbial antigens. A robust immune response against invading pathogens is critical for their clearance but an excessive or uncontrolled inflammation can result in chronic inflammation and lead to the development of inflammatory conditions such as IBD (**Figure 1**). The collected evidence to date suggest that the aberrant immune response in IBD patients is attributed to the dysregulated adaptive and innate

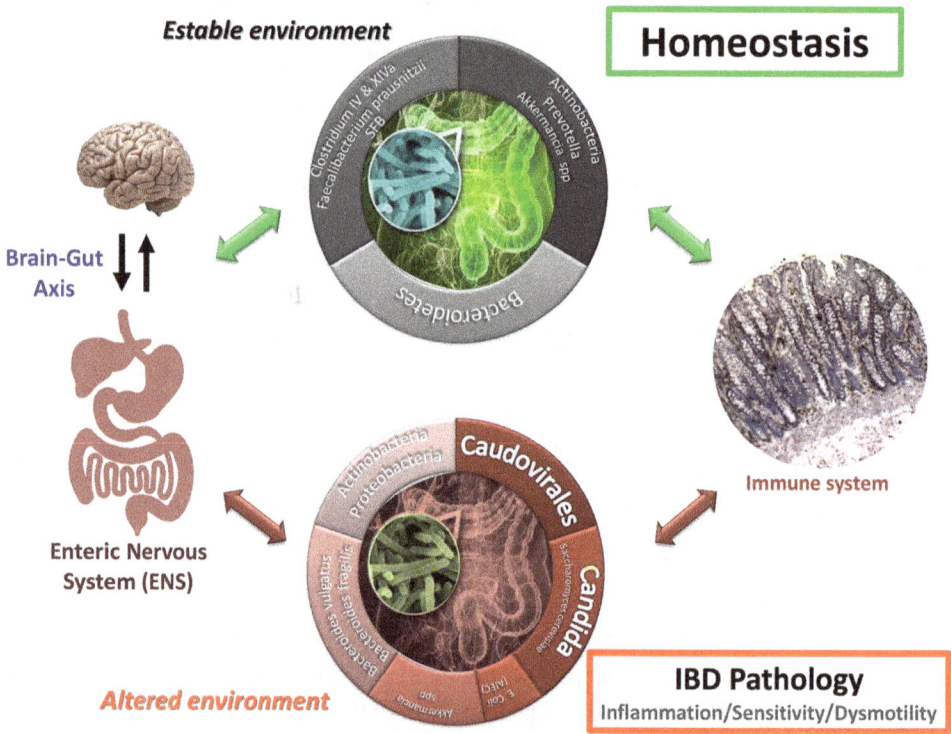

Figure 1. The gastrointestinal (GI) tract harbours up to 10^{14} bacteria, 10 times more than the number of cells of the human body. These bacteria include up to 1000 bacterial strains but are covered in few phyla. The most important ones in mammals are the Firmicutes (including Clostridium and Lactobacilli) and Bacteroidetes. Traditionally, it has been described that GI function is controlled by the intestinal immune system. Recent research has also highlighted that the enteric nervous system (ENS) and the gut commensal microbiota system play a crucial and an active role in influencing gut homeostasis. The ENS, mainly represented by the myenteric and the submucous plexus, Also known as the second brain due to it can work alone. The gut is connected to the CNS by the brain-gut axis, which maintains a bidirectional communication. When these three systems are balanced, there is a physiological homeostasis. An imbalance in any and/or all of these three systems can lead to the development of functional GI disorders and chronic inflammatory GI disorders such as IBD.

immune responses [7, 10]. The innate immune response is the first line of defence against harmful agents. Pattern recognition receptors (PRRs) detect microbial 'pathogen-associated molecular patterns' (PAMPs) or host-derived 'damage-associated molecular patterns' (DAMPs) inducing innate immune responses. Among PRRs, the intestinal Toll-like receptors (TLRs) are critical both in keeping intestinal homeostasis and in mounting innate immune responses. In humans, a total of 10 TLRs have been described, with the majority of them, except TLR3, signalling via the adaptor protein MyD88. Activation of TLRs via MyD88 induces several pathways including the transcription factor nuclear factor-kappa light-chain enhancer of activated B cells (NF-κB), mitogen-activated protein kinase (MAPK) and AP1, while the MyD88-independent pathway activates the interferon regulatory factor 3/7 (IRF-3/-7) signalling pathway [18]. In recent years, it has become evident that bacteria can penetrate/translocate through the intestinal barrier of IBD patients thereby inducing TLR-induced responses both by mucosal non-immune cells (e.g. epithelial cells) and innate immune cells (e.g. macrophages, dendritic cells). TLRs are expressed by

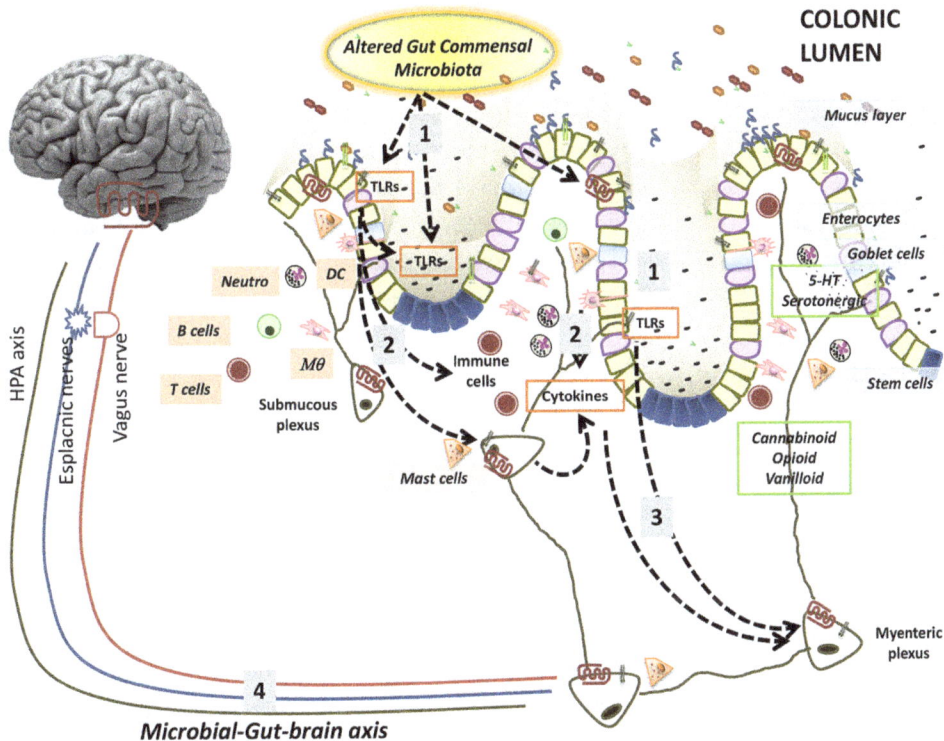

Figure 2. Representative schema of some of the putative mechanisms involved in IBD pathophysiology associated with microbial neuro-immune changes. The intestinal microbiota and microbial-derived products interact with the host bacterial recognition systems (such as TLRs) (1) generating a signalling cascade (2) that will lead to a local immune activation including mast cells, macrophages, T cells, neutrophils, dendritic cells and neuroendocrine systems (such as enterochromaffin cells) that seems to persist even when the overt inflammation is resolved. This persistent activation has the potential to influence sensory neural mechanisms within the gut depending upon the ENS (3) and the extrinsic innervation. In addition, the bidirectional communication between the gut and the CNS (4) is also altered that can offer an explanation for the altered perception of sensory signals and therefore altered manifestation of pain in patients suffering from IBD. Neutro—neutrophils; MΘ—macrophages; DC—dendritic cells; TLRs—Toll-like receptors.

both epithelial and immune cells, and alterations in TLRs expression have been reported in both UC and CD tissue including increase expression of TLR4, TLR2 and TLR5 [18]. Activation of TLRs, for example, TLR4, leads to the activation of NF-κB pathway, which is responsible for the transcription of various pro-inflammatory cytokines and chemokines associated with IBD pathology (**Figure 2**). Other PRRs involved in CD pathology include NOD2, which is a cytosolic receptor belonging to the nucleotide-binding domain and leucine-rich repeat containing family (NLRs). NOD2 recognizes muramyl dipeptide (MDP), present in both Gram-positive and Gram-negative bacteria and activates the NF-κB pathway. NOD2 has also been identified as a susceptible gene for CD with 3 SNPs linked to ileal CD, suggesting that a defect in recognition and clearance of bacteria might be associated with CD development. However, the specific inflammatory mechanisms associated with NOD2 mutations are still largely unknown [18].

The intestine of IBD patients presents a chronic inflammation that differs in terms of immune cell subsets and cytokine profile. The colons of UC patients are heavily infiltrated with neutrophils, T and B cells with high levels of several pro-inflammatory cytokines including IL-1β, IL-6 and TNF-α and an atypical T helper (Th2) profile (IL-5, IL-10 and IL-13) [7, 10, 19]. Other chemokines such as IL-8 and GRO-α are highly increased in UC mucosa, with IL-8 levels correlating with the degree of inflammation and disease activity [20, 21]. Although neutrophils are indispensable for eliminating pathogens, their excessive presence in the tissue and their resistance to apoptosis [22] can lead to extensive tissue damage in UC, which can be caused by the persistent release of cytokines (IL-17, IL-6), reactive oxygen species (ROS) and proteases, all of which highly associated with patients with active UC [7, 19, 23]. The intestinal wall of CD patients is highly infiltrated by macrophages and T cells. It is acknowledged that CD is primarily mediated by Th17/Th1 cells as well high levels of innate pro-inflammatory cytokines including IL-1β, IL-6 and TNF-α [6, 10]. Further, the elevated levels of circulating and tissue B cells as well as their activity have also been reported in IBD patients [24, 25].

3. Intestinal neural pathways and visceral pain in IBD

A particular characteristic of the GI tract is the presence of an intrinsic nervous system, the enteric nervous system (ENS) also known as the second brain. Within the intestine, the ENS presents a clear distribution in two neuronal plexuses localized within the submucosa (submucosal or Meissner's plexus) and between the circular and longitudinal smooth muscle layers (myenteric or Auerbach's plexus). The ENS can maintain GI functions alone by the network around the gut wall formed by both plexi. It is composed by around 10^8 neurons consisting of intrinsic primary afferents, interneurons and motor neurons [26–28]. Enteric neurons are supported by glial cells (counterparts of the central nervous system (CNS) astrocytes), which can communicate with the mucosal immune system and the intestinal epithelium by producing different mediators including cytokines. The ENS controls intestinal motility, secretion and absorption, mucosal growth, local blood flow, the immune and barrier function and also carries nociceptive (painful) stimuli to the CNS [29–31] (**Figure 2**).

The gut receives also extrinsic innervation from the autonomic nervous system (ANS) and the spinal afferent nerve fibres that coordinate its activity. The ANS is composed of the sympathetic nervous system (SNS) and the parasympathetic nervous system (PSNS). The extrinsic innervation consists of vagal and spinal sensory nerves, vagal and sacral parasympathetic motor neurons, and sympathetic neurons from prevertebral ganglia, and it plays a key role in maintaining the bidirectional communication with the CNS as well as it is the anatomical basis of the gut–brain–gut axis [32–34].

The vagus nerve (cranial nerve X interfacing with the PSNS) has a motor and a sensorial division and three different endings in the gut: the intraganglionic laminar endings within the myenteric plexus, the intramuscular arrays within the smooth muscle layers and the mucosal fibres within the mucosa [32]. The SNS suppresses GI functions under vagus nerve's activation, cell bodies arise from the paravertebral sympathetic chain ganglia, adjacent to the spinal column and innervating the GI vasculature, as well as the prevertebral (celiac and superior/inferior mesenteric) ganglia, which controls motility and secretomotor neurons. Axons extend to the gut by the mesenteric nerves but also by the vagus nerve, cranially, which also contacts with the ENS [32, 35]. The spinal innervation of the gut comes directly from the dorsal root ganglia (DRG) of the spinal cord, and it is less extensive when compared to the ANS. They extend to the gut by the splanchnic (cranially) and the parasympathetic pelvic nerves (distally). The colon, which harbours large amounts of bacteria, has specific DRG in their innervation [32].

4. Visceral hypersensitivity

Nociception is the neural processes of encoding and processing noxious stimuli that can be accompanied, or not, with pain [26, 36]. Visceral pain originates from the internal organs and is initiated by nociceptors, which can detect mechanical, thermal or chemical changes above a basal threshold [37]. Perception of visceral pain relies mainly in spinal C and Aδ afferents fibres from DRG although vagal afferent stimulation can also mediate pain [38]. The strong compression, as well as chemical stimuli or irritation, of the colon generates afferent signals that can hypersensitize afferent nerves and become nociceptive [39–41].

Although most of the intestinal functions can be carried out by the ENS, extrinsic innervation is necessary to maintain a coordinated activity with the rest of the body and for sensory functions related to visceral pain perception within the gut. This is particularly important because visceral pain and/or altered visceral sensitivity (hypersensitivity) are frequent symptoms in several GI diseases including irritable bowel syndrome (IBS) and IBD. Visceral hypersensitivity generally originates from a local inflammation leading to an enhanced response to a painful stimulus (hyperalgesia) as a result of activation of the immune system, stressful conditions and the intestinal microbiota [42–44] (**Figures 1** and **2**). Alterations in sympathetic neural activity have specifically been implicated in IBD [25, 45]. A decrease in noradrenaline release from sympathetic varicosities in inflamed and uninflamed regions of the GI tract has consistently been reported in animal models of colitis, which appears to be due to the inhibition of N-type voltage-gated Ca^{2+} current in postganglionic sympathetic neurons [46]. However, specific alterations of sympathetic function and its role in IBD remain unclear [25]. In the last two decades, numerous morphological, pharmacological and molecular studies have characterized sensory-related systems within the gut, among them the serotonergic system, the endocannabinoid system, endogenous opiates and the vanilloid system have received particular attention due to their potential benefit as pharmacological targets for the treatment of visceral pain. A short description of each of these systems is outlined below.

4.1. The intestinal serotonergic system

The serotonergic system involves the neurotransmitter serotonin (5-hydroxytryptamine; 5-HT), which is mainly stored in mucosal enterochromaffin (EC) cells and in a lesser extent within the enteric neurons (up to 95% of body 5-HT is present in the gut). Tryptophan hydroxylase (TPH) is the limiting enzyme mediating 5-HT synthesis. Two TPH isoforms exist, namely TPH1, mainly expressed in EC cells, and TPH2, expressed in central and enteric neurons. TPH expression/activity is regarded as a reliable indicator of 5-HT availability, whereby high expression levels are indicative of a high rate of serotonin production and release [47–49]. Within the GI tract, 5-HT participates in motor, sensory and secretory functions modifying gut motility/sensation in several ways [50]. For example, 5-HT present within the enteric nerves and acting on 5-HT3 receptors of the vagal afferent nerve fibres can stimulate intestinal secretion and motor reflexes. 5-HT can also act on the receptors 5-HT3, 5-HT4 and 5-HT1P present on enteric neurons, thereby contributing to peristalsis and stimulating intestinal transit [51]. Expression of 5-HT7 receptor has been found on intestinal immune cells and demonstrated a key role in development of experimental colitis [52]. Intestinal inflammation is accompanied by alterations in enteroendocrine cells, among which EC is the most abundant. These cells are distributed throughout the GI tract, with many of them concentrated in the small intestine and rectum and in between epithelial cells, where they act as sensors of the intraluminal milieu. 5-HT release from EC cells is mediated by luminal or neuronal stimuli including mucosal stroking and endogenous chemical stimuli such as adenosine. Changes in the content, release and reuptake of 5-HT as well as increase numbers of EC cells have been reported 8 in both inflamed and non-inflamed gut of IBD patients and in experimental models of IBD [53, 54]. Some studies have also shown that changes in the microbial composition or stressful conditions can induce 5-HT release from EC cells, leading to the initiation of intestinal inflammation and the generation of abnormal sensory-related responses (i.e. altered viscerosensitivity) [48, 55–57]. The sodium-dependent serotonin transporter (SERT), a member of the Na^+/Cl^- neurotransmitter transporter family, is expressed by epithelial cells and neurons in the gut [47] and is involved in the reuptake of 5-HT. SERT expression is reduced in the inflamed and in the healing colonic mucosa of UC patients, thereby increasing 5-HT levels [25, 58]. Furthermore, deletion of SERT increases the severity of 2,4,6-trinitrobenzenesulfonic acid (TNBS)-induced colitis in mice [59] and mice treated with the SERT inhibitor paroxetine presented alterations in GI motility and sensitivity [60]. Interestingly, the regulatory cytokine transforming growth factor-beta 1 (TGF-β1) was recently shown to stimulate SERT function suggesting a novel neuro-immune therapeutic strategy to treat GI disorders [61]. These findings implicate that 5-HT signalling and its SERT-mediated termination can contribute to the symptoms associated with IBD pathophysiology and suggest that drugs targeting this pathway may benefit patients suffering from IBD and other inflammation-related gut disorders [25, 62].

4.2. The intestinal opioid system

The endogenous opioid system is composed by three G protein-coupled receptors: μ, δ and k opioid receptors. Within the GI tract, intestinal opioids, ligands and receptors are found in myenteric and submucosal neurons and in epithelial, endocrine and immune cells (including myeloid and CD4+ T and CD8+ T cells). Opioids have a well-characterized analgesic activity in visceral sensitivity [63, 64], which is mainly linked to the activation of μ and, to a lesser extent, k receptors. The expression of δ opioid receptor together with μ receptor is increased after administration of the inflammatory irritant mustard oil, thereby evoking allodynia and visceral hyperalgesia [25, 65]. μ-Opioid receptors (MOR) are overexpressed in active IBD mucosa, most likely as a compensatory analgesic mechanism generated in states of potentially increased sensitivity. MOR are also significantly enhanced by pro-inflammatory cytokines and repressed by NF-κB inhibitors in myeloid and lymphocytic cell lines [66]. Increased numbers of β-endorphin immunoreactive CD4+ T cells and CD11b+ macrophages are found in murine colonic lamina propria in chronic dextran sodium sulphate (DSS)-induced colitis, where the release of endogenous opioids decreases nociceptive signalling through the activation of μ-opioid receptors [67]. Therefore, it is speculated that the anti-nociceptive actions of peripheral opioids in colitis may indirectly result from a reduction of the neurogenic 'pro-nociceptive' components of inflammation, by decreasing CGRP and Substance P (SP) release that could counteract the pro-nociceptive effects of inflammatory mediators such as TNF-α during inflammation [68]. Recent studies have suggested that probiotics and microbial-related products can also module the intestinal expression of MOR [66, 69–72].

4.3. The intestinal endocannabinoid system

The endocannabinoid (CB) system comprises of two main receptors, CB1 and CB2, their endogenous ligands and their metabolizing enzymes, Mainly the fatty acid amide hydrolase, FAAH. Because of their chemical characteristics, endocannabinoid ligands are difficult to determine; therefore, the expression of CB1, CB2 and the enzyme FAAH, are used to assess endocannabinoid functionality. Within the GI tract, the endocannabinoid system controls intestinal motility, nociception and intestinal inflammation. CB1 and CB2 receptors are expressed on intestinal ganglionic neural cells within the ENS, in epithelial cells and immune cells in the gut [73–76]. The CB1 receptor is predominantly found in neural and epithelial cells, whereas the CB2 receptors are predominantly expressed in immune cells [77]. Upon activation, both receptors mediate analgesic effects and appear to have anti-inflammatory properties [75, 77–80]. Probiotics, bacterial products and stressful stimuli have been postulated to influence the endocannabinoid system [70, 81–83]. In IBD, an increased in CB1 expression has been identified in inflamed mucosa, while a reduction in the endocannabinoid agonist anandamide and no increase in CB2 expression were found.

Ex vivo cultures of IBD biopsies and immune cells with the non-hydrolysable AEA ana-logue methanandamide (MAEA) resulted in a reduction in IFN-γ and TNF-α secretion [84]. In animal models of colitis, the CB2 agonist JWH-133 attenuates colitis in IL-10$^{-/-}$ mice and in DSS-induced colitis by decreasing the number of mucosal immune cells (in-cluding CD4$^+$ T cells, neutrophils, Mast cells and natural killer cells) [85]. Recent studies in humans and animals have identified a new strategy for the endocannabinoid system, whereby targeting of the enzyme FAAH can prove to be a better approach due to the potentially less side effects when compared to the currently available CB compounds [86–88]. Overall, the preclinical findings indicate that manipulating the endocannabinoid sys-tem can have beneficial effects in IBD patients, and therefore, the use of *Cannabis sativa* has also been studied, although further research is necessary in this context [89, 90].

4.4. The intestinal vanilloid system

The vanilloid system consists of one of six subfamilies of the transient receptor potential (TRP) channel family, with six types of transient receptor potential vanilloid (TRPV1-6) [91]. These receptors are calcium permeable, non-selective cation channels involved in thermo- and chemo-sensitive transduction [92]. In the intestine, TRPV1, 3 and 4 have been linked to viscerosensitivity and are characterized as pro-algesic receptors [79, 92–94]. TRPV are mainly expressed in intestinal afferent nerves, although they can also be found in EC cells as well as epithelial and immune cells [95–97]. In agreement with their pro-algesic effects, TRPV are upregulated in states of intestinal inflammation and visceral hypersensitivity; for example, TRPV1 is highly increased in immunoreactive nerves in IBD tissue and in quiescent IBD with IBS-like symptoms such as pain [98–102]. TRPV1 deletion prevented the development of post-inflammatory visceral hypersensitivity and pain-associated behaviours, while SP can sensitize TRPV1 function leading to a pro-algesic state [101, 103]. TRPV1 has been linked to the crosstalk between the microbiota and the neuro-immune response in the gut, because TRPV1 and CGRP can modulate cytokine response to lipopolysaccharide (LPS) independently of the adaptive immune response. It has been proposed that TLR4 can activate TRPV1 via intracellular signalling thereby inducing the subsequent release of anti-inflammatory CGRP to maintain mucosal homeostasis [104]. In addition, blocking of TRPV4 has also been shown to alleviate colitis and pain associated with the intestinal inflammation induced by TNBS in mice [105]. Similarly, intrathecal injection of antisense oligonucleotides to TRPA1, another member of the transient receptor potential channel family, decrease its expression and attenuates visceral hyperalgesia in TNBS-induced colitis [25, 65].

4.5. Neurotransmitters, neuropeptides and neurotrophins

More than two dozens of putative neurotransmitters have been described to date, with neurons usually expressing a combination thereof. Most of these mediators have been implicated in the neuro-immune communication associated with gut homeostasis and in the pathophysiology of intestinal inflammation but their specific functions are still to be established [106]. A short description of the most relevant mediators is outlined under this section.

Substance P (SP), an 11-amino acid peptide secreted by nerves and immune cells (including monocytes, macrophages, eosinophils and lymphocytes) belongs to the tachykinins family and acts by binding to the neurokinin-1 (NK-1) receptor. It functions in smooth muscle contraction, vasodilation and epithelial ion transport. It is a mediator of neurogenic inflammation due to stimulation of cytokine release from immune cells (e.g. macrophages, mast cells) and endothelium causing tissue damage and neurodegeneration [25, 107]. High expression of SP and NK-1 receptor was reported in the myenteric plexus and inflamed mucosa of patients with IBD. This is associated with a shift from mainly cholinergic innervation to a more extensive SP innervation, which correlates with the severity of UC and may be part of the neuronal basis for the observed altered motility disturbance seen in these patients [106, 108–110]. Antagonists of NK-1 receptors have been shown to ameliorate inflammation and protect from T-cell-induced colitis. Based on these findings, tachykinin antagonists have been proposed as potential anti-inflammatory treatment for IBD [25, 108, 111, 112].

Vasoactive intestinal polypeptide (VIP), a 28-amino acid peptide belonging to the pituitary adenylate cyclase-activating polypeptide (PACAP)/glucagon superfamily, is highly expressed in the myenteric plexus of the colon. VIP inhibits the peristaltic reflex in the circular muscle layer, controls intestinal blood flow and modulates the immune system by binding to both G protein-coupled VIP receptors 1 and 2. VIP is released from nerve terminals that contain nitric oxide synthase (NOS). These two peptides are thought to be the primary intestinal components of non-adrenergic, non-cholinergic nerve transmission. VIP expression is increased in colonic neurons of CD patients but not in UC patients [25, 113–115]. Treatment with VIP in murine TNBS-induced colitis reduces colitis severity and Th1-cell response [116, 117]. In addition, glucagon-like peptide 2 (GLP-2), a regulator of absorption with anti-inflammatory properties, decreases mucosal inflammation in TNBS-induced colitis in rats by activating VIP neurons of the submucosal plexus [118]. Neurotrophins are a family of proteins regulating neuronal activity in the CNS and PNS, belonging to a class of growth factors and playing a major role in visceral hypersensitivity in the inflamed gut. This is, partly linked to the effects of peripheral neurotrophic factors (NTFs) on local afferent neurons. Among these, nerve growth factor (NGF) is primarily involved in the regulation of growth, maintenance, proliferation and survival of certain target neurons and in innate and adaptive immune responses; brain-derived neurotrophic factor (BDNF) links the commensal microbiota and the CNS [119, 120]; and the family of glial cell line-derived NTFs (including GDNF, artemin and neurturin) are implicated in sensorial alterations observed in inflammatory and functional GI disorders [112].

5. Intestinal neuro-immune interactions

Intestinal inflammation, even if mild, causes significant alterations in neurally controlled gut functions including pain and altered motility. These symptoms are caused, in part, by persistent hyperexcitability of enteric neurons that can occur even after the resolution of colitis. Among cells generating inflammatory signals within the gut mucosa and affecting neural signalling in the ENS, mast cells and enterochromaffin cells seem to play a big role. Both of them are increased in the colonic mucosa of IBD patients [25]. The ENS and the mucosal immune system have the ability to regulate each other functions. In the intestinal wall, nerve cells are localized in close proximity to immune cells and they share several chemical mediators. The collected evidence point towards a major role of inflammatory signals affecting the enteric neurons and most likely generating IBD-associated symptoms [25, 121, 122] (**Figure 2**).

Inflammation-related alterations in the ENS are divided into those that alter the structural morphology of neurons and glial cells of the ENS and those that modify enteric neurotransmitters [25, 122–124]. During intestinal inflammation, morphological and functional alterations, including remodelling of visceral afferents, are also observed outside the primary region affected by the insult [112]. ENS structural changes are more marked in CD than in UC patients and are often associated with the extent of inflammatory infiltrate. In fact, it has been suggested that severe and extensive necrosis of gut axons may be a distinct feature in CD [25]. In support of this notion is the ablation of myenteric neurons, accompanied by a high neutrophil infiltration and an excessive production of the Th1 cytokines IFN-γ, TNF-α and IL-12 present in models of colitis. Interestingly, neuronal loss persisted for up to 56 days, that is when the inflammation had resolved in these models [125–128]. Others proposed mechanisms implicated in neuron loss, arisen from animal models and IBD patients, Which involve an increase in immune cell infiltrates, including eosinophils, lymphocytes, plasma cells and mast cells, in myenteric ganglia [25, 123, 126, 128, 129] as well as the activation of apoptotic pathways [130]. Furthermore, enteric glial cell ablation induces a significant decrease in the number of myenteric neurons, which appear to be associated with the loss of NOS-containing neurons in the myenteric plexus, likely underlying the alterations observed in smooth muscle relaxation and intestinal transit time [25, 131]. It is also believed that the reduced availability of neuroprotective factors due to neuronal cell loss may increase the susceptibility of enteric neurons to insults such as oxidative stress, which can have an important role in IBD pathophysiology. Overall, the collected data indicate that the loss of nerve cells is dependent on the time needed to develop inflammation, the type of inflammatory cells and the mediators profile required for nerve–immune interactions [107].

Immune cells found in the intestine, including dendritic and mast cells, lymphocytes and macrophages, express receptors for small molecule neurotransmitters and neuropeptides and produce cytokines targeting the enteric neurons [106]. Neuro-immune regulation includes degranulation of mast cells and influx of neutrophils due to neuronal activation. Neuropeptides released by enteric nerves including SP and VP can stimulate lymphocytes to induce their differentiation and alter immunoglobulin production. Signalling between immune cells and enteric neurons can also evoke alterations in gut function. Hyperexcitability of intrinsic primary afferent neurons may be secondary to activation of cyclooxygenase (COX)-2 and production of prostaglandins (PGE_2) from inflamed colon [25, 132]. Intestinal kinases have also been involved in intestinal inflammation. Protein kinase A activity in nerve terminals increases in previously inflamed colon and facilitates a fast synaptic transmission and the release-ready pool of synaptic vesicles [25, 133, 134]. There is also evidences that pro-inflammatory cytokines such as IL-1β and TNF-α exhibit pro-secretory effects in the human distal colon. Both IL-1β

and IL-6 are reported to increase excitability in submucous and myenteric neurons and to mediate effects on cholinergic and non-cholinergic transmission [135–137].

Mast cells are a major player in the innate immune response. Apart from their prominent role in immunoglobulin E (IgE)-dependent hypersensitivity, mast cells can release and modulate the release of several mediators including cytokines, growth factors, chemokines as well as histamine, proteases, and probably serotonin 22 receptors that regulate multiple important biological processes including neural actions in the human ENS [137]. Neuropeptides released from enteric and visceral afferent nerves regulate human intestinal mast cell mediator's release. In healthy individuals, mast cells are generally located in the lamina propria, in fewer amounts in the submucosa and sporadically found in the muscle layers or in the serosa. An estimated 70% of intestinal mucosal mast cells are in direct contact with nerves, and another 20% are within a 2-μm distance. Mast cells respond to neurotransmitters and nerves and can thereby regulate their activation threshold [137, 138], submucous neurons would respond with a transient excitation mediated primarily by 5-HT3 receptors [139]. Cytokines and chemokines can have different effect on mast cell functions. For example, the chemokine, macrophage inflammatory protein-1α (MIP-1α) is required for optimal mast cell degranulation in mice [140]. In contrast, the regulatory cytokine TGF-β1 can dose dependently inhibits stem cell factor-dependent growth of human intestinal mast cells by both enhancing apoptosis and decreasing proliferation [141] as well as it can influence mediator secretion by reducing histamine, cysteinyl leukotrienes and TNF-α release while prostaglandin D2 (PGD2) generation and COX1 and 2 expressions are upregulated. Mucosal mast cells can also respond to other mediators including adenosine triphosphate (ATP), somatostatin, calcitonin gene-related peptide (CGRP) and SP. Colorectal biopsies from patients with active CD or UC incubated with SP induce mast cell degranulation and histamine release [30, 142].

Histamine, proteases and TNF-α are stored as granules in mast cells and can be released within seconds. Other mediators such as lipid mediators and most cytokines are synthesized once the mast cells are activated. The most important mast cell mediator identified so far is histamine. Histamine influences fluid and ion transport, which is partly nerve mediated and directly excites submucous extrinsic sensory neurons [137, 142, 143]. There are four histamine receptors (H1, H2, H3 and H4), which are found as receptor clusters on submucous neurons, with the most frequent clusters being H1/H3 (29%), H2 (27%) and H1/H2/H3 (20%), respectively. The implication of histamine on sensory neurons comes from studies in rodents [142]. Rat dorsal root ganglion cells with projections to the viscera increased Ca^{2+} responses to a TRPV4 agonist and enhanced TRPV4 expression, when adding histamine or serotonin [144]. The pathophysiological relevance of histamine in both allergic and non-allergic conditions including IBD and IBS is established [141, 145]. In IBD, it has been reported that histamine secretion is increased in the jejunum of active CD and in urine of UC patients [146], although in a recent study, no differences in serum levels of histamine were identified [147].

Proteases, in particular the serine protease tryptase, are prominent mediators released from mast cells. Tryptase is present in almost all human mast cells, comprising up to 25% of their total proteins [148]. Proteases signal to nerves is mediated through protease-activated receptors (PARs), with four cloned PAR receptors identified in humans. PAR1, PAR3 and PAR4 are predominantly activated by thrombin, and PAR2 is activated by trypsin and mast cell tryptase [137]. In patients with UC, tryptase induces the release of inflammatory cytokines and chemokines, some of which may exert their effects through nerve pathways as outlined above [149]. Supernatants from stool of IBS and UC patients contain increased protease levels and when supernatants from UC patients were injected to mice, it promoted hypoalgesia, which was dependent on cathepsin-G-PAR4 activation [150]. PAR2 activation in mice increases intestinal permeability, which is mediated by SP and capsaicin-sensitive spinal afferent nerves while in rats PAR2 evoked visceral hypersensitivity [151]. Interestingly, PAR positive cells were increased in mucosa of UC patients and preferentially co-localized with tryptase+ cells suggesting that mast cells activation via PAR2 might be involved in the pathogenesis of UC [149]. Similarly, mucosal biopsy supernatants from UC patients can activate mouse DRG neurons innervating the colon, via TNF-α regulation [137, 152].

6. Microbial alterations in IBD

The microbial community of the GI tract is composed by bacteria, virus, fungi, protozoa and yeasts. Gut colonization starts at birth and, when completed, it harbours about 100 trillion microbial commensals and symbionts belonging approximately to 5000 distinct species divided in the phyla Firmicutes, Bacteriodetes, Proteobacteria, Verrucomicrobia, Actinobacteria, Fusobacteria and Cyanobacteria [153–155]. The intestinal microbiota is not homogenously distributed along the GI tract. For example, *Proteobacteria* spp. (mainly Enterobacteria) and Lactobacillales preferentially populate the small intestine while Bacteroidetes and Clostridia populate the large intestine. The density of bacterial cells in the gut increases caudally with the maximal counts (10^{11}–10^{12} cells/g of content in both human and rodents) localized in the ceco-colonic region [156–159]. Intestinal bacteria can be transient i.e. bacteria introduced during adult life; they do not permanently colonize the gut and can have positive (probiotics) or negative (pathogens) effects on the host, or be innocuous, or permanent. The latter ones are long-term colonists of the gut, the true commensals, and they can have immunostimulatory effects (so called authobionts), or they can confer detrimental effects under certain specific conditions (so called pathobionts) [160].

Overall, the commensal microbiota serves the host with protection against pathogens, metabolizing complex lipids and polysaccharides and neutralizing drugs and carcinogens; but it can also modulate intestinal motility, influence the maturation of the intestinal immune system and modulate visceral perception [33, 161]. Changes in the normal composition of the microbiota, termed generally in the literature as dysbiosis, have been associated with chronic inflammatory and functional GI disorders such as IBD and IBS [154, 162] (**Figure 1**). Dysbiosis can occur in parallel to intestinal pathogenesis and can be either a consequence or a cause of the disease [163]. In fact, the causal effects of the microbiota in IBD are still a matter of discussion, with some authors considering that dysbiotic state a consequence and/or a perpetuating factor, rather than a cause of the disease [164, 165].

Many pathogenic organisms have been investigated as causing agents of IBD, including *Mycobacterium avium* subsp paratuberculosis *Helicobacter* spp, non-jejuni/coli *campylobacter* and *Escherichia coli* as well as viruses including Epstein–Barr virus, cytomegalovirus, paramyxoviruses and others [166, 167]. However, to date any pathogenic organism has proven to be a causative agent or even correlate to IBD severity. Recently, the focus has shifted with the conception that the gut commensal microbiota as a whole and/or in relationship to the host can influence disease outcome. This shift has arisen from reports showing that distal ileum and colon (containing the highest microbiota loads) are most susceptible to inflammation and that germ-free animals do not develop inflammation. Similarly, antibiotics and certain probiotics have shown therapeutic efficacy in certain IBD cohorts. An altered bacterial composition (dysbiosis) is associated with IBD patients, characterized by a reduction in bacterial diversity, especially the alpha diversity, which denotes the numbers of bacterial species and their abundance [168, 169].

Pathobionts have been identified and linked to intestinal pathology. For example, *Bacteroides vulgatus* can induce colitis in HLA/B27-β2m rats, but not in IL-10$^{-/-}$ mice and it can even prevent colitis in IL-2$^{-/-}$ mice [170, 171]. In stool samples and mucosal specimens from IBD patients, an increased abundance of Enterobacteriaceae (belonging to Proteobacteria), especially *E. Coli*, is repeatedly observed. Among this, the adherent-invasive *E. coli* (AIEC), which selectively colonizes the ileum of up to 40% of CD patients, has been suggested to be a strain-specific microbial factor in the pathogenesis of CD (**Figure 1**). The definition of AIEC was based on the ability of the AIEC-LF82 strain to adhere and invade epithelial cells and to persist within macrophages without induction of cell death and by inducing the secretion of pro-inflammatory cytokines such as TNF-α [169, 172–175].

In terms of commensals, a reduction in Firmicutes and a spatial reorganization of the Bacteroidetes has been described in patients with IBD [176–178]. For example, *Bacteroides fragilis* is responsible for a greater proportion of the bacterial mass in these patients. Some specific strains of Bacteroidetes and their polysaccharide A have been linked to harbour immunomodulatory potential, as shown by their protective effect on intestinal inflammation by suppressing IL-17 production and enhancing the production of IL-10 by intestinal CD4$^+$Foxp3$^+$ T regulatory cells [156, 179–181]. A higher abundance of *Actinobacteria* and a loss of *Prevotella* spp are identified in CD patients. A loss of the commensal *Faecalibacterium prausnitzii* (belonging to Clostridia) abundance has been described in IBD [177, 182]. *F. prausnitzii* was shown to have beneficial immune-regulatory effects on the host, with the A2-165 strain ameliorating inflammation in experimental models. *F. prausnitzii* has also been linked with a new subset of CD4$^+$CD8$\alpha\alpha^+$ T cells with regulatory/suppressive functions, a cell type that is less abundant in IBD patients. In addition to the anti-inflammatory properties, *F. prausnitzii* is an important supplier of butyrate to the colonic epithelium and it is found adherent to the gut mucosa where oxygen diffuses from epithelial cells thereby improving barrier function [183]. The loss of *F. prausnitzii* is speculated to be an indicator for increased IBD risk [184–187]. *Clostridium* spp. constitutes one of the largest families of the commensal microbiota and, probably due to *C. difficile* infections, it has traditionally been regarded as a pathogenic bacteria. However, recent data suggest that some members of the Clostridia group, , *Clostridium IV* and *Clostridium XIVa*, might have an anti-inflammatory potential in immune responses [180, 188] (**Figure 1**). Moreover, the Clostridia-related group of segmented filamentous bacteria (SFB) has been associated with both intestinal inflammation and immune regulation [180], but their role in human IBD pathogenesis is uncovered. Other commensal strains such as Lactobacilli and Bifidobacteria strains are typically considered to confer health benefits to the host and are frequently used as probiotics [189]. Interestingly, *L. acidophilus* seems to modulate sensory mechanisms leading to visceral analgesia [70] while Bifidobacteria can act as immunostimulants [190]. Probiotic treatment in IBD patients has, to date, not being as successful as in, for example, patients with pouchitis when compared to current treatments in UC patients. In CD patients, probiotic treatment appears to be even less beneficial [191–193]. Verrucomicrobia are a mucus-degrading group of bacteria that seems to affect intestinal barrier function through the degradation of the epithelial mucus layer [194] and some Verrucobacteria spp such as *Akkermancia muciniphila* alleviate experimental colitis and can also mediate intestinal immune tolerance [195, 196]. A reduction in *Akkermansia* spp has been identified in IBD patients [197] (**Figure 1**).

Recent research has identified diet as a major factor influencing commensal microbiota composition. Dietary fibres are often associated with reducing the risk of IBD as well as alterations in bacterial carbohydrate metabolism [177]. Fibres are metabolized to short-chain fatty acids (SCFA) by commensal microbiota in the distal GI tract. SCFA can influence the growth of pathogens, increase intestinal barrier function, influence visceral sensitivity and serve as energy source for colonocytes, and they can facilitate the generation and differentiation of intestinal regulatory T cells [198, 199]. Patients with CD and UC are associated with impairment in SCFA production [185], which is linked to a reduction in butyrate-producing bacteria, including *Roseburia inulinivorans*, *Ruminococcus torques*, *C. lavalense*, *B. uniformis* and *F. prausnitzii* as well as a reduction in butyrate levels. Less butyrate is linked to changes in visceral hypersensitivity [169, 200]. In contrast to dietary fibres, Westernized high-fat diet, full of refined carbohydrates, is strongly associated with the development of colitis in different IBD animal models, contrary to a diet highly based on fruits, vegetables and polyunsaturated fatty acid-3, which has a protective effect against disease progression in these models. Recent data have also revealed that specific changes in dietary intake, for example, feeding of milk-fat diet, can modify the composition of the gut microbiota, resulting in the emergence of pathobionts (*Bilophila wadsworthia*). The correlations of these 'Westernized' diets and blooming of pathobionts in human IBD onset, development and/or relapse are Still to be further investigated [201–203].

The composition of the gut microbiota has recently been linked to the uptake and signalling effects of bile acids. Some members of the *Eubacterium* and *Clostridium* XIVa clusters possess the ability to 7α-dehydroxylate which are involved in secondary bile acid production. In fact, alteration in bile acid profiles may have the potential to protect against pathogens (such as *C. difficile*) [204] or pathobionts (such as *B. wadsworthia*). The latter one exacerbates colitis in IL-10$^{-/-}$ mice and is known to respond to alterations in bile acid profiles [201, 205].

Apart from bacteria, there are also alterations in the commensal fungi composition as well as the virome. Fungal microbiota is skewed in IBD; for example, CD patients show reduced fungal diversity together with an increased *Candida* taxa [206] and an increased Basidiomycota/Ascomycota ratio, and a decreased proportion of *Saccharomyces cerevisiae* has also been reported. Overall, the data indicate that the IBD gut environment might favour fungi at the expenses of bacteria [207]. An increase abundance of *Caudovirales* bacteriophages has also been reported in IBD patients. Some authors are suggesting that viral dysbiosis *per se* contributes to IBD pathology and changes in the bacterial ecosystem due to their predator–prey relationship [207, 208] (**Figure 1**).

7. Microbiota–gut–brain axis and IBD

There is a bidirectional signalling pathway between the GI and the brain, mainly through the vagus nerve, in which the commensal microbiota have an active role, denoted as the 'microbiota-gut-brain axis'. This axis is vital for maintaining homeostasis and it may be also involved in the aetiology of intestinal dysfunctions/disorders (**Figures 1** and **2**). There are evidences of the ability of the gut microbiota to communicate with the brain and thus modulate behaviour and pain and also transfer and eliminate micro-organisms for selecting the commensal profile. The proposal of a 'microbiota-gut-brain' implies that through a dynamic alignment, the microbiota inhabiting the intestinal lumen will affect the host's superior functions by changing CNS activity and vice versa, that is the brain activity and will also impact on microbiota development and composition. Apart from cognitive and vegetative functions, the 'microbiota-gut-brain axis' has been studied in visceral pain [209–212]. Although it has been traditionally studied in the context of IBS pathology, some of those findings can be translated to IBD, since IBD shares some overlapping mechanisms with IBS [161, 213, 214]. This includes the dysfunction of the brain-gut axis, the implication of TNFSF gene, the abnormal microbial composition and altered host functions, the low-grade inflammation and the presence of IBS symptoms in patients with IBD in remission [215]. Overall, there is evidence that host–microbe alterations might be not only divergent regarding the abundance of microbial community members but also in their metabolic activity.

The intestinal TLRs are critical for bacterial recognition and initiation of innate immune responses. In particular, TLR2, 4 and 7 have been directly implicated in the modulation of nociceptive markers and visceral hypersensitivity and pain [72, 104, 210, 216–221]. It has also been proposed that a neurochemical 'delivery system' exists whereby gut bacteria can send messages to the brain. This delivery system links the commensal gut microbiota to a number of neurotransmitters including GABA, serotonin, noradrenaline, dopamine, acetylcholine and melatonin, all of which are crucial for brain-regulated functions including visceral pain, brain development, anxiety or behaviour [33, 222, 223].

Some of the mechanisms described in the microbiota-gut-brain axis imply the activation of TLRs. Among them, TLR2, expressed in enteric neurons, glia and smooth muscle cells of the intestinal wall appear to regulate intestinal inflammation by controlling ENS structure and neurochemical coding, along with intestinal neuromuscular function. Colitis in Tlr2$^{-/-}$ mice is more severe compared to wild-type mice that is associated with altered ENS architecture and neurochemical profile, intestinal dysmotility, abnormal mucosal secretion, reduced levels of GDNF and impaired signalling via Ret-GFR-α1. Treatment with GDNF to Tlr2$^{-/-}$ mice led to improved colitis [219].

TLR4, increased in IBD patients, has also been associated with severe colitis with impaired epithelial barrier, altered expression of anti-microbial peptide genes and altered epithelial cell differentiation [221]. A putative LPS–TLR4–TRPV1 axis has been described, directly implicating microbiota in changes of the nervous system by means of the innate immune system, that is the TLRs. In line with this notion, the local stimulation of TLR4 but also TLR7, both expressed in epithelial, immune and neural cells, can induce an immune activation that leads to changes in different nociceptive markers, implicating mainly the cannabinoid and the vanilloid system, without having an overt inflammatory response [216, 217]. These findings address some of the putative mechanisms associated with microbial neuro-immune responses, which can contribute to IBD pathophysiology (**Figure 2**).

8. Conclusions and perspectives

The intestinal immune system has as its main function to protect the host against invading pathogens as well as to tolerate the myriad of our commensal micro-organisms. If this crosstalk is altered due to genetic predisposition and/or environmental factors, the steady state will be broken and it will result in the development of chronic inflammation such as IBD. Recent research has also identified a third player, the nervous system consisting of both the ENS and the CNS, which can directly regulate the intestinal immune system (**Figure 1**). In this chapter, It is summarized the findings linking the intestinal neuronal pathways with the intestinal immune system and the microbiota in IBD patients. In several cases, the degree of inflammation appears to determine the alteration in neuronal pathways, for example, serotonin, the endocannabinoid system, the loss of neural axons, or the increase in EC and lía cell numbers [25, 26, 84, 106, 224–226]. However, it is worthy to note that an altered neuronal signalling can persist long after inflammation is apparently resolved in patients with inactive disease and in animal models after disease is resolved [227].

In conclusion, further studies addressing the triad gut microbiota nerves will be a major challenge in the future. Fundamental understanding of neuronal pathways in inflammatory conditions such as IBD is crucial for the discovery of future target strategies. These will in particular target the regulation of functional bowel symptoms such as abdominal pain, visceral sensitivity, which are prevalent in IBD patients with quiescent disease and are regulated by several of the outlined pathways. To date, the evidence on the gut–brain–microbiota axis in human IBD is scarce but future research will aim to delineate this axis in depth, with the goal to evolve our understanding on GI function, to elucidate the complex interaction of this axis with systemic organs and to cover new potential treatments.

Acknowledgements

This publication has emanated from the financial support of Science Foundation Ireland (SFI) under Grant Number SFI/12/RC/2273. The authors want to thank Dr Vicente Martinez for helpful discussions and valuable comments on the content of this chapter.

Author details

Mònica Aguilera and Silvia Melgar*

*Address all correspondence to: s.melgar@ucc.ie

APC Microbiome Institute, University College Cork, National University of Ireland, Cork, Ireland

References

[1] Wilks S. Lectures on Pathological Anatomy. London: Churchill; 1875.

[2] Crohn BB, Ginzburg L, Oppenheimer GD. Regional ileitis: a pathologic and clinical entity. 1932. Mt Sinai J Med 2000;67:263–8.

[3] Kaplan GG. The global burden of IBD: from 2015 to 2025. Nat Rev Gastroenterol Hepatol 2015;12:720–7.

[4] Kelsen J, Baldassano RN. Inflammatory bowel disease: the difference between children and adults. Inflamm Bowel Dis 2008;14 Suppl 2:S9–11.

[5] Betteridge JD, Armbruster SP, Maydonovitch C, Veerappan GR. Inflammatory bowel disease prevalence by age, gender, race, and geographic location in the U.S. military health care population. Inflamm Bowel Dis 2013;19:1421–7.

[6] Baumgart DC, Sandborn WJ. Crohn's disease. Lancet 2012;380:1590–605.

[7] Melgar S, Shanahan F. Inflammatory bowel disease—from mechanisms to treatment strategies. Autoimmunity 2010;43:463–77.

[8] Parray FQ, Wani ML, Bijli AH, Thakur N, Irshad I. Crohn's disease: a surgeon's perspective. Saudi J Gastroenterol 2011;17:6–15.

[9] Loftus E V. Management of extraintestinal manifestations and other complications of inflammatory bowel disease. Curr Gastroenterol Rep 2004;6:506–13.

[10] de Souza HSP, Fiocchi C. Immunopathogenesis of IBD: current state of the art. Nat Rev Gastroenterol Hepatol 2015;13:13–27.

[11] Anderson CA, Boucher G, Lees CW, Franke A, D'Amato M, Taylor KD, et al. Meta-analysis identifies 29 additional ulcerative colitis risk loci, increasing the number of confirmed associations to 47. Nat Genet 2011;43:246–52.

[12] Lees CW, Satsangi J. Genetics of inflammatory bowel disease: implications for disease pathogenesis and natural history. Expert Rev Gastroenterol Hepatol 2009;3:513–34.

[13] Rivas MA, Beaudoin M, Gardet A, Stevens C, Sharma Y, Zhang CK, et al. Deep resequencing of GWAS loci identifies independent rare variants associated with inflammatory bowel disease. Nat Genet 2011;43:1066–73.

[14] Turner JR. Intestinal mucosal barrier function in health and disease. Nat Rev Immunol 2009;9:799–809.

[15] Atreya R, Neurath MF. IBD pathogenesis in 2014: Molecular pathways controlling barrier function in IBD. Nat Rev Gastroenterol Hepatol 2015;12:67–8.

[16] Merga Y, Campbell BJ, Rhodes JM. Mucosal barrier, bacteria and inflammatory bowel disease: possibilities for therapy. Dig Dis 2014;32:475–83.

[17] Keita A V, Söderholm JD. Barrier dysfunction and bacterial uptake in the follicle-associated epithelium of ileal Crohn's disease. Ann N Y Acad Sci 2012;1258:125–34.

[18] Walsh D, McCarthy J, O'Driscoll C, Melgar S. Pattern recognition receptors—molecular orchestrators of inflammation in inflammatory bowel disease. Cytokine Growth Factor Rev 2013;24:91–104.

[19] Ordás I, Eckmann L, Talamini M, Baumgart DC, Sandborn WJ. Ulcerative colitis. Lancet 2012;380:1606–19.

[20] Mazzucchelli L, Hauser C, Zgraggen K, Wagner H, Hess M, Laissue JA, et al. Expression of interleukin-8 gene in inflammatory bowel disease is related to the histological grade of active inflammation. Am J Pathol 1994;144:997–1007.

[21] Daig R, Andus T, Aschenbrenner E, Falk W, Schölmerich J, Gross V. Increased inter-leukin 8 expression in the colon mucosa of patients with inflammatory bowel disease. Gut 1996;38:216–22.

[22] Brannigan AE, O'Connell PR, Hurley H, O'Neill A, Brady HR, Fitzpatrick JM, et al. Neutrophil apoptosis is delayed in patients with inflammatory bowel disease. Shock 2000;13:361–6.

[23] Naito Y, Takagi T, Yoshikawa T. Molecular fingerprints of neutrophil-dependent oxidative stress in inflammatory bowel disease. J Gastroenterol 2007;42:787–98.

[24] Noronha AM, Liang Y, Hetzel JT, Hasturk H, Kantarci A, Stucchi A, et al. Hyperacti-vated B cells in human inflammatory bowel disease. J Leukoc Biol 2009;86:1007–16.

[25] Lakhan SE, Kirchgessner A. Neuroinflammation in inflammatory bowel disease. J Neuroinflammation 2010;7:37.

[26] Vermeulen W, De Man JG, Pelckmans PA, De Winter BY. Neuroanatomy of lower gastrointestinal pain disorders. World J Gastroenterol 2014;20:1005–20.

[27] Sharkey K. Neuroimmune and epithelial interactions in intestinal inflammation. Curr Opin Pharmacol 2002;2:669–77.

[28] Sharkey KA, Savidge TC. Role of enteric neurotransmission in host defense and protection of the gastrointestinal tract. Auton Neurosci 2014;181:94–106.

[29] Costa M, Glise H, Sjodahl R. The enteric nervous system in health and disease. Gut 2000;47:iv1.

[30] Kraneveld AD, Rijnierse A, Nijkamp FP, Garssen J. Neuro-immune interactions in inflammatory bowel disease and irritable bowel syndrome: future therapeutic targets. Eur J Pharmacol 2008;585:361–74.

[31] Furness JB, Clerc N, Kunze WA. Memory in the enteric nervous system. Gut 2000;47 Suppl 4:iv60–2; discussion iv76.

[32] Ratcliffe EM. Molecular development of the extrinsic sensory innervation of the gastrointestinal tract. Auton Neurosci 2011;161:1–5.

[33] Collins SM, Bercik P. The relationship between intestinal microbiota and the central nervous system in normal gastrointestinal function and disease. Gastroenterology 2009;136:2003–14.

[34] Collins SM, Surette M, Bercik P. The interplay between the intestinal microbiota and the brain. Nat Rev Microbiol 2012;10:735–42.

[35] Jänig W. Encyclopedia of Neuroscience. Berlin Heidelberg, Elsevier; 2009.

[36] Loeser JD, Treede R-D. The Kyoto protocol of IASP Basic Pain Terminology. Pain 2008;137:473–7.

[37] Sikandar S, Dickenson AH. Visceral pain: the ins and outs, the ups and downs. Curr Opin Support Palliat Care 2012;6:17–26.

[38] Blackshaw LA, Brookes SJH, Grundy D, Schemann M. Sensory transmission in the gastrointestinal tract. Neurogastroenterol Motil 2007;19:1–19.

[39] Sushil K. Sarna. Colonic Motility From Bench Side to Bedside. University of Texas Medical Branch. San Rafael (CA): Morgan & Claypool Life Sciences; 2010.

[40] Reigstad CS, Kashyap PC. Beyond phylotyping: understanding the impact of gut microbiota on host biology. Neurogastroenterol Motil 2013;25:358–72.

[41] Spencer NJ. Control of migrating motor activity in the colon. Curr Opin Pharmacol 2001;1:604–10.

[42] Fukudo S. Stress and visceral pain: focusing on irritable bowel syndrome. Pain 2013;154 Suppl :S63–70.

[43] de Jonge WJ. The gut's little brain in control of intestinal immunity. ISRN Gastroenterol 2013;2013:630159.

[44] Srinath A, Young E, Szigethy E. Pain management in patients with inflammatory bowel disease: translational approaches from bench to bedside. Inflamm Bowel Dis 2014;20:2433–49.

[45] Tougas G. The autonomic nervous system in functional bowel disorders. Gut 2000;47:78iv – 80.

[46] Motagally MA, Neshat S, Lomax AE. Inhibition of sympathetic N-type voltage-gated Ca^{2+} current underlies the reduction in norepinephrine release during colitis. Am J Physiol Gastrointest Liver Physiol 2009;296:G1077–84.

[47] Gershon MD, Tack J. The serotonin signaling system: from basic understanding to drug development for functional GI disorders. Gastroenterology 2007;132:397–414.

[48] Ghia J-E, Li N, Wang H, Collins M, Deng Y, El-Sharkawy RT, et al. Serotonin has a key role in pathogenesis of experimental colitis. Gastroenterology 2009;137:1649–60.

[49] Cremon C, Carini G, Wang B, Vasina V, Cogliandro RF, De Giorgio R, et al. Intestinal serotonin release, sensory neuron activation, and abdominal pain in irritable bowel syndrome. Am J Gastroenterol 2011;106:1290–8.

[50] Camilleri M. Serotonin in the gastrointestinal tract. Curr Opin Endocrinol Diabetes Obes 2009;16:53–9.

[51] Gershon MD. Enteric serotonergic neurones ... finally! J Physiol 2009;587:507.

[52] Kim JJ, Khan WI. 5-HT7 receptor signaling: improved therapeutic strategy in gut disorders. Front Behav Neurosci 2014;8:396.

[53] O'Hara JR, Ho W, Linden DR, Mawe GM, Sharkey KA. Enteroendocrine cells and 5-HT availability are altered in mucosa of guinea pigs with TNBS ileitis. Am J Physiol Gastrointest Liver Physiol 2004;287:G998–1007.

[54] Spiller R. Serotonin and GI clinical disorders. Neuropharmacology 2008;55:1072–80.

[55] Kidd M, Gustafsson BI, Drozdov I, Modlin IM. IL1beta- and LPS-induced serotonin secretion is increased in EC cells derived from Crohn's disease. Neurogastroenterol Motil 2009;21:439–50.

[56] Julio-Pieper M, O'Mahony CM, Clarke G, Bravo JA, Dinan TG, Cryan JF. Chronic stress-induced alterations in mouse colonic 5-HT and defecation responses are strain de-pendent. Stress 2012;15:218–26.

[57] Margolis KG, Stevanovic K, Li Z, Yang QM, Oravecz T, Zambrowicz B, et al. Pharma-cological reduction of mucosal but not neuronal serotonin opposes inflammation in mouse intestine. Gut 2014;63:928–37.

[58] Bischoff SC. Physiological and pathophysiological functions of intestinal mast cells. Semin Immunopathol 2009;31:185–205.

[59] Bischoff SC, Mailer R, Pabst O, Weier G, Sedlik W, Li Z, et al. Role of serotonin in intestinal inflammation: knockout of serotonin reuptake transporter exacerbates 2,4,6-trinitrobenzene sulfonic acid colitis in mice. Am J Physiol Gastrointest Liver Physiol 2009;296:G685–95.

[60] Coates MD, Johnson AC, Greenwood-Van Meerveld B, Mawe GM. Effects of serotonin transporter inhibition on gastrointestinal motility and colonic sensitivity in the mouse. Neurogastroenterol Motil 2006;18:464–71.

[61] Nazir S, Kumar A, Chatterjee I, Anbazhagan AN, Gujral T, Priyamvada S, et al. Mechanisms of intestinal serotonin transporter (SERT) upregulation by TGF-β1 induced non-Smad pathways. PLoS One 2015;10:e0120447.

[62] Makharia GK. Understanding and treating abdominal pain and spasms in organic gastrointestinal diseases: inflammatory bowel disease and biliary diseases. J Clin Gastroenterol 2011;45 Suppl:S89–93.

[63] Holzer P. Opioid receptors in the gastrointestinal tract. Regul Pept 2009;155:11–7.

[64] Gray AC, Coupar IM, White PJ. Comparison of opioid receptor distributions in the rat ileum. Life Sci 2006;78:1610–6.

[65] Yang J, Li Y, Zuo X, Zhen Y, Yu Y, Gao L. Transient receptor potential ankyrin-1 participates in visceral hyperalgesia following experimental colitis. Neurosci Lett 2008;440:237–41.

[66] Philippe D, Chakass D, Thuru X, Zerbib P, Tsicopoulos A, Geboes K, et al. Mu opioid receptor expression is increased in inflammatory bowel diseases: implications for homeostatic intestinal inflammation. Gut 2006;55:815–23.

[67] Boué J, Basso L, Cenac N, Blanpied C, Rolli-Derkinderen M, Neunlist M, et al. Endogenous regulation of visceral pain via production of opioids by colitogenic CD4(+) T cells in mice. Gastroenterology 2014;146:166–75.

[68] Valdez-Morales E, Guerrero-Alba R, Ochoa-Cortes F, Benson J, Spreadbury I, Hurlbut D, et al. Release of endogenous opioids during a chronic IBD model suppresses the excitability of colonic DRG neurons. Neurogastroenterol Motil 2013;25:39–46.e4.

[69] Pol O, Alameda F, Puig MM. Inflammation enhances mu-opioid receptor transcription and expression in mice intestine. Mol Pharmacol 2001;60:894–9.

[70] Rousseaux C, Thuru X, Gelot A, Barnich N, Neut C, Dubuquoy L, et al. Lactobacillus acidophilus modulates intestinal pain and induces opioid and cannabinoid receptors. Nat Med 2007;13:35–7.

[71] Hutchinson MR, Lewis SS, Coats BD, Skyba DA, Crysdale NY, Berkelhammer DL, et al. Reduction of opioid withdrawal and potentiation of acute opioid analgesia by systemic AV411 (ibudilast). Brain Behav Immun 2009;23:240–50.

[72] Sauer R-S, Hackel D, Morschel L, Sahlbach H, Wang Y, Mousa SA, et al. Toll like receptor (TLR)-4 as a regulator of peripheral endogenous opioid-mediated analgesia in inflammation. Mol Pain 2014;10:10.

[73] Storr MA, Yüce B, Andrews CN, Sharkey KA. The role of the endocannabinoid system in the pathophysiology and treatment of irritable bowel syndrome. Neurogastroenterol Motil 2008;20:857–68.

[74] Wright K, Rooney N, Feeney M, Tate J, Robertson D, Welham M, et al. Differential expression of cannabinoid receptors in the human colon: cannabinoids promote epithelial wound healing. Gastroenterology 2005;129:437–53.

[75] Wright KL, Duncan M, Sharkey KA. Cannabinoid CB2 receptors in the gastrointestinal tract: a regulatory system in states of inflammation. Br J Pharmacol 2008;153:263–70.

[76] Aguilera M, Vergara P, Martínez V. Environment-related adaptive changes of gut commensal microbiota do not alter colonic toll-like receptors but modulate the local expression of sensory-related systems in rats. Microb Ecol 2013;66:232–43.

[77] Brusberg M, Arvidsson S, Kang D, Larsson H, Lindström E, Martinez V. CB1 receptors mediate the analgesic effects of cannabinoids on colorectal distension-induced visceral pain in rodents. J Neurosci 2009;29:1554–64.

[78] Petrella C, Agostini S, Alema' GS, Casolini P, Carpino F, Giuli C, et al. Cannabinoid agonist WIN55,212 in vitro inhibits interleukin-6 (IL-6) and monocyte chemo-attractant protein-1 (MCP-1) release by rat pancreatic acini and in vivo induces dual effects on the course of acute pancreatitis. Neurogastroenterol Motil 2010;22:1248–56, e323.

[79] De Petrocellis L, Orlando P, Moriello AS, Aviello G, Stott C, Izzo AA, et al. Cannabinoid actions at TRPV channels: effects on TRPV3 and TRPV4 and their potential relevance to gastrointestinal inflammation. Acta Physiol (Oxf) 2012;204:255–66.

[80] Zoppi S, Madrigal JLM, Pérez-Nievas BG, Marín-Jiménez I, Caso JR, Alou L, et al. Endogenous cannabinoid system regulates intestinal barrier function in vivo through cannabinoid type 1 receptor activation. Am J Physiol Gastrointest Liver Physiol 2012;302:G565–71.

[81] Kuiken SD, Tytgat GN, Boeckxstaens GE. Review article: drugs interfering with visceral sensitivity for the treatment of functional gastrointestinal disorders—the clinical evidence. Aliment Pharmacol Ther 2005;21:633–51.

[82] Alhouayek M, Muccioli GG. The endocannabinoid system in inflammatory bowel diseases: from pathophysiology to therapeutic opportunity. Trends Mol Med 2012;18:615–25.

[83] Hong S, Fan J, Kemmerer ES, Evans S, Li Y, Wiley JW. Reciprocal changes in vanilloid (TRPV1) and endocannabinoid (CB1) receptors contribute to visceral hyperalgesia in the water avoidance stressed rat. Gut 2009;58:202–10.

[84] Di Sabatino A, Battista N, Biancheri P, Rapino C, Rovedatti L, Astarita G, et al. The endogenous cannabinoid system in the gut of patients with inflammatory bowel disease. Mucosal Immunol 2011;4:574–83.

[85] Singh UP, Singh NP, Singh B, Price RL, Nagarkatti M, Nagarkatti PS. Cannabinoid receptor-2 (CB2) agonist ameliorates colitis in IL-10(−/−) mice by attenuating the activation of T cells and promoting their apoptosis. Toxicol Appl Pharmacol 2012;258:256–67.

[86] Sałaga M, Sobczak M, Fichna J. Inhibition of fatty acid amide hydrolase (FAAH) as a novel therapeutic strategy in the treatment of pain and inflammatory diseases in the gastrointestinal tract. Eur J Pharm Sci 2014;52:173–9.

[87] Tourteau A, Leleu-Chavain N, Body-Malapel M, Andrzejak V, Barczyk A, Djouina M, et al. Switching cannabinoid response from CB(2) agonists to FAAH inhibitors. Bioorg Med Chem Lett 2014;24:1322–6.

[88] Sałaga M, Mokrowiecka A, Zakrzewski PK, Cygankiewicz A, Leishman E, Sobczak M, et al. Experimental colitis in mice is attenuated by changes in the levels of endocannabinoid metabolites induced by selective inhibition of fatty acid amide hydrolase (FAAH). J Crohns Colitis 2014;8:998–1009.

[89] Esposito G, Filippis D De, Cirillo C, Iuvone T, Capoccia E, Scuderi C, et al. Cannabidiol in inflammatory bowel diseases: a brief overview. Phytother Res 2013;27:633–6.

[90] Naftali T, Mechulam R, Lev LB, Konikoff FM. Cannabis for inflammatory bowel disease. Dig Dis 2014;32:468–74.

[91] Nilius B, Mahieu F. A road map for TR(I)Ps. Mol Cell 2006;22:297–307.

[92] Venkatachalam K, Montell C. TRP channels. Annu Rev Biochem 2007;76:387–417.

[93] Izzo AA, Sharkey KA. Cannabinoids and the gut: new developments and emerging concepts. Pharmacol Ther 2010;126:21–38.

[94] Phillis BD, Martin CM, Kang D, Larsson H, Lindström EA, Martinez V, et al. Role of TRPV1 in high-threshold rat colonic splanchnic afferents is revealed by inflammation. Neurosci Lett 2009;459:57–61.

[95] Ueda T, Yamada T, Ugawa S, Ishida Y, Shimada S. TRPV3, a thermosensitive channel is expressed in mouse distal colon epithelium. Biochem Biophys Res Commun 2009;383:130–4.

[96] Blackshaw LA. TRPs in visceral sensory pathways. Br J Pharmacol 2014;171:2528–36.

[97] Blackshaw LA. Transient receptor potential cation channels in visceral sensory pathways. Br J Pharmacol 2014;171:2528–36.

[98] Boesmans W, Owsianik G, Tack J, Voets T, Vanden Berghe P. TRP channels in neuro-gastroenterology: opportunities for therapeutic intervention. Br J Pharmacol 2011;162:18–37.

[99] Vergnolle N. TRPV4: new therapeutic target for inflammatory bowel diseases. Biochem Pharmacol 2014;89:157–61.

[100] Holzer P. TRPV1: a new target for treatment of visceral pain in IBS? Gut 2008;57:882–4.

[101] Akbar A, Yiangou Y, Facer P, Brydon WG, Walters JRF, Anand P, et al. Expression of the TRPV1 receptor differs in quiescent inflammatory bowel disease with or without abdominal pain. Gut 2010;59:767–74.

[102] de Fontgalland D, Brookes SJ, Gibbins I, Sia TC, Wattchow DA. The neurochemical changes in the innervation of human colonic mesenteric and submucosal blood vessels in ulcerative colitis and Crohn's disease. Neurogastroenterol Motil 2014;26:731–44.

[103] Lapointe TK, Basso L, Iftinca MC, Flynn R, Chapman K, Dietrich G, et al. TRPV1 sensitization mediates postinflammatory visceral pain following acute colitis. Am J Physiol Gastrointest Liver Physiol 2015;309:G87–99.

[104] Assas BM, Miyan JA, Pennock JL. Cross-talk between neural and immune receptors provides a potential mechanism of homeostatic regulation in the gut mucosa. Mucosal Immunol 2014.

[105] Fichna J, Mokrowiecka A, Cygankiewicz AI, Zakrzewski PK, Małecka-Panas E, Janecka A, et al. Transient receptor potential vanilloid 4 blockade protects against experimental colitis in mice: a new strategy for inflammatory bowel diseases treatment? Neurogastroenterol Motil 2012;24:e557–60.

[106] Margolis KG, Gershon MD. Neuropeptides and inflammatory bowel disease. Curr Opin Gastroenterol 2009;25:503–11.

[107] Taylor CT, Keely SJ. The autonomic nervous system and inflammatory bowel disease. Auton Neurosci 2007;133:104–14.

[108] Bernstein CN, Robert ME, Eysselein VE. Rectal substance P concentrations are in-creased in ulcerative colitis but not in Crohn's disease. Am J Gastroenterol 1993;88:908–13.

[109] ter Beek WP, Biemond I, Muller ESM, van den Berg M, Lamers CBHW. Substance P receptor expression in patients with inflammatory bowel disease. Determination by three different techniques, i.e., storage phosphor autoradiography, RT-PCR and immunohistochemistry. Neuropeptides 2007;41:301–6.

[110] Neunlist M, Aubert P, Toquet C, Oreshkova T, Barouk J, Lehur PA, et al. Changes in chemical coding of myenteric neurones in ulcerative colitis. Gut 2003;52:84–90.

[111] Gad M, Pedersen AE, Kristensen NN, Fernandez C de F, Claesson MH. Blockage of the neurokinin 1 receptor and capsaicin-induced ablation of the enteric afferent nerves protect SCID mice against T-cell-induced chronic colitis. Inflamm Bowel Dis 2009;15:1174–82.

[112] Jardí F, Fernández-Blanco JA, Martínez V, Vergara P. Persistent alterations in colonic afferent innervation in a rat model of postinfectious gut dysfunction: Role for changes in peripheral neurotrophic factors. Neurogastroenterol Motil 2016.

[113] Belai A, Boulos PB, Robson T, Burnstock G. Neurochemical coding in the small intestine of patients with Crohn's disease. Gut 1997;40:767–74.

[114] Mazumdar S, Das KM. Immunocytochemical localization of vasoactive intestinal peptide and substance P in the colon from normal subjects and patients with inflammatory bowel disease. Am J Gastroenterol 1992;87:176–81.

[115] Schneider J, Jehle EC, Starlinger MJ, Neunlist M, Michel K, Hoppe S, et al. Neurotransmitter coding of enteric neurones in the submucous plexus is changed in non-inflamed rectum of patients with Crohn's disease. Neurogastroenterol Motil 2001;13:255–64.

[116] Arranz A, Juarranz Y, Leceta J, Gomariz RP, Martínez C. VIP balances innate and adaptive immune responses induced by specific stimulation of TLR2 and TLR4. Peptides 2008;29:948–56.

[117] Arranz A, Abad C, Juarranz Y, Leceta J, Martinez C, Gomariz RP. Vasoactive intestinal peptide as a healing mediator in Crohn's disease. Neuroimmunomodulation 2008;15:46–53.

[118] Sigalet DL, Wallace LE, Holst JJ, Martin GR, Kaji T, Tanaka H, et al. Enteric neural pathways mediate the anti-inflammatory actions of glucagon-like peptide 2. Am J Physiol Gastrointest Liver Physiol 2007;293:G211–21.

[119] Delafoy L, Gelot A, Ardid D, Eschalier A, Bertrand C, Doherty AM, et al. Interactive involvement of brain derived neurotrophic factor, nerve growth factor, and calcitonin gene related peptide in colonic hypersensitivity in the rat. Gut 2006;55:940–5.

[120] Bercik P, Denou E, Collins J, Jackson W, Lu J, Jury J, et al. The intestinal microbiota affect central levels of brain-derived neurotropic factor and behavior in mice. Gastroenterology 2011;141:599–609, 609.e1–3.

[121] Beyak MJ, Vanner S. Inflammation-induced hyperexcitability of nociceptive gastrointestinal DRG neurones: the role of voltage-gated ion channels. Neurogastroenterol Motil 2005;17:175–86.

[122] Geboes K, Collins S. Structural abnormalities of the nervous system in Crohn's disease and ulcerative colitis. Neurogastroenterol Motil 1998;10:189–202.

[123] De Giorgio R, Camilleri M. Human enteric neuropathies: morphology and molecular pathology. Neurogastroenterol Motil 2004;16:515–31.

[124] Villanacci V, Bassotti G, Nascimbeni R, Antonelli E, Cadei M, Fisogni S, et al. Enteric nervous system abnormalities in inflammatory bowel diseases. Neurogastroenterol Motil 2008;20:1009–16.

[125] Linden DR, Couvrette JM, Ciolino A, McQuoid C, Blaszyk H, Sharkey KA, et al. Indiscriminate loss of myenteric neurones in the TNBS-inflamed guinea-pig distal colon. Neurogastroenterol Motil 2005;17:751–60.

[126] Sanovic S, Lamb DP, Blennerhassett MG. Damage to the enteric nervous system in experimental colitis. Am J Pathol 1999;155:1051–7.

[127] Aulí M, Nasser Y, Ho W, Burgueño JF, Keenan CM, Romero C, et al. Neuromuscular changes in a rat model of colitis. Auton Neurosci 2008;141:10–21.

[128] Wang X-Y, Vannucchi M-G, Nieuwmeyer F, Ye J, Faussone-Pellegrini M-S, Huizinga JD. Changes in interstitial cells of Cajal at the deep muscular plexus are associated with loss of distention-induced burst-type muscle activity in mice infected by Trichinella spiralis. Am J Pathol 2005;167:437–53.

[129] Pontell L, Castelucci P, Bagyánszki M, Jovic T, Thacker M, Nurgali K, et al. Structural changes in the epithelium of the small intestine and immune cell infiltration of enteric ganglia following acute mucosal damage and local inflammation. Virchows Arch 2009;455:55–65.

[130] Sarnelli G, De Giorgio R, Gentile F, Calì G, Grandone I, Rocco A, et al. Myenteric neuronal loss in rats with experimental colitis: role of tissue transglutaminase-induced apoptosis. Dig Liver Dis 2009;41:185–93.

[131] Bush TG, Savidge TC, Freeman TC, Cox HJ, Campbell EA, Mucke L, et al. Fulminant jejuno-ileitis following ablation of enteric glia in adult transgenic mice. Cell 1998;93:189–201.

[132] Linden DR, Sharkey KA, Ho W, Mawe GM. Cyclooxygenase-2 contributes to dysmotility and enhanced excitability of myenteric AH neurones in the inflamed guinea pig distal colon. J Physiol 2004;557:191–205.

[133] Krauter EM, Strong DS, Brooks EM, Linden DR, Sharkey KA, Mawe GM. Changes in colonic motility and the electrophysiological properties of myenteric neurons persist following recovery from trinitrobenzene sulfonic acid colitis in the guinea pig. Neurogastroenterol Motil 2007;19:990–1000.

[134] Chen Z, Suntres Z, Palmer J, Guzman J, Javed A, Xue J, et al. Cyclic AMP signaling contributes to neural plasticity and hyperexcitability in AH sensory neurons following intestinal Trichinella spiralis-induced inflammation. Int J Parasitol 2007;37:743–61.

[135] Xia Y, Hu HZ, Liu S, Ren J, Zafirov DH, Wood JD. IL-1beta and IL-6 excite neurons and suppress nicotinic and noradrenergic neurotransmission in guinea pig enteric nervous system. J Clin Invest 1999;103:1309–16.

[136] Kelles A, Janssens J, Tack J. IL-1beta and IL-6 excite neurones and suppress cholinergic neurotransmission in the myenteric plexus of the guinea pig. Neurogastroenterol Motil 2000;12:531–8.

[137] Buhner S, Schemann M. Mast cell-nerve axis with a focus on the human gut. Biochim Biophys Acta 2012;1822:85–92.

[138] Bienenstock J. From IgA to neuro-immunomodulation: a travelogue through immunology. Neth J Med 1991;39:183–7.

[139] Michel K, Zeller F, Langer R, Nekarda H, Kruger D, Dover TJ, et al. Serotonin excites neurons in the human submucous plexus via 5-HT3 receptors. Gastroenterology 2005;128:1317–26.

[140] Miyazaki D, Nakamura T, Toda M, Cheung-Chau K-W, Richardson RM, Ono SJ. Macrophage inflammatory protein-1alpha as a costimulatory signal for mast cell-mediated immediate hypersensitivity reactions. J Clin Invest 2005;115:434–42.

[141] Gebhardt T, Lorentz A, Detmer F, Trautwein C, Bektas H, Manns MP, et al. Growth, phenotype, and function of human intestinal mast cells are tightly regulated by transforming growth factor beta1. Gut 2005;54:928–34.

[142] Van Nassauw L, Adriaensen D, Timmermans J-P. The bidirectional communication between neurons and mast cells within the gastrointestinal tract. Auton Neurosci 2007;133:91–103.

[143] Breunig E, Michel K, Zeller F, Seidl S, Weyhern CWH, Schemann M. Histamine excites neurones in the human submucous plexus through activation of H1, H2, H3 and H4 receptors. J Physiol 2007;583:731–42.

[144] Vergnolle N, Cenac N, Altier C, Cellars L, Chapman K, Zamponi GW, et al. A role for transient receptor potential vanilloid 4 in tonicity-induced neurogenic inflammation. Br J Pharmacol 2010;159:1161–73.

[145] He S-H. Key role of mast cells and their major secretory products in inflammatory bowel disease. World J Gastroenterol 2004;10:309–18.

[146] Xie H, He S-H. Roles of histamine and its receptors in allergic and inflammatory bowel diseases. World J Gastroenterol 2005;11:2851–7.

[147] Hagel AF, de Rossi T, Konturek PC, Albrecht H, Walker S, Hahn EG, et al. Plasma histamine and tumour necrosis factor-alpha levels in Crohn's disease and ulcerative colitis at various stages of disease. J Physiol Pharmacol 2015;66:549–56.

[148] Schwartz LB, Lewis RA, Austen KF. Tryptase from human pulmonary mast cells. Purification and characterization. J Biol Chem 1981;256:11939–43.

[149] Kim J-A, Choi S-C, Yun K-J, Kim D-K, Han M-K, Seo G-S, et al. Expression of protease-activated receptor 2 in ulcerative colitis. Inflamm Bowel Dis 2003;9:224–9.

[150] Annaházi A, Gecse K, Dabek M, Ait-Belgnaoui A, Rosztóczy A, Róka R, et al. Fecal proteases from diarrheic-IBS and ulcerative colitis patients exert opposite effect on visceral sensitivity in mice. Pain 2009;144:209–17.

[151] Cenac N, Garcia-Villar R, Ferrier L, Larauche M, Vergnolle N, Bunnett NW, et al. Proteinase-activated receptor-2-induced colonic inflammation in mice: possible involvement of afferent neurons, nitric oxide, and paracellular permeability. J Immunol 2003;170:4296–300.

[152] Ibeakanma C, Vanner S. TNFalpha is a key mediator of the pronociceptive effects of mucosal supernatant from human ulcerative colitis on colonic DRG neurons. Gut 2010;59:612–21.

[153] Qin J, Li R, Raes J, Arumugam M, Burgdorf KS, Manichanh C, et al. A human gut microbial gene catalogue established by metagenomic sequencing. Nature 2010;464:59–65.

[154] Kamdar K, Nguyen V, DePaolo RW. Toll-like receptor signaling and regulation of intestinal immunity. Virulence 2013;4:207–12.

[155] Sommer F, Bäckhed F. The gut microbiota – masters of host development and physiology. Nat Rev Microbiol 2013;11:227–38.

[156] Swidsinski A, Loening-Baucke V, Lochs H, Hale L-P. Spatial organization of bacterial flora in normal and inflamed intestine: a fluorescence in situ hybridization study in mice. World J Gastroenterol 2005;11:1131–40.

[157] Dinoto A, Suksomcheep A, Ishizuka S, Kimura H, Hanada S, Kamagata Y, et al. Modulation of rat cecal microbiota by administration of raffinose and encapsulated Bifidobacterium breve. Appl Environ Microbiol 2006;72:784–92.

[158] Sekirov I, Russell SL, Antunes LCM, Finlay BB. Gut microbiota in health and disease. Physiol Rev 2010;90:859–904.

[159] Kamada N, Chen GY, Inohara N, Núñez G. Control of pathogens and pathobionts by the gut microbiota. Nat Immunol 2013;14:685–90.

[160] Ivanov II, Honda K. Intestinal commensal microbes as immune modulators. Cell Host Microbe 2012;12:496–508.

[161] Montiel-Castro AJ, González-Cervantes RM, Bravo-Ruiseco G, Pacheco-López G. The microbiota-gut-brain axis: neurobehavioral correlates, health and sociality. Front Integr Neurosci 2013;7:70.

[162] Simrén M, Barbara G, Flint HJ, Spiegel BMR, Spiller RC, Vanner S, et al. Intestinal microbiota in functional bowel disorders: a Rome foundation report. Gut 2013;62:159–76.

[163] Salzman NH, Bevins CL. Dysbiosis—a consequence of Paneth cell dysfunction. Semin Immunol 2013;25:334–41.

[164] Comito D, Romano C. Dysbiosis in the pathogenesis of pediatric inflammatory bowel diseases. Int J Inflam 2012;2012:687143.

[165] Carding S, Verbeke K, Vipond DT, Corfe BM, Owen LJ. Dysbiosis of the gut microbiota in disease. Microb Ecol Health Dis 2015;26:26191.

[166] De Hertogh G, Aerssens J, Geboes KP, Geboes K. Evidence for the involvement of infectious agents in the pathogenesis of Crohn's disease. World J Gastroenterol 2008;14:845–52.

[167] Berg AM, Dam AN, Farraye FA. Environmental influences on the onset and clinical course of Crohn's disease – part 2: infections and medication use. Gastroenterol Hepatol (N Y) 2013;9:803–10.

[168] Sokol H. Probiotics and antibiotics in IBD. Dig Dis 2014;32 Suppl 1:10–7.

[169] Buttó LF, Schaubeck M, Haller D. Mechanisms of microbe-host interaction in Crohn's disease: dysbiosis vs. pathobiont selection. Front Immunol 2015;6:555.

[170] Rath HC, Wilson KH, Sartor RB. Differential induction of colitis and gastritis in HLA-B27 transgenic rats selectively colonized with Bacteroides vulgatus or Escherichia coli. Infect Immun 1999;67:2969–74.

[171] Waidmann M, Bechtold O, Frick J-S, Lehr H-A, Schubert S, Dobrindt U, et al. Bacteroides vulgatus protects against Escherichia coli-induced colitis in gnotobiotic interleukin-2-deficient mice. Gastroenterology 2003;125:162–77.

[172] Baumgart M, Dogan B, Rishniw M, Weitzman G, Bosworth B, Yantiss R, et al. Culture independent analysis of ileal mucosa reveals a selective increase in invasive Escherichia coli of novel phylogeny relative to depletion of Clostridiales in Crohn's disease involving the ileum. ISME J 2007;1:403–18.

[173] Walters WA, Xu Z, Knight R. Meta-analyses of human gut microbes associated with obesity and IBD. FEBS Lett 2014;588:4223–33.

[174] Boudeau J, Glasser AL, Masseret E, Joly B, Darfeuille-Michaud A. Invasive ability of an Escherichia coli strain isolated from the ileal mucosa of a patient with Crohn's disease. Infect Immun 1999;67:4499–509.

[175] Willot S, Gauthier C, Patey N, Faure C. Nerve growth factor content is increased in the rectal mucosa of children with diarrhea-predominant irritable bowel syndrome. Neurogastroenterol Motil 2012;24:734–9, e347.

[176] Peterson DA, Frank DN, Pace NR, Gordon JI. Metagenomic approaches for defining the pathogenesis of inflammatory bowel diseases. Cell Host Microbe 2008;3:417–27.

[177] Marchesi JR, Adams DH, Fava F, Hermes GDA, Hirschfield GM, Hold G, et al. The gut microbiota and host health: a new clinical frontier. Gut 2015;65:330–9.

[178] Manichanh C, Rigottier-Gois L, Bonnaud E, Gloux K, Pelletier E, Frangeul L, et al. Reduced diversity of faecal microbiota in Crohn's disease revealed by a metagenomic approach. Gut 2006;55:205–11.

[179] Round JL, Mazmanian SK. Inducible Foxp3+ regulatory T-cell development by a commensal bacterium of the intestinal microbiota. Proc Natl Acad Sci U S A 2010;107:12204–9.

[180] Barnes MJ, Powrie F. Immunology. The gut's Clostridium cocktail. Science 2011;331:289–90.

[181] Walker AW, Sanderson JD, Churcher C, Parkes GC, Hudspith BN, Rayment N, et al. High-throughput clone library analysis of the mucosa-associated microbiota reveals dysbiosis and differences between inflamed and non-inflamed regions of the intestine in inflammatory bowel disease. BMC Microbiol 2011;11:7.

[182] Hansen R, Russell RK, Reiff C, Louis P, McIntosh F, Berry SH, et al. Microbiota of de-novo pediatric IBD: increased Faecalibacterium prausnitzii and reduced bacterial diversity in Crohn's but not in ulcerative colitis. Am J Gastroenterol 2012;107:1913–22.

[183] Khan MT, Duncan SH, Stams AJM, van Dijl JM, Flint HJ, Harmsen HJM. The gut anaerobe Faecalibacterium prausnitzii uses an extracellular electron shuttle to grow at oxic-anoxic interphases. ISME J 2012;6:1578–85.

[184] Sokol H, Pigneur B, Watterlot L, Lakhdari O, Bermúdez-Humarán LG, Gratadoux J-J, et al. Faecalibacterium prausnitzii is an anti-inflammatory commensal bacterium identified by gut microbiota analysis of Crohn disease patients. Proc Natl Acad Sci U S A 2008;105:16731–6.

[185] Machiels K, Joossens M, Sabino J, De Preter V, Arijs I, Eeckhaut V, et al. A decrease of the butyrate-producing species Roseburia hominis and Faecalibacterium prausnitzii defines dysbiosis in patients with ulcerative colitis. Gut 2014;63:1275–83.

[186] Cao Y, Shen J, Ran ZH. Association between Faecalibacterium prausnitzii reduction and inflammatory bowel disease: a meta-analysis and systematic review of the literature. Gastroenterol Res Pract 2014;2014:872725.

[187] Sarrabayrouse G, Alameddine J, Altare F, Jotereau F. Microbiota-specific CD4CD8αα Tregs: role in intestinal immune homeostasis and implications for IBD. Front Immunol 2015;6:522.

[188] Lopetuso LR, Scaldaferri F, Petito V, Gasbarrini A. Commensal Clostridia: leading players in the maintenance of gut homeostasis. Gut Pathog 2013;5:23.

[189] Turroni F, Ventura M, Buttó LF, Duranti S, O'Toole PW, Motherway MO, et al. Molecular dialogue between the human gut microbiota and the host: a Lactobacillus and Bifidobacterium perspective. Cell Mol Life Sci 2014;71:183–203.

[190] Grangette C. Bifidobacteria and subsets of dendritic cells: friendly players in immune regulation! Gut 2012;61:331–2.

[191] Gionchetti P, Rizzello F, Lammers K-M, Morselli C, Sollazzi L, Davies S, et al. Antibiotics and probiotics in treatment of inflammatory bowel disease. World J Gastroenterol 2006;12:3306–13.

[192] Veerappan GR, Betteridge J, Young PE. Probiotics for the treatment of inflammatory bowel disease. Curr Gastroenterol Rep 2012;14:324–33.

[193] Quigley EMM. Therapies aimed at the gut microbiota and inflammation: antibiotics, prebiotics, probiotics, synbiotics, anti-inflammatory therapies. Gastroenterol Clin North Am 2011;40:207–22.

[194] Derrien M, Vaughan EE, Plugge CM, de Vos WM. Akkermansia muciniphila gen. nov., sp. nov., a human intestinal mucin-degrading bacterium. Int J Syst Evol Microbiol 2004;54:1469–76.

[195] Derrien M, Van Baarlen P, Hooiveld G, Norin E, Müller M, de Vos WM. Modulation of mucosal immune response, tolerance, and proliferation in mice colonized by the Mucin-Degrader Akkermansia muciniphila. Front Microbiol 2011;2:166.

[196] Kang C-S, Ban M, Choi E-J, Moon H-G, Jeon J-S, Kim D-K, et al. Extracellular vesicles derived from gut microbiota, especially Akkermansia muciniphila, protect the progression of dextran sulfate sodium-induced colitis. PLoS One 2013;8:e76520.

[197] Png CW, Lindén SK, Gilshenan KS, Zoetendal EG, McSweeney CS, Sly LI, et al. Mucolytic bacteria with increased prevalence in IBD mucosa augment in vitro utilization of mucin by other bacteria. Am J Gastroenterol 2010;105:2420–8.

[198] Clausen MR. Butyrate and colorectal cancer in animals and in humans (mini-symposium: butyrate and colorectal cancer). Eur J Cancer Prev 1995;4:483–90.

[199] Smith PM, Howitt MR, Panikov N, Michaud M, Gallini CA, Bohlooly-Y M, et al. The microbial metabolites, short-chain fatty acids, regulate colonic Treg cell homeostasis. Science 2013;341:569–73.

[200] Takahashi K, Nishida A, Fujimoto T, Fujii M, Shioya M, Imaeda H, et al. Reduced abundance of butyrate-producing bacteria species in the fecal microbial community in Crohn's disease. Digestion 2016;93:59–65.

[201] Devkota S, Wang Y, Musch MW, Leone V, Fehlner-Peach H, Nadimpalli A, et al. Dietary-fat-induced taurocholic acid promotes pathobiont expansion and colitis in Il10–/– mice. Nature 2012;487:104–8.

[202] Leone V, Chang EB, Devkota S. Diet, microbes, and host genetics: the perfect storm in inflammatory bowel diseases. J Gastroenterol 2013;48:315–21.

[203] Legaki E, Gazouli M. Influence of environmental factors in the development of inflammatory bowel diseases. World J Gastrointest Pharmacol Ther 2016;7:112–25.

[204] Buffie CG, Bucci V, Stein RR, McKenney PT, Ling L, Gobourne A, et al. Precision microbiome reconstitution restores bile acid mediated resistance to Clostridium difficile. Nature 2014;517:205–8.

[205] Joyce SA, Gahan CGM. Bile acid modifications at the microbe-host interface: potential for nutraceutical and pharmaceutical interventions in host health. Annu Rev Food Sci Technol 2016;7:313-33. doi: 10.1146/annurev-food-041715-033159. Epub 2016 Jan 11. Review.

[206] Chehoud C, Albenberg LG, Judge C, Hoffmann C, Grunberg S, Bittinger K, et al. Fungal signature in the gut microbiota of pediatric patients with inflammatory bowel disease. Inflamm Bowel Dis 2015;21:1948–56.

[207] Sokol H, Leducq V, Aschard H, Pham H-P, Jegou S, Landman C, et al. Fungal microbiota dysbiosis in IBD. Gut 2016 Feb 3. pii: gutjnl-2015-310746. doi: 10.1136/gutjnl-2015-310746. [Epub ahead of print].

[208] Norman JM, Handley SA, Baldridge MT, Droit L, Liu CY, Keller BC, et al. Disease-specific alterations in the enteric virome in inflammatory bowel disease. Cell 2015;160:447–60.

[209] Aguilera M, Vergara P, Martínez V. Stress and antibiotics alter luminal and wall-adhered microbiota and enhance the local expression of visceral sensory-related systems in mice. Neurogastroenterol Motil 2013;25:e515–29.

[210] Aguilera M, Cerdà-Cuéllar M, Martínez V. Antibiotic-induced dysbiosis alters host-bacterial interactions and leads to colonic sensory and motor changes in mice. Gut Microbes 2014;6:1–14.

[211] Verdú EF, Bercik P, Verma-Gandhu M, Huang X-X, Blennerhassett P, Jackson W, et al. Specific probiotic therapy attenuates antibiotic induced visceral hypersensitivity in mice. Gut 2006;55:182–90.

[212] O'Mahony SM, Felice VD, Nally K, Savignac HM, Claesson MJ, Scully P, et al. Disturbance of the gut microbiota in early-life selectively affects visceral pain in adulthood without impacting cognitive or anxiety-related behaviors in male rats. Neuroscience 2014;277C:885–901.

[213] El Aidy S, Dinan TG, Cryan JF. Immune modulation of the brain-gut-microbe axis. Front Microbiol 2014;5:146.

[214] Mayer EA, Savidge T, Shulman RJ. Brain-gut microbiome interactions and functional bowel disorders. Gastroenterology 2014 May;146(6):1500-12. doi: 10.1053/j.gastro. 2014.02.037. Epub 2014 Feb 28.

[215] Barbara G, Cremon C, Stanghellini V. Inflammatory bowel disease and irritable bowel syndrome: similarities and differences. Curr Opin Gastroenterol 2014;30:352–8.

[216] Aguilera M, Pla J, Martinez V. Tu1723 stimulation of colonic toll-like receptor 4 (TLR4) with LPS enhances host-bacterial interactions and leads to a local immune activation and an up-regulation of sensory-related systems in rats. Gastroenterology 2013;144:S–831.

[217] Aguilera M, Martínez V. STIMULATION OF COLONIC TOLLLIKE RECEPTORS 4 AND 7 INDUCES A SPECIFIC NEUROIMMUNE ACTIVATION IN RATS. Oral sessions. Acta Physiol 2016;216:34–84.

[218] Qi J, Buzas K, Fan H, Cohen JI, Wang K, Mont E, et al. Painful pathways induced by TLR stimulation of dorsal root ganglion neurons. J Immunol 2011;186:6417–26.

[219] Brun P, Giron MC, Qesari M, Porzionato A, Caputi V, Zoppellaro C, et al. Toll-like receptor 2 regulates intestinal inflammation by controlling integrity of the enteric nervous system. Gastroenterology 2013;145:1323–33.

[220] Tramullas M, Finger BC, Moloney RD, Golubeva A V, Moloney G, Dinan TG, et al. Toll-like receptor 4 regulates chronic stress-induced visceral pain in mice. Biol Psychiatry 2014;76:340–8.

[221] Dheer R, Santaolalla R, Davies JM, Lang JK, Phillips MC, Pastorini C, et al. Intestinal epithelial TLR4 signaling affects epithelial function, colonic microbiota and promotes risk for transmissible colitis. Infect Immun 2016 Jan 11;84(3):798-810. doi: 10.1128/IAI. 01374-15.

[222] Bailey MT, Dowd SE, Galley JD, Hufnagle AR, Allen RG, Lyte M. Exposure to a social stressor alters the structure of the intestinal microbiota: implications for stressor-induced immunomodulation. Brain Behav Immun 2011;25:397–407.

[223] Harris J, Hartman M, Roche C, Zeng SG, O'Shea A, Sharp FA, et al. Autophagy controls IL-1beta secretion by targeting pro-IL-1beta for degradation. J Biol Chem 2011;286:9587–97.

[224] Tada Y, Ishihara S, Kawashima K, Fukuba N, Sonoyama H, Kusunoki R, et al. Down-regulation of serotonin reuptake transporter gene expression in healing colonic mucosa in presence of remaining low grade inflammation in ulcerative colitis. J Gastroenterol Hepatol 2015 Dec 16. doi: 10.1111/jgh.13268. [Epub ahead of print].

[225] Stoyanova II, Gulubova M V. Mast cells and inflammatory mediators in chronic ulcerative colitis. Acta Histochem 2002;104:185–92.

[226] Holzer P, Hassan AM, Jain P, Reichmann F, Farzi A. Neuroimmune pharmacological approaches. Curr Opin Pharmacol 2015;25:13–22.

[227] Lomax AE, Linden DR, Mawe GM, Sharkey KA. Effects of gastrointestinal inflammation on enteroendocrine cells and enteric neural reflex circuits. Auton Neurosci 2006;126–127:250–7.

8

Inflammation as a Potential Therapeutic Target in IBS

Alexandra Chira, Romeo Ioan Chira and
Dan Lucian Dumitrascu

Abstract

The pathogenesis of irritable bowel syndrome (IBS) has been intensively researched, and despite a long journey for unraveling all the structures and the pathways involved, it still remains partially obscure. Inflammation was the first to be hypothesized as a potential pathway for the pathogenesis of IBS. It remains a keystone in the complex machinery of the pathogenesis that is currently considered multifactorial. Elucidating the pathogenesis of IBS is crucial for a targeted therapy of the disease. In this chapter, we review information regarding gut inflammation in IBS, underlining some of the newest data or the cornerstones. Additionally, our aim was also to review treatment currently available and future perspectives regarding anti-inflammatory treatments for IBS. Newer techniques allow detection and research of mediators involved in inflammation, as well as their potential role to be targeted by pharmacological agents. Recent data supports not only further research of the newer agents that are currently being developed but also some of the available ones that do not have sufficient evidence. Emerging therapies that target inflammation are under evaluation, in trials. A multidrug or a multidisciplinary approach needs to be considered in some cases that fail to respond to current treatment.

Keywords: anti-inflammatory, inflammation, irritable bowel syndrome, IBS treatment, postinfectious

1. Introduction

Despite the intensive research on irritable bowel syndrome (IBS) is being conducted, the pathogenesis still remains partially obscure. Since the description of this syndrome, many researchers have questioned the cause of IBS, which is currently being considered as multifactorial [1–3] with increasing evidence that support the concept [4, 5], since there are multiple mechanisms that could trigger the clinical complaints.

Not just one structure or system is involved in the occurrence of IBS, and there is a complex network already described and currently referred to as brain-gut axis [6–9] with multiple directions and ways to communicate or interrelate between these structures and paths [10] that are reflected also in the heterogeneity of the subtypes of IBS.

Although IBS is a functional gastrointestinal disorder [11] with no structural or biochemical abnormalities, there is some evidence suggesting that in some subtypes of IBS, inflammation might play a key role in generating a low-grade inflammatory response and a spectrum of symptoms that sometimes overlap with those of inflammatory bowel diseases in remission [12, 13], leading to difficulties in establishing the diagnosis in clinical practice.

In this chapter, we will review literature data concerning inflammation and its relation to IBS underlining some of the newest data or the key ones. Our aim was also to review treatment currently available and future perspectives regarding anti-inflammatory treatments for IBS.

2. Inflammation in IBS

Inflammation, defined as the answer of the immune system to various triggers, was first described by Celsus [14], who has assigned to it the four signs: *dolor* (pain), *rubor* (redness), *tumor* (swelling), *calor* (heat), and to which Rudolf Virchow [15] added *functio laesa* (functional impairment). All the characteristics that define inflammation are induced by a complex set of mediators [16]. In addition, the triggers that could initiate inflammatory responses are numerous and diverse [17]. The inflammatory responses may be acute or chronic [16, 17].

Inflammation was one of the first hypothesised causes of IBS [18]. Intestinal inflammation was proposed as a potential mechanism involved in the pathogenesis of IBS since 1960s, when Hiatt et al. [18] described mast cells in the muscularis externa of the terminal colon and cecum. Discovered by Paul Ehrlich, mast cells are the precursors of CD34+ hematopoietic stem cells [19]. Due to the diversity of functions of mast cells, they have been a cornerstone in the study of multiple conditions, being intensively researched in the last decades. Mast cells have multiple functions [20], some of them involving the gut: neuroimmune interactions, epithelial secretion and permeability, and visceral sensation [20, 21]. In addition, it can express receptors for several cytokines that are involved in immunity [19] or release key mediators [22]. Numerous studies assessed the presence and/or the role of mast cells in IBS [23–25]. There are also rigorous papers that reviewed studies investigating mast cells and/or the mast cell mediators in IBS [26].

Other types of mediators, such as immunoglobulin (Ig) E and atopia, have been investigated in IBS and linked to mast cells [27, 28]. Degranulation of mast cells and, subsequently, the release of mast cell mediators can also be induced by IgE [28]. There are few data regarding IgE levels in IBS. Vara et al. [29] showed higher levels of IgE in IBS compared with healthy controls.

Besides mast cells, there are data indicating that inflammatory cells are present in colonic mucosa in IBS patients [23]. They showed on colonic biopsies multiple types of cells such as neutrophils and T lymphocytes besides mast cells, all of which may support the role of the immune system in the ethiopathogenesis of IBS [23, 30]. If most of the studies examined mucosa of the rectum [31, 32], there are few studies that assessed also the deeper layers of the enteral wall [33]. There is a complex local response when triggers are detected [16, 34].

The balance of pro-inflammatory and anti-inflammatory responses and the mediators that are involved in the complex interactions have also been the subject of many studies. There is evidence of sustained inflammation in IBS supported by numerous studies that have detected low anti-inflammatory cytokines in IBS patients [35] or others that found high levels of those pro-inflammatory ones or a misbalance of the pro- and anti-inflammatory cytokine proportion [36, 37]. The complex dialogue between the structures involved in maintaining the homeostasis includes interrelation of nervous, immune, and endocrine systems [30, 34], where a pivotal piece is the brain that governs the humoral and neurological systems [34, 38, 39], in a complex network with multidirectional communicating systems [10]. Not only the anatomical integrity but also the functional status of all the systems is of major importance [40].

Psychological factors can participate in this mechanism, maintaining a state of low inflammation [41]. Inflammation in the gut might be responsible also for hyperalgesia [42] present in some patients with IBS contributing to the maintenance of the complaints.

2.1. Postinfectious IBS

Postinfectious IBS (PI-IBS) is a more recently coined type of IBS, initially identified as post-dysenteric IBS (PD-IBS) [43]. PI-IBS is defined as a subset of IBS in which the onset of IBS symptoms develops after an infectious episode and was first described by Chaudhary and Truelove [43]. This entity was confirmed by other studies [44]. The incidence of PI-IBS varies between 4 and 32% [45–47]. More frequently, PI-IBS was described and studied after an enteral infection [44, 48]. Pathogens already recognized to be involved in enteral infections are the following:

- bacteria: *Campylobacter jejuni* [31], *Salmonella enterica* [45], *Shigella* [49], *Escherichia coli* [50–52], *Clostridium difficile* [53]

- viruses: *Norovirus* [50, 54]

- parasites: *Giardia lamblia* [50, 55], *Blastocystis* spp. [56], *Dientamoeba fragilis* [57]

This subset of IBS patients offers a strong support emphasizing the importance of inflammation as one of the main paths to IBS. Enteral pathogens may induce pathological changes [31]. Spiller et al. [31] reported an imbalance of the enteroendocrine cells and of T lymphocytes, these two being assessed by histopathological examination of the rectal biopsies of the PI-IBS when compared with controls. There can be at least three scenarios: a prolonged normal inflammatory response, an augmented pathological inflammatory response in these patients, or there is a certain group of patients with particular characteristics that have a higher susceptibility [44, 58–60]. Anyway, there is not yet a firm conclusion.

2.2. Barrier function

The gut barrier function is important in modulating the gut inflammation [26, 61]. The barrier has multiple roles and its integrity is essential for a normal functionality of the digestive system [61]. An impaired barrier could facilitate the passage of inflammatory triggers that might induce changes in the gut. An increased permeability of the barrier might expose various structures to antigen contact [31].

2.3. Cholinergic system

There is another important piece in the complex domino of Inflammation – the so-called "cholinergic anti-inflammatory pathway" [34, 62, 63]. We did not intend to review the data regarding this system as there are multiple reviews [34] that have already analyzed the evidence, but to find the studies that support the interrelation with inflammation in IBS. Dinan et al. [64] investigated several cytokines, such as interleukin (IL): IL-6, IL-8, IL-10, and the growth hormone in the two arms of the study. They found that only IL-6 and the growth hormone in the group of IBS patients were overproduced when compared with controls after the administration of pyridostigmine that might suggest the implication of the cholinergic system [64].

2.4. Low-grade inflammation

More and more data sustain the hypotheses of a low-grade inflammation in IBS [65–67]. The fine line between normal to a pathological inflammatory response is still difficult to set. There is a low-grade inflammation of the gut that has been already acknowledged and literature data supports the putative role of the low-grade inflammation in IBS [65–68]. Several articles addressed this issue, some authors investigated tissue samples [23], while others assessed blood or stool samples [69–72] in order to detect and determine the inflammation status in IBS patients.

There are already numerous studies that assessed erythrocyte sedimentation rate, C-reactive protein (CRP) from blood sample, fecal calprotectin, and/or lactoferin in order to detect their presence in IBS and/or to calculate their predictive values [71–73]. Valuable information was provided by a meta-analysis, although that assessed their cut-off values in order to exclude inflammatory bowel diseases [74].

There are limited data regarding the presence of high-sensibility CRP [69] in IBS, but results indicate that when compared with healthy subjects, levels of high sensibility CRP are statistically significantly higher in IBS patients ($P < 0.001$) [69]. So literature data supports the presence of low-grade inflammation in IBS since the levels of high-sensibility CRP, though were still within the normal range, were higher in IBS than in controls [69].

A similar situation is for calprotectin, which is used mainly for differential diagnosis of inflammatory bowel diseases [73], but there are also studies that showed increased levels of calprotectin in IBS patients when comparing the values of those of healthy controls [72].

In the search to quantify the levels of inflammation, many authors proposed various biomarkers, and others proposed multiple biomarkers such as a panel or a set of markers [75, 76].

2.5. Genes and inflammation in IBS

Genetic factors have also been suspected as being involved in the inflammation in IBS.

Regarding genes and polymorphism, there are several studies that have assessed gene polymorphism, of which IL-10 and α tumor necrosis factor are some of the ones that are being intensively investigated [77–79].

As for the other studies that addressed IBS, their findings are inconsistent since some of the studies that assessed IL-10 genotypes in IBS patients versus controls showed high-producer genotype for IL-10 had a lower frequency statistically significant in IBS than in controls ($P = 0.003$) [79], and other studies did not find statistically significant difference of IL-10 polymorphism in IBS patients [78]. Schmulson et al. [78] assessed two polymorphisms: IL-10 (-1082G/A) and α tumor necrosis factor (-308G/A) in IBS patients and compared them with controls. There were no statistically significant differences between IBS and controls regarding either of the two polymorphisms.

There are also other studies besides these that assessed single nucleotide polymorphisms and more complex studies such as genome-wide association studies [80].

2.6. New hypotheses

There is a growing interest in applying the latest techniques used in molecular biology also for the study of IBS, such as the study of microRNA—miRNAs [81], small interfering RNA—siRNAs [82] or new approaches such as meta-omics [83].

Recently, new directions have been proposed in the study of the etiopathogenesis of IBS [81, 84]. The role of stem cells has been already intensively researched [85, 86], even in inflammatory bowel diseases [87], but these potent cells have raised interest about their role or potential use in IBS.

Very recent data advances the hypotheses that intestinal stem cells might be involved in the inflammatory paths discussed in IBS [84, 88]. Due to their properties, stem cells not only are able to respond to pathogens but also may modulate the spectrum of answers by their secretory functions [84, 89]. These stem cells might also represent therapeutic targets [84], but future studies to identify a specific target, either structural or functional, of the stem cells are mandatory.

The scientific community is eager to develop and improve current technologies, both for identifying new therapeutic targets and also for new treatment.

3. Anti-inflammatory treatment

Treatment of IBS still represents a challenge for clinicians. Due to the marked heterogeneity of the IBS subtypes, we will address anti-inflammatory agents used or those with potential use in IBS. Considering the multifactorial etiology, there are authors who propose a treatment determined by the main pathological path that led to IBS [4]. Literature data are limited concerning pharmacological anti-inflammatory classes studied in IBS as well as for the number of the members of these pharmacological classes that were investigated. Since we cannot still establish the main cause that led to IBS, an etiopathogenetic treatment is not possible, and some are currently being developed; a main aim in the treatment of IBS still is to alleviate the symptoms [1]. Though there are few studies that assessed anti-inflammatory classes or members of these classes in IBS, there is an intensive research activity into unraveling new targets and new treatments [90]. There are ongoing trials [91] and research programs and networks [92] that bring valuable information for a deeper understanding of IBS.

4. Aminosalicylic acid agents

Since the discovery of 5-aminosalicylic acid agents (5-ASA) by Svartz [93] and afterward with their active properties being described by Azad et al. [94], these agents were intensively researched as well as used in clinical practice [95]. The 5-ASA derivates have been used in several inflammatory conditions such as the inflammatory bowel disorders [95]. There are already consistent data regarding the efficacy of 5-ASA in ulcerative colitis [95] as well as regarding their safety. The rationale for prescribing 5-ASA agents in IBS is represented by their anti-inflammatory properties and is the result of several mechanisms [96].

Article	Type of article	Conclusions
Min et al. [97]	Letter	In selected subgroups of IBS might be efficient
Törnblom et al. [98]	Commentaries	In selected subgroups of IBS might be efficient
Lazaraki et al. [99]	Review	Inconclusive regarding the use of mesalasine in IBS
Camilleri et al. [100]	Review	Inconclusive, though some studies show a positive effect on pain, results were not replicated by others
Xue et al. [101]	Letter	Inconclusive—analyzed impact of mesalazine on gut microbiota
Hanevik et al. [102]	Letter + pilot CT	Inefficient
Farup et al. [103]	Letter	Inconclusive – authors underline that Andrews et al. [108] did not analyze drop out patients in their study

Table 1. Articles reviewing the use of 5-ASA in IBS.

Though there are few original studies, there are also reviews that analyze the use of 5-ASA in IBS (**Table 1**). Literature data indicate that in certain group of patients such as those with

PI-IBS, especially the IBS with diarrhoea (IBS-D) subtype could benefit, at least for a certain period of the anti-inflammatory effects of this class (see **Tables 1** and **2**). Regarding the length of treatment, dosing, and schemes of treatment, there are few data in the literature, and there is no study to assess all of this. Future studies are required in order to configure an a priori set of features regarding what type of IBS patient is likely to respond to 5-ASA treatment, as well as the regimen and dosing.

Article	Type of article, type of IBS	Dose and time of treatment	Conclusions
Barbara et al. [104]	Placebo-controlled trial (CT), multicentre IBS	800 mg tid, 12 weeks	Mesalazine treatment was not statistically significant or more efficient than placebo (P = 0.870). In certain groups of patients, it might be useful.
Lam et al. [105]	CT, IBS-D	2 g/day—2 weeks, if tolerated 2 g bid—11 weeks	In certain groups of selected IBS-D patients, it might be efficient, although there is no clear evidence of it being useful.
Bafutto et al. [106]	Pilot study, IBS-D	Various dosing—in the fourth groups	May be useful in certain groups of patients.
Tuteja et al. [107]	CT, PI-IBS	1.6 g bid, 12 weeks	No statistically significant improvement of symptoms ($P \geq 0.11$) nor QOL ($P \geq 0.16$).
Andrews et al. [108]	Pilot study, IBS-D	1.5 g bid, 4 weeks	Significant improvement of pain.
Bafutto et al. [109]	CT, IBS-D	800 mg tid, 30 days	Significant improvement of total symptom score, inclusive of pain. ($P < 0.0001$)
Dorofeyev et al. [110]	CT, IBS, all subtypes	500 mg qid, 28 days	Statistical improvement of abdominal pain ($P < 0.01$) as well as some histopathological aspects.
Hanevik et al. [102]	Letter + pilot CT	800 mg bid, 6 weeks	Inefficient.
Corinaldesi et al. [111]	CT, IBS	800 mg tid, 8 weeks	Mesalazine significantly improved only general well-being ($P = 0.038$), having no significant statistic effect regarding bloating ($P = 0.177$), abdominal pain ($P = 0.084$), or bowel habits.
Preobrazhenskii [112]*	Study	4–6 g daily, not shown	Efficient.

*Articles in other languages (Russian) or full text could not be retrieved.

Table 2. Studies assessing 5-ASA agents in IBS.

4.1. Acetylsalicylic acid

Regarding the use of acetylsalicylic acid, we have identified just one study that assessed it in relation to IBS, but the purpose of the study was to determine if certain anti-inflammatory drugs could induce constipation [113]. In fact, the study assessed that the use of some anti-inflammatory drugs among acetylsalicylic acid was related to constipation. [113].

4.2. Mast cell stabilizers

Mast cell stabilizers (cromoglycate and ketotifen) have been tested in IBS, but there are very few literature data concerning this class of drugs. Also, the criteria used for diagnosing IBS were different; therefore, there is no uniformity when comparing these studies. Subsequent studies are mandatory in order to have the answer: which IBS patients are suited to a mast cell stabilizer treatment and what is the dosing, or what is a suitable regimen.

4.3. Ketotifen

Klooker et al. [114] investigated ketotifen, suggesting that it can reduce visceral hypersensitivity and improve the quality of life. Though there is just one study to investigate ketotifen in IBS patients, there has already been questions about its safety [115]. For certain other studies, to assess this class for IBS treatment is mandatory in order to grade the levels of evidence. Although there is just one study with positive results, we also consider encouraging these results [33], and we strongly feel that there are more therapeutic options that have not yet been explored.

4.4. Cromoglycate

Regarding cromoglycate, there are several studies that assessed it in IBS patients. Literature data suggest that they could have a beneficial role in certain groups of patients, especially in those who have also food allergies or intolerances (see **Table 3**). There are methodological issues concerning these studies; so in order to reduce some of the biases, rigorous parallel studies are needed.

Article	Conclusion
Leri et al. [116]	Efficient (in conjunction with dietary exclusions in IBS patients with food intolerance)
Stefanini et al. [117]	Efficient (in IBS patients with food intolerance)
Grazioli et al. [118]	Efficient (in pediatric IBS patients with food intolerance)
Stefanini et al. [119]	Efficient (in IBS patients with food intolerance)
Lunardi et al. [120]	Efficient (in IBS patients with food intolerance)
Paganelli et al. [121]	Inconclusive
Antico et al. [122]*	—
Stefanini et al. [123]	Efficient
Tomecki et al.* [124]	Inefficient

*Article in other languages than English (Polish, Italian) also could not be retrieved.

Table 3. Articles that assessed cromoglycate in IBS.

4.5. Montelukast

There is just one report of the use of montelukast in IBS stating a positive effect [125]. Considering the pathways that are involved in the pathogenesis of IBS, it seems reasonable that the authors proposed and used it. The wonder is that there are so few data regarding it, though there are data regarding IBS and allergies [29]. Montelukast might be an option for the patients who have IBS and allergic conditions, but there is a lack of studies to address this issue. Rigorous trials with such drugs are needed in order to conclude about their use in IBS.

4.6. Corticosteroids

Some authors even proposed corticosteroids as anti-inflammatory agents in IBS [126]. A short course-3 weeks, 30 mg prednisolone/day was administered to PI-IBS patients and compared with placebo. There was no statistically significant difference between the number of enterochromaffin cells between patients treated with prednisolone and those that received placebo ($P = 0.5$). Though for the reduction of the number of T lymphocytes in the lamina propria. Dunlop et al. [126] found a statistically significant difference that favors prednisolone, there was no improvement regarding several symptoms of IBS.

Due to their known side effects, one study investigated the impact of using oral steroids, showing that they do not have a higher risk for inducing IBS symptoms in adults under 40 years [127].

We conducted a search on PubMed search motor between 1–21st July 2016 using multiple strategies as seen in **Table 4**. There is just one study that assessed the corticoid therapy in IBS, though there are several authors who consider corticosteroids as a reasonable treatment option in certain subgroups of IBS patients (**Table 4**).

Strategy	Results	Appropriate	Inappropriate
"Corticosteroids, irritable bowel syndrome"	91	2 [127, 128]	89
"Corticosteroids, IBS"	64	1 [128]	63
"Prednisone, irritable bowel syndrome"	5	0	5
"Prednisolone, irritable bowel syndrome"	12	1 [126]	11
"Prednisolone, IBS"	5	1 [127]	4
"Budesonide, irritable bowel syndrome"	10	1 [128]	9

Table 4. Results retrieved by several search strategies on PubMed search motor.

4.7. Imunglobulin E antibody (Omalizumab)

There is just one study that addresses this issue [28], which presents a case of a patient that had concurrently IBS and asthma. The patient received an IgE antibody with a major improvement of IBS symptoms. These results suggest that in certain subgroups of patients with concurrent diseases as IBS and atopic status, or extra-intestinal symptoms, IgE antibodies might be useful.

5. Conclusions

Inflammation remains an important pathway involved in the pathogenesis of IBS. Despite the high interest in the field of functional gastrointestinal disorders, till now, researchers have not entirely discovered all the pieces of the complex puzzle that is the etiopathogenesis of IBS, or all of the components of the pathways that finally lead to IBS.

Newer techniques allow detection and promote research of mediators that are involved in inflammation, even in low amounts. Also, the new technologies are able to identify new structures, as well as their potential role to be targeted by pharmacotherapeutic agents.

Results suggest that there are potential pharmacological classes, alongside with potential therapeutic targets that deserve to be reassessed for IBS.

Recent data supports further research of the pathways and structures involved, as well as assessment of not only the newer agents that are currently being developed but also of some of the available ones that do not have sufficient evidence. Emerging therapies that target inflammation are under evaluation, in trials. A multidrug or a multidisciplinary approach needs to be considered in cases that fail to respond to current treatment or to a single therapy, heading toward the current trend, of a personalized medicine.

Abbreviations

5-Aminosalicylic acid agents: 5-ASA

Bis in die: bid

C reactive protein: CRP

Irritable bowel syndrome: IBS

IBS with diarrhoea: IBS-D

Immunoglobulin: Ig

Interleukin: IL

Quarter in die: qid

Quality of life: QOL

Placebo-controlled trial: CT

Postinfectious IBS: PI-IBS

Postdysenteric IBS: PD-IBS

Ter in die: tid

Author details

Alexandra Chira[1], Romeo Ioan Chira[2] and Dan Lucian Dumitrascu[1*]

*Address all correspondence to: ddumitrascu@umfcluj.ro

1 - 2nd Medical Clinic, Department of Internal Medicine, "Iuliu Hatieganu" University of Medicine and Pharmacy Cluj-Napoca, Romania

2 - 1st Medical Clinic, Department of Internal Medicine, Div. Gastroenterology, "Iuliu Hatieganu" University of Medicine and Pharmacy Cluj-Napoca, Romania

References

[1] Drossman DA, Camilleri M, Mayer EA, Whitehead WE. AGA technical review on irritable bowel syndrome. Gastroenterology. 2002;123(6):2108–31.

[2] Bellini M, Gambaccini D, Stasi C, Urbano MT, Marchi S, Usai-Satta P. Irritable bowel syndrome: a disease still searching for pathogenesis, diagnosis and therapy. World J Gastroenterol. 2014;20(27):8807–20.

[3] Barbara G, De Giorgio R, Stanghellini V, Cremon C, Corinaldesi R. A role for inflammation in irritable bowel syndrome? Gut. 2002;51 Suppl 1:i41–4.

[4] Malagelada JR, Malagelada C. Mechanism-oriented therapy of irritable bowel syndrome. Adv Ther. 2016;33(6):877–93.

[5] Chumpitazi BP, Shulman RJ. Underlying molecular and cellular mechanisms in childhood irritable bowel syndrome. Mol Cell Pediatr. 2016;3(1):11.

[6] Mayer EA. Gut feelings: the emerging biology of gut-brain communication. Nat Rev Neurosci. 2011;12(8):453–66.

[7] Jones MP, Dilley JB, Drossman D, Crowell MD. Brain-gut connections in functional GI disorders: anatomic and physiologic relationships. Neurogastroenterol Motil. 2006;18(2):91–103.

[8] James W. What is an emotion? Mind. 1884;9:188–205.

[9] Fichna J, Storr MA. Brain-gut interactions in IBS. Front Pharmacol. 2012;3:127.

[10] Koloski NA, Jones M, Talley NJ. Evidence that independent gut-to-brain and brain-to-gut pathways operate in the irritable bowel syndrome and functional dyspepsia: a 1-year population-based prospective study. Aliment Pharmacol Ther. 2016;44(6):592–600.

[11] Longstreth GF, Thompson WG, Chey WD, Houghton LA, Mearin F, Spiller RC. Functional bowel disorders. Gastroenterology. 2006;130(5):1480–91.

[12] Grover M, Herfarth H, Drossman DA. The functional-organic dichotomy: postinfectious irritable bowel syndrome and inflammatory bowel disease-irritable bowel syndrome. Clin Gastroenterol Hepatol. 2009;7(1):48–53.

[13] Berrill JW, Green JT, Hood K, Campbell AK. Symptoms of irritable bowel syndrome in patients with inflammatory bowel disease: examining the role of sub-clinical inflammation and the impact on clinical assessment of disease activity. Aliment Pharmacol Ther. 2013;38(1):44–51.

[14] Celsus AC. De Medicina, praef. iii. 4.

[15] Rather LJ. Disturbance of function (functio laesa): the legendary fifth cardinal sign of inflammation, added by Galen to the four cardinal signs of Celsus. Bull N Y Acad Med 1971;47:303–322.

[16] Baumann H, Gauldie J. The acute phase response. Immunol Today. 1994;15:74–80.

[17] Sell S, editor. Immunology, Immunopathology, and Immunity. 6th ed. Washington, DC: ASM Press; 2001.

[18] Hiatt RB, Katz L. Mast cells in inflammatory conditions of the gastrointestinal tract. Am J Gastroenterol. 1962;37:541–5.

[19] Shea-Donohue T, Stiltz J, Zhao A, Notari L. Mast cells. Curr Gastroenterol Rep. 2010;12(5):349–57.

[20] Zhang L, Song J, Hou X. Mast cells and irritable bowel syndrome: from the bench to the bedside. J Neurogastroenterol Motil. 2016; 22(2):181–92.

[21] Bischoff SC, Kramer S. Human mast cells, bacteria, and intestinal immunity. Immunol Rev. 2007; 217:329–37.

[22] Barbara G, Stanghellini V, De Giorgio R, Cremon C, Cottrell GS, Santini D, et al. Activated mast cells in proximity to colonic nerves correlate with abdominal pain in irritable bowel syndrome. Gastroenterology. 2004;126(3):693–702.

[23] Chadwick VS, Chen W, Shu D, Paulus B, Bethwaite P, Tie A, et al. Activation of the mucosal immune system in irritable bowel syndrome. Gastroenterology. 2002; 122(7): 1778–83.

[24] O'Sullivan M, Clayton N, Breslin NP, Harman I, Bountra C, McLaren A, et al. Increased mast cells in the irritable bowel syndrome. Neurogastroenterol Motil. 2000;12(5):449–57.

[25] Cremon C, Gargano L, Morselli-Labate AM, Santini D, Cogliandro RF, De Giorgio R, et al. Mucosal immune activation in irritable bowel syndrome: gender-dependence and association with digestive symptoms. Am J Gastroenterol. 2009; 104(2):392–400.

[26] Camilleri M, Lasch K, Zhou W. Irritable bowel syndrome: methods, mechanisms, and pathophysiology. The confluence of increased permeability, inflammation, and pain in

irritable bowel syndrome. Am J Physiol Gastrointest Liver Physiol. 2012; 303(7):G775–85.

[27] Coca A, Cooke R. On the classification of the phenomena of hypersensitiveness. J Immunol; 1923 8: 163–182.

[28] Pearson JS, Niven RM, Meng J, Atarodi S, Whorwell PJ. Immunoglobulin E in irritable bowel syndrome: another target for treatment? A case report and literature review. Therap Adv Gastroenterol. 2015;8(5):270–7.

[29] Vara EJ, Valeur J, Hausken T, Lied GA. Extra-intestinal symptoms in patients with irritable bowel syndrome: related to high total IgE levels and atopic sensitization? Scand J Gastroenterol. 2016;51(8):908–13.

[30] Ohman L, Simren M. Pathogenesis of IBS: role of inflammation, immunity and neuroimmune interactions. Nat Rev Gastroenterol Hepatol. 2010;7(3):163–73.

[31] Spiller RC, Jenkins D, Thornley JP, Hebden JM, Wright T, Skinner M, et al. Increased rectal mucosal enteroendocrine cells, T lymphocytes, and increased gut permeability following acute *Campylobacter enteritis* and in post-dysenteric irritable bowel syndrome. Gut. 2000;47(6):804–11.

[32] Goral V, Kucukoner M, Buyukbayram H. Mast cells count and serum cytokine levels in patients with irritable bowel syndrome. Hepatogastroenterology. 2010;57(101):751–4.

[33] O'Sullivan M. Therapeutic potential of ketotifen in irritable bowel syndrome (IBS) may involve changes in mast cells at sites beyond the rectum. Gut. 2011;60(3):423; author reply.

[34] Pavlov VA, Wang H, Czura CJ, Friedman SG, Tracey KJ. The cholinergic anti-inflammatory pathway: a missing link in neuroimmunomodulation. Mol Med. 2003;9(5-8):125–34.

[35] Schmulson M, Pulido-London D, Rodriguez O, Morales-Rochlin N, Martinez-Garcia R, Gutierrez-Ruiz MC, et al. Lower serum IL-10 is an independent predictor of IBS among volunteers in Mexico. Am J Gastroenterol. 2012;107(5):747–53.

[36] Bashashati M, Rezaei N, Shafieyoun A, McKernan DP, Chang L, Ohman L, et al. Cytokine imbalance in irritable bowel syndrome: a systematic review and meta-analysis. Neurogastroenterol Motil. 2014;26(7):1036–48.

[37] Macsharry J, O'Mahony L, Fanning A, Bairead E, Sherlock G, Tiesman J, et al. Mucosal cytokine imbalance in irritable bowel syndrome. Scand J Gastroenterol. 2008;43(12):1467–76.

[38] Watkins LR, Maier SF, Goehler LE. Cytokine-to-brain communication: a review and analysis of alternative mechanisms. Life Sci 57:1011–26. 1995.

[39] Elmquist JK, Scammell TE, Saper CB. Mechanisms of CNS response to systemic immune challenge: the febrile response. Trends Neurosci 20:565–9.

[40] Posserud I, Ersryd A, Simren M. Functional findings in irritable bowel syndrome. World J Gastroenterol. 2006;12(18):2830–8.

[41] Tanaka Y, Kanazawa M, Fukudo S, Drossman DA. Biopsychosocial model of irritable bowel syndrome. J Neurogastroenterol Motil. 2011;17(2):131–9.

[42] Farzaei MH, Bahramsoltani R, Abdollahi M, Rahimi R. The role of visceral hypersensitivity in irritable bowel syndrome: pharmacological targets and novel treatments. J Neurogastroenterol Motil. 2016;22(4):558–574.

[43] Chaudhary NA, Truelove SC. The irritable colon syndrome. A study of the clinical features, predisposing causes, and prognosis in 130 cases. Q J Med. 1962;31:307–22.

[44] Gwee KA, Collins SM, Read NW, Rajnakova A, Deng Y, Graham JC, et al. Increased rectal mucosal expression of interleukin 1beta in recently acquired post-infectious irritable bowel syndrome. Gut. 2003;52(4):523–6.

[45] Rodriguez LA, Ruigomez A. Increased risk of irritable bowel syndrome after bacterial gastroenteritis: cohort study. BMJ. 1999;318(7183):565–6.

[46] Thabane M, Kottachchi DT, Marshall JK. Systematic review and meta-analysis: The incidence and prognosis of post-infectious irritable bowel syndrome. Aliment Pharmacol Ther. 2007;26(4):535–44.

[47] McKendrick MW, Read NW. Irritable bowel syndrome—post salmonella infection. J Infect. 1994;29(1):1–3.

[48] Spiller R, Garsed K. Postinfectious irritable bowel syndrome. Gastroenterology. 2009;136(6):1979–88.

[49] Kim HS, Lim JH, Park H, Lee SI. Increased immunoendocrine cells in intestinal mucosa of postinfectious irritable bowel syndrome patients 3 years after acute Shigella infection—an observation in a small case control study. Yonsei Med J. 2010;51(1):45–51.

[50] Grover M. Role of gut pathogens in development of irritable bowel syndrome. Indian J Med Res. 2014;139(1):11–8.

[51] Okhuysen PC, Jiang ZD, Carlin L, Forbes C, DuPont HL. Post-diarrhea chronic intestinal symptoms and irritable bowel syndrome in North American travelers to Mexico. Am J Gastroenterol. 2004;99(9):1774–8.

[52] Andresen V, Lowe B, Broicher W, Riegel B, Fraedrich K, von Wulffen M, et al. Postinfectious irritable bowel syndrome (PI-IBS) after infection with Shiga-like toxin-producing Escherichia coli (STEC) O104:H4: a cohort study with prospective follow-up. United Eur Gastroenterol J. 2016;4(1):121–31.

[53] Wadhwa A, Al Nahhas MF, Dierkhising RA, Patel R, Kashyap P, Pardi DS, et al. High risk of post-infectious irritable bowel syndrome in patients with Clostridium difficile infection. Aliment Pharmacol Ther. 2016;44(6):576–82.

[54] Marshall JK, Thabane M, Borgaonkar MR, James C. Postinfectious irritable bowel syndrome after a food-borne outbreak of acute gastroenteritis attributed to a viral pathogen. Clin Gastroenterol Hepatol. 2007;5(4):457–60.

[55] Wensaas KA, Langeland N, Hanevik K, Morch K, Eide GE, Rortveit G. Irritable bowel syndrome and chronic fatigue 3 years after acute giardiasis: historic cohort study. Gut. 2012;61(2):214–9.

[56] Azizian M, Basati G, Abangah G, Mahmoudi MR, Mirzaei A. Contribution of Blasto-cystishominis subtypes and associated inflammatory factors in development of irritable bowel syndrome. Parasitol Res. 2016;115(5):2003–9.

[57] Borody TJ, Warren EF, Wettstein A, Robertson G, Recabarren P, Fontella A, et al. Eradication of Dientamoeba fragilis can resolve IBS-like symptoms. J Gastroenterol Hepatol 17(Suppl):A103. 2002.

[58] Wouters MM, Van Wanrooy S, Nguyen A, Dooley J, Aguilera-Lizarraga J, Van Brabant W, et al. Psychological comorbidity increases the risk for postinfectious IBS partly by enhanced susceptibility to develop infectious gastroenteritis. Gut. 2016;65(8):1279–88.

[59] Collins SM, Piche T, Rampal P. The putative role of inflammation in the irritable bowel syndrome. Gut. 2001;49(6):743–5.

[60] Spiller RC. Postinfectious irritable bowel syndrome. Gastroenterology. 2003;124(6): 1662–71.

[61] Martinez C, Gonzalez-Castro A, Vicario M, Santos J. Cellular and molecular basis of intestinal barrier dysfunction in the irritable bowel syndrome. Gut Liver. 2012;6(3):305–15.

[62] Tracey KJ. The inflammatory reflex. Nature 2002;420:853–9..

[63] Blalock JE. Harnessing a neural-immune circuit to control inflammation and shock. J Exp Med 2002;195:F25–8.

[64] Dinan TG, Clarke G, Quigley EM, Scott LV, Shanahan F, Cryan J, et al. Enhanced cholinergic-mediated increase in the pro-inflammatory cytokine IL-6 in irritable bowel syndrome: role of muscarinic receptors. Am J Gastroenterol. 2008;103(10):2570–6.

[65] Akiho H, Ihara E, Nakamura K. Low-grade inflammation plays a pivotal role in gastrointestinal dysfunction in irritable bowel syndrome. World J Gastrointest Pathophysiol. 2010;1(3):97–105.

[66] Lee E, Schiller LR, Fordtran JS. Quantification of colonic lamina propria cells by means of a morphometric point-counting method. Gastroenterology. 1988;94(2):409–18.

[67] Sinagra E, Pompei G, Tomasello G, Cappello F, Morreale GC, Amvrosiadis G, et al. Inflammation in irritable bowel syndrome: myth or new treatment target? World J Gastroenterol. 2016;22(7):2242–55.

[68] Barbara G, Cremon C, Carini G, Bellacosa L, Zecchi L, De Giorgio R, et al. The immune system in irritable bowel syndrome. J Neurogastroenterol Motil. 2011;17(4):349–59.

[69] Hod K, Dickman R, Sperber A, Melamed S, Dekel R, Ron Y, et al. Assessment of high-sensitivity CRP as a marker of micro-inflammation in irritable bowel syndrome. Neurogastroenterol Motil. 2011;23(12):1105–10.

[70] Hod K, Ringel-Kulka T, Martin CF, Maharshak N, Ringel Y. High-sensitive C-reactive protein as a marker for inflammation in irritable bowel syndrome. J Clin Gastroenterol. 2015.

[71] Chang MH, Chou JW, Chen SM, Tsai MC, Sun YS, Lin CC, et al. Faecal calprotectin as a novel biomarker for differentiating between inflammatory bowel disease and irritable bowel syndrome. Mol Med Rep. 2014;10(1):522–6.

[72] David LE, Surdea-Blaga T, Dumitrascu DL. Semiquantitative fecal calprotectin test in postinfectious and non-postinfectious irritable bowel syndrome: cross-sectional study. Sao Paulo Med J. 2014:0.

[73] Otten CM, Kok L, Witteman BJ, Baumgarten R, Kampman E, Moons KG, et al. Diagnostic performance of rapid tests for detection of fecal calprotectin and lactoferrin and their ability to discriminate inflammatory from irritable bowel syndrome. Clin Chem Lab Med. 2008;46(9):1275–80.

[74] Menees SB, Powell C, Kurlander J, Goel A, Chey WD. A meta-analysis of the utility of C-reactive protein, erythrocyte sedimentation rate, fecal calprotectin, and fecal lactoferrin to exclude inflammatory bowel disease in adults with IBS. Am J Gastroenterol. 2015;110(3):444–54.

[75] Lembo AJ, Neri B, Tolley J, Barken D, Carroll S, Pan H. Use of serum biomarkers in a diagnostic test for irritable bowel syndrome. Aliment Pharmacol Ther. 2009;29(8):834–42.

[76] Jones MP, Chey WD, Singh S, Gong H, Shringarpure R, Hoe N, et al. A biomarker panel and psychological morbidity differentiates the irritable bowel syndrome from health and provides novel pathophysiological leads. Aliment Pharmacol Ther. 2014;39(4):426–37.

[77] Olivo-Diaz A, Romero-Valdovinos M, Gudino-Ramirez A, Reyes-Gordillo J, Jimenez-Gonzalez DE, Ramirez-Miranda ME, et al. Findings related to IL-

8 and IL-10 gene polymorphisms in a Mexican patient population with irritable bowel syndrome infected with blastocystis. Parasitol Res. 2012;111(1): 487–91.

[78] Schmulson M, Pulido-London D, Rodriguez O, Morales-Rochlin N, Martinez-Garcia R, Gutierrez-Ruiz MC, et al. IL-10 and TNF-alpha polymorphisms in subjects with irritable bowel syndrome in Mexico. Rev Esp Enferm Dig. 2013;105(7):392–9.

[79] Gonsalkorale WM, Perrey C, Pravica V, Whorwell PJ, Hutchinson IV. Interleukin 10 genotypes in irritable bowel syndrome: evidence for an inflammatory component? Gut. 2003;52(1):91–3.

[80] Ek WE, Reznichenko A, Ripke S, Niesler B, Zucchelli M, Rivera NV, et al. Exploring the genetics of irritable bowel syndrome: a GWA study in the general population and replication in multinational case-control cohorts. Gut. 2015;64(11): 1774–82.

[81] Zhou Q, Souba WW, Croce CM, Verne GN. MicroRNA-29a regulates intestinal membrane permeability in patients with irritable bowel syndrome. Gut. 2010;59(6):775–84.

[82] Cenac N, Bautzova T, Le Faouder P, Veldhuis NA, Poole DP, Rolland C, et al. Quantification and potential functions of endogenous agonists of transient receptor potential channels in patients with irritable bowel syndrome. Gastroenterology. 2015;149(2):433–44 e7.

[83] Mondot S, Lepage P. The human gut microbiome and its dysfunctions through the meta-omics prism. Ann N Y Acad Sci. 2016;1372(1):9–19.

[84] Ratanasirintrawoot S, Israsena N. Stem cells in the intestine: possible roles in pathogenesis of irritable bowel syndrome. J Neurogastroenterol Motil. 2016;22(3): 367–82.

[85] Ozkul Y, Galderisi U. The impact of epigenetics on mesenchymal stem cell biology. J Cell Physiol. 2016;231(11):2393–401.

[86] Wang Q, Ding G, Xu X. Immunomodulatory functions of mesenchymal stem cells and possible mechanisms. Histol Histopathol. 2016;31(9):949–59.

[87] De Francesco F, Romano M, Zarantonello L, Ruffolo C, Neri D, Bassi N, et al. The role of adipose stem cells in inflammatory bowel disease: from biology to novel therapeutic strategies. Cancer Biol Ther. 2016;17(9):889–898.

[88] Roostaee A, Benoit YD, Boudjadi S, Beaulieu JF. Epigenetics in intestinal epithelial cell renewal. J Cell Physiol. 2016;231(11):2361–7.

[89] Owens BM. Inflammation, innate immunity, and the intestinal stromal cell niche: opportunities and challenges. Front Immunol. 2015;6:319.

[90] Corsetti M, Whorwell P. Novel pharmacological therapies for irritable bowel syndrome. Expert Rev Gastroenterol Hepatol. 2016;10(7):807–15.

[91] International Foundation for Functional Gastrointestinal Disorders, Inc. (IFFGD) [Internet]. 1998–2016. Available from: http://www.aboutibs.org/take-part-in-online-studies.html [Accessed: 2016-07-21]

[92] GENIEUR.EU [Internet]. 2012. Available from: https://genieur.eu/ [Accessed: 2016-06-12]

[93] Svartz N. Salazopyrin, a new sulfanilamide preparation: A. Therapeutic results in rheumatic polyarthritis. B. Therapeutic results in ulcerative colitis. C. Toxic manifestations in treatment with sulfanilamide preparation. Acta Med Scand 1942;11:557–590.

[94] Azad Khan AK, Piris J, Truelove SC. An experiment to determine the active therapeutic moiety of sulphasalazine. Lancet. 1977;2(8044):892-5.

[95] Bohm SK, Kruis W. Long-term efficacy and safety of once-daily mesalazine granules for the treatment of active ulcerative colitis. Clin Exp Gastroenterol. 2014;7:369–83.

[96] Desreumaux P. Understanding the mechanism of 5-ASA in treating colonic inflammation. Gastroenterol Hepatol (N Y). 2008;4(5):319–20.

[97] Min T, Ford AC. Efficacy of mesalazine in IBS. Gut. 2016;65(1):187–8.

[98] Törnblom H, Simren M. In search for a disease-modifying treatment in irritable bowel syndrome. Gut. 2016;65(1):2–3.

[99] Lazaraki G, Chatzimavroudis G, Katsinelos P. Recent advances in pharmacological treatment of irritable bowel syndrome. World J. Gastroenterol. 2014;20(27):8867–85.

[100] Camilleri M. Pharmacological agents currently in clinical trials for disorders in neurogastroenterology. J Clin Invest. 2013;123(10):4111–20.

[101] Xue L, Huang Z, Zhou X, Chen W. The possible effects of mesalazine on the intestinal microbiota. Aliment Pharmacol Ther. 2012;36(8):813–4.

[102] Hanevik K, Dizdar V, Langeland N, Eide GE, Hausken T. Tolerability and effect of mesalazine in postinfectious irritable bowel syndrome. Aliment Pharmacol Ther. 2011;34(2):259–60.

[103] Farup PG. Questions about mesalazine and the irritable bowel syndrome. Aliment Pharmacol Ther. 2011;34(8):1036–7; author reply 7–8.

[104] Barbara G, Cremon C, Annese V, Basilisco G, Bazzoli F, Bellini M, et al. Randomised controlled trial of mesalazine in IBS. Gut. 2016;65(1):82–90.

[105] Lam C, Tan W, Leighton M, Hastings M, Lingaya M, Falcone Y, et al. A mechanistic multicentre, parallel group, randomised placebo-controlled trial of mesalazine for the treatment of IBS with diarrhoea (IBS-D). Gut. 2016;65(1):91-9.

[106] Bafutto M, Almeida JR, Leite NV, Costa MB, Oliveira EC, Resende-Filho J. Treatment of diarrhea-predominant irritable bowel syndrome with mesalazine and/or *Saccharomyces boulardii*. Arq Gastroenterol. 2013;50(4):304–9.

[107] Tuteja AK, Fang JC, Al-Suqi M, Stoddard GJ, Hale DC. Double-blind placebo-controlled study of mesalamine in post-infective irritable bowel syndrome—a pilot study. Scand J Gastroenterol. 2012;47(10):1159–64.

[108] Andrews CN, Griffiths TA, Kaufman J, Vergnolle N, Surette MG, Rioux KP. Mesalazine (5-aminosalicylic acid) alters faecal bacterial profiles, but not mucosal proteolytic activity in diarrhoea-predominant irritable bowel syndrome. Aliment Pharmacol Ther. 2011;34(3):374–83.

[109] Bafutto M, Almeida JR, Leite NV, Oliveira EC, Gabriel-Neto S, Rezende-Filho J. Treatment of postinfectious irritable bowel syndrome and noninfective irritable bowel syndrome with mesalazine. Arq Gastroenterol. 2011;48(1):36–40.

[110] Dorofeyev AE, Kiriyan EA, Vasilenko IV, Rassokhina OA, Elin AF. Clinical, endoscopical and morphological efficacy of mesalazine in patients with irritable bowel syndrome. Clin Exp Gastroenterol. 2011;4:141–53.

[111] Corinaldesi R, Stanghellini V, Cremon C, Gargano L, Cogliandro RF, De Giorgio R, et al. Effect of mesalazine on mucosal immune biomarkers in irritable bowel syndrome: a randomized controlled proof-of-concept study. Aliment Pharmacol Ther. 2009;30(3):245–52.

[112] Preobrazhenskii VN. Salozinal in the treatment of the irritable bowel syndrome in young persons. Ter Arkh. 1999;71(2):37–9.

[113] Chang JY, Locke GR, Schleck CD, Zinsmeister AR, Talley NJ. Risk factors for chronic constipation and a possible role of analgesics. Neurogastroenterol Motil. 2007;19(11):905-11.

[114] Klooker TK, Braak B, Koopman KE, Welting O, Wouters MM, van der Heide S, et al. The mast cell stabiliser ketotifen decreases visceral hypersensitivity and improves intestinal symptoms in patients with irritable bowel syndrome. Gut. 2010;59(9):1213–21.

[115] Reisinger KW, de Haan JJ, Schreinemacher MH. Word of caution before implementing ketotifen for gastrointestinal transit improvement. World J. Gastroenterol. 2013;19(27):4445–6.

[116] Leri O, Tubili S, De Rosa FG, Addessi MA, Scopelliti G, Lucenti W, et al. Management of diarrhoeic type of irritable bowel syndrome with exclusion diet and disodium cromoglycate. Inflammopharmacology. 1997;5(2):153–8.

[117] Stefanini GF, Saggioro A, Alvisi V, Angelini G, Capurso L, di Lorenzo G, et al. Oral cromolyn sodium in comparison with elimination diet in

the irritable bowel syndrome, diarrheic type. Multicenter study of 428 patients. Scand J Gastroenterol. 1995;30(6):535–41.

[118] Grazioli I, Melzi G, Balsamo V, Castellucci G, Castro M, Catassi C, et al. Food intolerance and irritable bowel syndrome of childhood: clinical efficacy of oral sodium cromoglycate and elimination diet. Minerva Pediatr. 1993;45(6):253–8.

[119] Stefanini GF, Prati E, Albini MC, Piccinini G, Capelli S, Castelli E, et al. Oral disodium cromoglycate treatment on irritable bowel syndrome: an open study on 101 subjects with diarrheic type. Am J Gastroenterol. 1992;87(1):55–7.

[120] Lunardi C, Bambara LM, Biasi D, Cortina P, Peroli P, Nicolis F, et al. Double-blind cross-over trial of oral sodium cromoglycate in patients with irritable bowel syndrome due to food intolerance. Clin Exp Allergy. 1991;21(5):569–72.

[121] Paganelli R, Fagiolo U, Cancian M, Sturniolo GC, Scala E, D'Offizi GP. Intestinal permeability in irritable bowel syndrome. Effect of diet and sodium cromoglycate administration. Ann Allergy. 1990;64(4):377–80.

[122] Antico A, Soana R, Clivio L, Baioni R. Irritable colon syndrome in intolerance to food additives. Minerva Dietol Gastroenterol. 1989;35(4):219–24.

[123] Stefanini GF, Bazzocchi G, Prati E, Lanfranchi GA, Gasbarrini G. Efficacy of oral disodium cromoglycate in patients with irritable bowel syndrome and positive skin prick tests to foods. Lancet. 1986;1(8474):207–8.

[124] Tomecki R. Ineffectiveness of disodium cromoglycate in the treatment of a diarrheal form of irritable bowel syndrome. Pol Tyg Lek. 1985;40(7):181–2.

[125] Fee WH. Irritable bowel syndrome helped by montelukast. Chest. 2002;122(4):1497.

[126] Dunlop SP, Jenkins D, Neal KR, Naesdal J, Borgaonker M, Collins SM, et al. Randomized, double-blind, placebo-controlled trial of prednisolone in post-infectious irritable bowel syndrome. Aliment Pharmacol Ther. 2003;18(1):77–84.

[127] Huerta C, Garcia Rodriguez LA, Wallander MA, Johansson S. Users of oral steroids are at a reduced risk of developing irritable bowel syndrome. Pharmacoepidemiol Drug Saf. 2003;12(7):583–8.

[128] Crentsil V. Will corticosteroids and other anti-inflammatory agents be effective for diarrhea-predominant irritable bowel syndrome? Med Hypotheses. 2005;65(1):97–102.

9

Autologous and Allogeneic Stem Cell Transplantation for Treatment of Crohn's Fistulae

Fernando de la Portilla, Ana M. García-Cabrera,
Rosa M. Jiménez-Rodríguez, Maria L. Reyes and
Damian García-Olmo

Abstract

Up to 20% of patients with Crohn's disease (CD) may have perianal fistula disease. Classically, surgery has played an important role; in recent years, medical treatment has taken a leading role. Immunosuppressants and biological trea tments have proven beneficial in many patients, but still, the percentage of patients who do not respond remains significant. In this scenario, cell therapy is envisaged as an effective alternative to surgery. The promising preclinical and clinical data that we review below suggest that cell therapy could represent a major advance in the clinical management of this difficult problem.

Keywords: stem cells, allogenic, autologous, transplantation, Crohn, fistulas

1. Introduction

Up to 20% of patients with Crohn's disease (CD) may have perianal fistula disease, which is frequently associated with perianal collections [1–3]. Classically, surgery has played an important role, by the placement of drains or setons creation of ostomies, and in severe cases, even proctectomy [4]. However, in recent years, medical treatment with or without the temporary placement of drains has taken a leading role. Immunosuppressants such as azathioprine, 6-mercaptopurine, methotrexate and cyclosporine have proven beneficial in many patients. In more complicated cases where these drugs are ineffective, biological treatments based on monoclonal antibodies have been shown to have some success for the induction and maintenance of remission of perianal fistula disease and associated proctitis [5–11]. Still, the percentage of patients who do not respond or do so only partially remains significant. Furthermore, the existence of serious complications associated with treatment should not be overlooked [9, 12, 13].

It is as a result of these inadequacies in current treatment strategies that cell therapy has arisen as a complementary option [14]. The promising results published in recent years, both with autologous and in allogeneic cells, highlight a need for greater understanding of the basic principles of this new route and for clarification of the current state of the topic.

2. Basic concepts of cell therapy

Stem cells have both the capacity for self-renewal or self-replication and for production of daughter cells that proceed along specific developmental pathways that will eventually lead to differentiation into specialised cell types [15].

Embryonic stem cells are obtained from the inner cell mass of the embryo at the blastocyst stage. They are able to generate cell lines derived from any of the three embryonic germ layers (ectoderm, mesoderm and endoderm), giving them great therapeutic potential. In mature adult tissues, we find adult multipotent stem cells, which are generally only able to renew and regenerate tissues from the embryonic layer of which they come. However, based on the so-called phenomenon of cellular plasticity, in some instances, they can differentiate into cell populations different to those of their embryonic origin, providing many therapeutic options [16].

Finally, we have the so-called induced pluripotent stem cells (iPS), which are somatic cells that have been subjected to a process of nuclear reprogramming by ectopic expression of specific transcription factors. These acquire molecular and functional characteristics of pluripotency that make them akin to embryonic stem cells. They also display similar characteristics to these in terms of morphology, proliferation, gene expression, epigenetic status of pluripotent genes and their ability to differentiate *in vivo* and *in vitro* [17].

Although embryonic stem cells and iPS have great potential for cell-based therapies, there are several limitations to their use, including regulatory, ethical and genetic engineering considerations. As a result, there are currently no clinical trials evaluating their use [18].

On the other hand, adult stem cells can be obtained using much simpler methods and have no restrictions or ethical considerations. Furthermore, because of their autologous origin, they are not immunoreactive. Early studies using adult stem cells have focused on mesenchymal stem cells (MSCs). These can be found in the stroma of virtually every organ, for example, in subcutaneous adipose tissue and bone marrow. Being fibroblastoid cells, they are the precursors of all types of non-haematopoietic connective tissues (bone, fat, cartilage, etc.). MSCs are generally obtained by selection through adherence to tissue culture plastic, as they are able to adhere and grow in conditions where other cell types do not usually proliferate [19]. They are required to meet minimal criteria defined by the International Society for Cellular Therapy, namely, more than 95% of cells must express CD105, CD73 and CD90, as measured by flow cytometry; and <2% must be positive for CD45, CD34, CD14, CD11b, CD79a or CD19 and human leukocyte antigen (HLA) Class II. Moreover, they should be able to differentiate into osteoblasts, chondroblasts and adipocytes under standard *in vitro* differentiation conditions [20].

MSCs have a high capacity for proliferation and differentiation. Furthermore, under certain experimental conditions, they have displayed the ability to differentiate into non-connective cell lineages, such as neuronal and endothelial. Finally, as a particularly interesting property for the use at hand, they are capable, both *in vitro* and *in vivo*, of inhibiting immune response. This ability to immunoregulate includes inhibition of the activation of T, B and NKcells, the maturation of dendritic cells, as well as protecting against inflammatory and/or autoimmune pathologies, including transplant rejection [21].

3. Mesenchymal stem cells as therapies

Early studies with adult stem cells focused on MSCs isolated from bone marrow stroma, which have demonstrated adipogenic, osteogenic, chondrogenic, myogenic and neurogenic potential *in vitro*. However, obtaining stem cells from this source is painful for the patient and only provides a small number of cells [22]. Recently, methods of harvesting adult stem cells from adipose tissue by simple liposuction have been developed. Adipose tissue is rich in such cells, and their preparation is easier than that from bone marrow. Although there is some debate about whether stem cells originate in the fat tissue itself, or if perhaps they are mesenchymal or even peripheral blood stem cells passing through the fat, it is clear that adipose tissue represents a valuable source of potentially useful stem cells. These adipose-derived stem cells (ASCs) have been shown to have an inherent ability to self-renew, proliferate and differentiate into mature tissues, depending on the microenvironment that surrounds them. Such characteristics, intrinsic to all stem cells, make them highly attractive for use in cell therapy and regenerative medicine [23].

Interest in multipotent ASCs is increasing, owing to the ability to harvest large quantities of tissue under local anaesthesia via the liposuction process. Indeed, from just 1 g of adipose tissue, 5×10^3 stem cells can be obtained, which is much greater than the amount that can be acquired from bone marrow. Furthermore, compared to bone marrow MSCs, in the early stages, ASCs express CD34 to a greater extent (100–500 times higher) [24].

The terms adipose tissue-derived stromal cell (ADSC), adipose stromal–vascular cell fraction (SVF) and adipose-derived regenerative cells (ADRC) all correspond to cells obtained immediately after digestion of adipose tissue by collagenase. On the other hand, the terms processed lipoaspirate cells (PLA) and plastic-adherent adipose-derived stem cells (ASCS) describe those that are obtained after culturing those produced by the digestion process. As a unifying term, we refer to these cell types as adipose-derived stem cells (ASC), in accordance with the International Fat Applied Technology Society Consensus [25].

4. Utilisation of MSCs in the treatment of perianal fistula disease

The precise mechanism of the therapeutic action of MSCs is not fully understood, but is likely to reflect their inherent characteristics, in particular their differentiation potential [26, 27]. MSCs have the ability to migrate to the site of a lesion or inflammatory process, stimulate the proliferation and differentiation of resident stem cells through the secretion of growth factors, remodel the matrix and exert an immunomodulatory and anti-inflammatory effect. Together, these properties aid help the healing of tissues [28–31]. It has also been demonstrated that MSCs can induce an increase in epithelialisation and angiogenesis through a process of differentiation and paracrine interaction with skin cells [32–34].

Today, we know that Crohn's disease delays T-cell apoptosis [35, 36], and a mechanism of action of ASCs when injected into the inflammation site in the fistula tract has been postulated. Initially, the cells recognise proinflammatory cytokines such as IFN-γ, followed by activation of the indoleamine 2,3-dioxygenase (IDO) enzyme, which is ultimately responsible for creating a microenvironment—lymphocyte freezing by inhibition of phosphorylation. This results in a reduction in the release of proinflammatory mediators (TNF-α, IL-6, etc.) and an increase in that of anti-inflammatory species such as IL-10 [37].

5. Treatment protocol for anal fistulae

The protocol for stem cell treatment of anal fistulae inevitably starts with the harvesting of the MSCs, either from the patient's bone marrow or their fat (autologous), or from a healthy donor (allogeneic). Bone marrow cells are harvested by aspiration, and then, the MSCs are expanded *ex vivo* for subsequent use in the fistula tract [38, 39]. Although there are various protocols for expansion and differentiation of cells obtained from adipose tissue (with a consequent variation in results), ASCs are normally used after digestion with collagenase under constant stirring. The obtained solution is then centrifuged at low speed, and the resultant is filtered through a nylon mesh of 40–200 μm. The new solution is then centrifuged again, and the cells are re-suspended in fresh expansion medium. It is important to stress that this procedure must be carried out in extremely sterile conditions [40].

As for the route of administration, there is a single study in which allogeneic bone marrow MSCs were given intravenously, with the closure of fistulas being a secondary objective of the study [41]; all other published studies have employed the intralesional route [38, 39, 42–50].

Before intralesional injection of the isolated MSCs, the lesion site must be prepared with similarly intensive curettage, avoiding the use of cytolytic substances (hydrogen peroxide). The inner fistula orifice can then be sealed with an absorbable suture. At this point, half of the cell preparation is administered to the tissue around the inner hole, making small submucosal wheals. The other half is applied along the walls of the fistula tract, if possible along its whole length, while taking care not to go deeper than a few millimetres, again in small wheals (**Figure 1**). Several studies have investigated the use of fibrin glue as an adjuvant or scaffold, in order to enhance the attachment of cells in the fistula tract [43, 45–47]. The dose of cells required for optimum results remains to be determined; in published studies, this ranges from 3.5×10^6 to 40×10^6 cells [39–50].

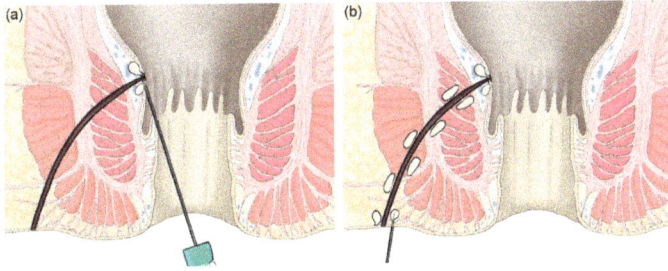

Figure 1. Implant points. (a) Wheal in the internal fistula orifice; (b) injection in the fistula tract at a depth of no more than 2 mm (courtesy of Tigenix).

Most studies have used ASCs, but there are also some that have evaluated the use of bone marrow cells. As for the cell source, the advantages of an allogeneic source (from healthy donors) are innumerable in comparison with those of an autologous source, especially in terms of greater accessibility, easy expandability and good stability. Their use is possible because of their low immunogenicity and limited persistence, which reduce the chances of provoking an adverse effect in the host [51].

6. Safety and efficacy of MSCs in the treatment of anal fistulae

The first experience with stem cells in the treatment of anal fistulae was reported by García-Olmo et al. [52]. Several studies have since been published, the majority of which are from Spanish groups. The MSCs used have mainly originated from adipose tissue, with only two studies using bone marrow MSCs. In these latter cases, both allogeneic and autologous cells have been used. In all studies, administration was intralesional, with fibrin glue often used [38, 39].

Today, any questions as to the feasibility and safety of such treatment seem to have been resolved, at least within the range of doses used. A retrospective study evaluating whether MSC treatment has any influence on fertility, course of pregnancy, birthweight or physical status was recently published [53]. Five patients with fistula associated with Crohn's disease treated with ASCs, and who indicated their intention to have children after completion of treatment, were tracked. Fertility and pregnancy course were not found to be affected by this therapy. Furthermore, no treatment-related malformations in newborns were observed. Therefore, it was concluded that in the patients analysed in the study, local injection of ASCs was not associated with adverse effects on the ability to conceive, pregnancy course or the newborn's condition.

In the published literature, there are differences in cure rate depending on the follow-up, but in general, it is estimated to be between 50 and 70% (**Table 1**).

Authors, year	Study design	Source of cells	Results
Garcia-Olmo et al., 2005 (Spain) [42]	Phase I clinical study ($n = 4$)	ASCs (autologous)	Complete closure: 50% of patients; 75% fistulas
Garcia-Olmo et al., 2009 (Spain) [42]	Open-label, multicenter, phase II study ($n = 14$)	ASCs (autologous); fibrin glue	Fistula healing: 71 vs 14%
Ciccocioppo et al., 2011 (Italy) [38]	Prospective study ($n = 10$)	MSCs (autologous)	Reduction in CDAI, PDAI and pain/discharge PDAI scores
Guadalajara et al., 2012 (Spain) [43]	Retrospective follow-up of Garcia-Olmophase II study ($n = 5$)	ASCs (autologous); fibrin glue	58% sustained fistula closure at end of follow-up by mean 3 years No safety problem
Cho et al., 2013 (Korea) [47]	Open-label, multicentre, dose escalationphase I study ($n = 10$)	ASCs (autologous); fibrin glue	Healing in 50% in the group with 2×10^7 cells
Lee et al., 2013 (Korea) [45]	Open-label, multicentre, phase II study ($n = 42$; 33 completed follow-up)	ASCs (autologous); fibrin glue	Fistula closure in 79%, recidive 11%
de la Portilla et al., 2013 (Spain) [48]	Open-label pilot study ($n = 24$)	ASCs (allogeneic)	Complete closure: 56.3% at 24 weeks
Ciccocioppo et al., 2015 (Italy) [44]	5-year follow-up of 2011 study ($n = 10$)	MSCs (autologous)	37% fistula relapse-free 4 years later
Cho et al., 2013 (Korea) [46]	Retrospective, 1-year follow-up from 2013 study	ASCs (autologous); fibrin glue	Complete closure maintained in 75% at 2 years ITT analysis; 80% PP analysis
Garcia-Olmo et al., 2015 (Spain) [49]	Retrospective, open-label ($n = 3$ with CD)	ASCs (allogeneic andautologous)	Healing in 2/3 CD fistula patients
Molendijk et al., 2015 (The Netherlands) [39]	Double-blind, placebo-controlledphase II study ($n = 21$)	MSCs (allogeneic)	Healing up to 85%
Park et al., 2015 (Korea) [50]	Multicentre, open-label, dose escalation pilot study ($n = 6$)	ASCs (allogeneic); fibrin glue	Group 1 (1×10^7 cells/ml); healing 100% Group 2 (3×10^7 cells/ml); healing 100%

ASCs, adipose-derived stem cells; CD, Crohn's disease; CDAI, Crohn's disease activity index; ITT, intention to treat; IV, intravenous; MSCs, mesenchymal stem cells/mesenchymal stromal cells; PDAI, Pouchitis disease activity index; PP, per protocol; SC, stem cells.

Table 1. Published studies using MSCs to treat Crohn's disease patients with perianal fistulas.

Ciccocioppo et al. evaluated the long-term safety and efficacy of the use of bone-marrow-derived MSCs. In their study, 8 patients were followed prospectively for 72 months. These patients were part of a phase I/II trial previously conducted, in which a cure rate of 70% per year was reported, with improvement observed in the remaining 30% [44]. Patients received serialised injections of MSCs (4 on average) at intervals of 4 weeks. Secondary endpoints were the time patients remained without fistula and the time they were free of medical or surgical treatment. The Chrohn's Disease Activity Index (CDAI) increased over the first 2 years, followed by a gradual decline in the third year, and stabilisation at the end of follow-up at figures similar to those of the first year. The probability of remaining without fistula was 88% for the first year, 50% at 2 years and 37% over the next 4 years. The probability of patients being free from surgery was 100% for the first year, 75% for years 2–4 and 63% at years 5 and 6. Finally, the probability of patients being free from medical treatment was 88% for the first year, 25% at years 2–4 and 25% at years 5 and 6. No adverse effects related to treatment in these follow-up periods were recorded. The authors conclude that the fact that the activity indices increase again in the second year might suggest that this therapy is not curative, but that it does improve the remission rate in patients with refractory disease. Moreover, almost all patients required the reintroduction of biological or immunosuppressive therapy after the second year [44].

We are currently awaiting the publication of the results of a phase III, randomised, placebo, double-blind, multicentre, and international clinical trial employing Cx601, a preparation of allogeneic ASCs. It has recently been reported that, after 24 weeks, Cx601 was statistically superior to placebo in achieving the combined response (clinical and imaging) of complex perianal fistulas in Crohn's disease patients whose response to previous treatment, including anti-TNFs, had been inadequate.

7. Future perspectives

There is no doubt that a new avenue has opened for the treatment of Crohn's disease patients suffering from fistulae refractory to conventional therapy. Since the first description of the treatment, interest in this therapy has grown, so that in addition to the 11 studies published to date, at the time we write this chapter, there are more than a dozen clinical trials in recruitment or in the results publication phase.

While the safety of ASC therapy seems to have been well established, the optimal dosage, route of administration (intravenous versus intralesional), administration technique (alone or together with fibrin glue), among other matters, are yet to be adequately determined. However, these should be investigated and resolved in the coming years.

Acknowledgements

Tigenix SAU thank for the help in the writing of this chapter and easy editing of figures and particularly Dra. Mary Carmen Díaz

Author details

Fernando de la Portilla[1*], Ana M. García-Cabrera[1], Rosa M. Jiménez-Rodríguez[1], Maria L. Reyes[1] and Damian García-Olmo[2]

*Address all correspondence to: fportilla@us.es

1 Department of General and Digestive Surgery, Colorectal Surgery Unit, "Virgen del Rocío" University Hospital/IBiS/CSIC/University of Seville, Seville, Spain

2 Department of Surgery (Fundacion Jimenez Diaz), Universidad Autonoma de Madrid, Madrid, Spain

References

[1] Schwartz DA, Loftus EV, Tremaine WJ. The natural history of fistulizing Crohn's disease in Olmsted Country, Minnesota. Gastroenterology. 2002;122:875–880. doi:10.1053/gast. 2002.32362

[2] Ardizzone S, Bianchi-Porro G. Perianal Crohn's disease: overview. Dig Liver Dis. 2007;39:957–958. doi:10.1016/j.dld.2007.07.152

[3] Ingle SB, Loftus EV. The natural history of perianal Crohn's disease. Dig Liver Dis. 2007;39:963–969. doi:10.1016/j.dld.2007.07.154

[4] Singh B, George BD, Mortensen NJ. Surgical therapy of perianal Crohn's disease. Dig Liver Dis. 2007;39:988–992. doi:10.1016/j.dld.2007.07.157

[5] Sandborn WJ, Fazio VW, Feagan BG. AGA technical review on perianal Crohn's disease. Gastroenterology. 2003;125:1508–1530. doi:10.1016/j.gastro.2003.08.025

[6] Griggs L, Schwartz DA. Medical options for treating perianal Crohn's disease. Dig Liver Dis. 2007;39:979–987. doi:10.1016/j.dld.2007.07.156

[7] Present DH, Rutgeerts P, Targan S. Infliximab for the treatment of fistulas in patients with Crohn's disease. N Engl J Med. 1999;340:1398–1405. doi:10.1056/ NEJM199905063401804

[8] Sands BE, Anderson FH, Bernstein CN. Infliximab maintenance therapy for fistulizing Crohn's disease. N Engl J Med. 2004;350:876–885. doi:10.1056/NEJMoa030815

[9] Rutgeerts P, Feagan BG, Lichtenstein GR. Comparison of scheduled and episodic treatment strategies of infliximab in Crohn's disease. Gastroenterology.2004;126:402–413. doi:10.1053/j.gastro.2003.11.014

[10] Van der Hagen SJ, Baeten CG, Soeters PB. Anti-TNFalpha (infliximab) used as induction treatment of active proctitis in a multistep strategy followed by definitive surgery of

complex anal fistulas in Crohn's disease: a preliminary report. Dis Colon Rectum. 2005;48:758–767. doi:10.1007/s10350-004-0828-0

[11] Schroder O, Blumenstein I, Schulte-Bockholt A. Combining infliximab and methotrexate in fistulizing Crohn's disease resistant or intolerant to azathioprine. Aliment Pharmacol Ther. 2004;19:295–301. doi:10.1111/j.1365-2036.2004.01850.x

[12] Ochsenkuhn T, Goke B, Sackmann M. Combining infliximab with 6-mercaptopurine/azathioprine for fistula therapy in Crohn's disease. Am J Gastroenterol. 2002;97:2022–2025. doi:10.1111/j.1572-0241.2002.05918.x

[13] Baert F, Noman M, Vermeire S. Influence of immunogenicity on the long-term efficacy of infliximab in Crohn's disease. N Engl J Med. 2003;348:601–608. doi:10.1056/NEJMoa020888

[14] García-Olmo D, García-Arranz M, Herreros D, Pascual I, Peiro C, Rodríguez-Montes JA. A phase I clinical trial of the treatment of Crohn's fistula by adipose mesenchymal stem cell transplantation. Dis Colon Rectum. 2005;48:1416–1423. doi:10.1007/s10350-005-0052-6

[15] Gardner RL. Stem cells and regenerative medicine: principles, prospects and problems. C R Biol. 2007;330:465–473. doi:10.1016/j.crvi.2007.01.005

[16] Marshak DR, Gardner RL, Gottlieb D. Stem cell biology. New York: Cold Spring Harbor Laboratory Press; 2001. 550 p. doi:10-87969-575-7/01

[17] Yamanaka S. Pluripotency and nuclear reprogramming. Phil Trans R Soc Lond B Biol Sci. 2008;363:2079–2087. doi:10.1098/rstb.2008.2261

[18] Trebol Lopez J, Georgiev Hristov T, García-Arranz M, García-Olmo D. Stem cell therapy for digestive tract diseases: current state and future perspectives. Stem Cells Dev. 2011;20:1113–1129. doi:10.1089/scd.2010.0277

[19] Verfaillie CM. Adult stem cells: assessing the case for pluripotency. Trends Cell Biol. 2002;12:502–508.doi:10.1016/S0962-8924(02)02386-3

[20] Chamberlain G, Fox J, Ashton B, Middleton J. Concise review: mesenchymal stem cells: their phenotype, differentiation capacity, immunological features, and potential for homing. Stem Cells. 2007;25:2739–2749.doi:10.1634/stemcells.2007-0197

[21] García-Gómez I, Elvira G, Zapata AG, et al. Mesenchymal stem cells: biological properties and clinical applications. Expert Opin Biol Ther. 2010;10(10):1453–1468. doi:10.1517/14712598.2010.519333

[22] Singer AJ, Clark RAF. Cutaneous wound healing. N Engl J Med. 1999;341:738–746. doi:10.1056/NEJM199909023411006

[23] Stappenbeck TS, Miyoshi H. The role of stromal stem cells in tissue regeneration and wound repair. Science. 2009;324:1666–1669.doi:10.1126/science.1172687

[24] Keating A. Mesenchymal stromal cells. Curr Opin Hematol. 2006;13:419–425. doi: 10.1097/01.moh.0000245697.54887.6f

[25] Dominici M, Le Blanc K, Mueller I, et al. Minimal critering for definig multipotent mesenchymal stromal cells. The International Society for Cellular Therapy position statement. Cytotherapy. 2006;83:15. doi:10.1080/14653240600855905

[26] Gimble JM, Guilak, F. Adipose-derived adult stem cells: isolation, characterization, and differentiation potential. Cytotherapy.2003;5:362–369. doi:10.1080/14653240310003026

[27] Gimble, JM, Katz AJ, Bunnell BA. Adipose-derived stem cells for regenerative medicine. Circ Res.2007;100:1249–1260. doi:10.1161/01.RES.0000265074.83288.09

[28] Chapel A, Bertho JM, Bensidhoum M, et al. Mesenchymal stem cells home to injured tissues when co-infused with hematopoietic cells to treat a radiation-induced multi-organ failure syndrome. J Gene Med. 2003;5:1028–1038. doi:10.1002/jgm.452

[29] Le Blanc, K. Mesenchymal stromal cells: tissue repair and immune modulation. Cytotherapy.2006;8:559–561. doi:10.1080/14653240601045399

[30] Yagi H, Soto-Gutierrez A, Parekkadan B, et al. Mesenchymal stem cells: mechanisms of immunomodulation and homing. Cell Transplant. 2010;19:667–679. doi: 10.3727/096368910X508762

[31] Yoo KH, Jang IK, Lee MW, et al. Comparison of immunomodulatory properties of mesenchymal stem cells derived from adult human tissues. Cell Immunol. 2009;259:150–156. doi:10.1016/j.cellimm.2009.06.010

[32] Falanga V, Iwamoto S, Chartier M, et al. Autologous bone marrow derived cultured mesenchymal stem cells delivered in a fibrin spray accelerate healing in murine and human cutaneous wounds. Tissue Eng. 2007;13:1299–1312. doi:10.1038/jid.2012.77

[33] McFarlin K, Gao X, Liu YB, et al. Bone marrow- derived mesenchymal stromal cells accelerate wound healing in the rat. Wound Repair Regen. 2006;14:471–478. doi: 10.1111/j.1743-6109.2006.00153.x

[34] Wu Y, Chen L, Scott PG, et al. Mesenchymal stem cells enhance wound healing through differentiation and angiogenesis. Stem Cells. 2007;25:2648–2659. doi:10.1634/stemcells. 2007-0226

[35] Ina K, Itoh J, Fukushima K, et al. Resistance of Crohn's disease T cells to multiple apoptotic signals is associated with a Bcl-2/Bax mucosal imbalance. J Immunol. 1999;163:1081–1090. doi:10.0022-1767/99/02.00

[36] Mudter J, Neurath MF. Apoptosis of T cells and the control of inflammatory bowel disease: therapeutic implications. Gut. 2007;56:293–303.doi:10.1136/gut. 2005.090464

[37] De la Rosa O, Lombardo E, Beraza A, et al. Requirement of IFN-gamma-mediated indoleamine 2,3-dioxygenase expression in the modulation of lymphocyte prolifera-

tion by human adipose-derived stem cells. Tissue Eng Part A. 2009;15:2795–2806. doi: 10.1089/ten.TEA.2008.0630

[38] Ciccocioppo R, Bernardo ME, Sgarella A, Maccario R, Avanzini MA, Ubezio C, Minelli A, Alvisi C, Vanoli A, Calliada F, Dionigi P, Perotti C, Locatelli F, Corazza GR. Autologous bone marrow derived mesenchymal stromal cells in the treatment of fistulising Crohn's disease. Gut. 2011;60:788–798. doi:10.1136/gut.2010.214841

[39] Molendijk I, Bonsing BA, Roelofs H, Peeters KC, Wasser MN, Dijkstra G, van der Woude CJ, Duijvestein M, Veenendaal RA, Zwaginga JJ, Verspaget HW, Fibbe WE, van der Meulen-de Jong AE, Hommes DW. Allogeneic bone marrow-derived mesenchymal stromal cells promote healing of refractory perianal fistulas in patients with Crohn's disease. Gastroenterology. 2015;149(4):918–927.e6. doi: 10.1053/j.gastro.2015.06.014

[40] Casteilla L, Planat-Benard V, Bourin P, Laharrague P, Cousin B. Use of adipose tissue in regenerative medicine. Transfus Clin Biol. 2011;18:124–128. doi:10.1016/j.tracli. 2011.01.008

[41] Mannon PJ. Remestemcel-L: human mesenchymal stem cells as an emerging therapy for Crohn's disease. Expert Opin Biol Ther.2011;11:1249–1256. doi: 10.1517/14712598.2011.602967

[42] Garcia-Olmo D, Herreros D, Pascual I, Pascual JA, Del-Valle E, Zorrilla J, De-La-Quintana P, Garcia-Arranz M, Pascual M. Expanded adipose-derived stem cells for the treatment of complex perianal fistula: a phase II clinical trial. Dis Colon Rectum. 2009;52:79–86. doi:10.1007/DCR. 0b013e3181973487

[43] Guadalajara H, Herreros D, De-La-Quintana P, Trebol J, Garcia-Arranz M, Garcia-Olmo D. Long-term follow-up of patients undergoing adipose derived adult stem cell administration to treat complex perianal fistulas. Int J Colorectal Dis. 2012;27:595–600. doi:10.1007/s00384-011-1350-1

[44] Ciccocioppo R, Gallia A, Sgarella A, Kruzliak P, Gobbi PG, Corazza GR. Long-term follow-up of Crohn disease fistulas after local injections of bone marrow-derived mesenchymal stem cells. Mayo Clin Proc. 2015;90:747–755. doi:10.1016/j.mayocp. 2015.03.023

[45] Lee WY, Park KJ, Cho YB, Yoon SN, Song KH, Kim do S, Jung SH, Kim M, Yoo HW, Kim I, Ha H, Yu CS. Autologous adipose tissue-derived stem cells treatment demonstrated favorable and sustainable therapeutic effect for Crohn's fistula. Stem Cells. 2013;31:2575–2581. doi:10.1002/stem.1357

[46] Cho YB, Lee WY, Park KJ, Kim M, Yoo HW, Yu CS. Autologous adipose tissue-derived stem cells for the treatment of Crohn's fistula: a phase I clinical study. Cell Transplant. 2013;22:279–285. doi:10.3727/096368912X656045

[47] Cho YB, Park KJ, Yoon SN, Song KH, Kim do S, Jung SH, Kim M, Jeong HY, Yu CS. Long-term results of adipose-derived stem cell therapy for the treatment of Crohn's fistula. Stem Cells Transl Med. 2015;4:532–537. doi:10.5966/sctm.2014-0199

[48] de la Portilla F, Alba F, García-Olmo D, Herrerías JM, González FX, Galindo A. Expanded allogeneic adipose-derived stem cells (eASCs) for the treatment of complex perianal fistula in Crohn's disease: results from a multicenter phase I/IIa clinical trial. Int J Colorectal Dis. 2013;28:313–323. doi:10.1007/s00384-012-1581-9

[49] Garcia-Olmo D, Guadalajara H, Rubio-Perez I, Herreros MD, de-la-Quintana P,Garcia-Arranz M. Recurrent anal fistulae: limited surgery supported by stem cells. World J Gastroenterol. 2015 Mar 21;21(11):3330–6. doi:10.3748/wjg.v21.i11.3330.

[50] Park KJ, Ryoo SB, Kim JS, Kim TI, Baik SH, Kim HJ, Lee KY, Kim M, Kim WH. Allogeneic adipose-derived stem cells for the treatment of perianal fistula in Crohn's disease: a pilot clinical trial. Colorectal Dis. 2015. doi:10.1111/codi.13223

[51] Barkholt L, Flory E, Jekerle V, Lucas-Samuel S, Ahnert P, Bisset L, Büscher D, Fibbe W, Foussat A, Kwa M, Lantz O, Mačiulaitis R, Palomäki T, Schneider CK, Sensebé L, Tachdjian G, Tarte K, Tosca L, Salmikangas P. Risk of tumorigenicity in mesenchymal stromal cell-based therapies--bridging scientific observations and regulatory viewpoints. Cytotherapy. 2013;15(7):753–759. doi:10.1016/j.jcyt.2013.03.005

[52] García-Olmo D, García-Arranz M, García LG, Cuellar ES, Blanco IF, Prianes LA, Montes JA, Pinto FL, Marcos DH, García-Sancho L. Autologous stem cell transplantation for treatment of rectovaginal fistula in perianal Crohn's disease: a new cell-based therapy. Int J Colorectal Dis. 2003;18(5):451–454. doi:10.1007/s00384-003-0490-3

[53] Sanz-Baro R, García-Arranz M, Guadalajara H, de la Quintana P, Herreros MD, García-Olmo D. First-in-human case study: pregnancy in women with Crohn's perianal fistula treated with adipose-derived stem cells: a safety study. Stem Cells Transl Med. 2015;4(6):598–602. doi:10.5966/sctm.2014-0255

10

Inflammatory Bowel Disease: The Association of Inflammatory Cytokine Gene Polymorphisms

Abdulrahman Al-Robayan, Misbahul Arfin,
Ebtissam Saleh Al-Meghaiseeb, Reem Al-Amro and
Abdulrahman K Al-Asmari

Abstract

The frequencies of alleles and genotypes of *TNF-α*, *TNF-β*, and *IL-10* genes were examined in Saudi subjects including IBD patients (UC and CD) and matched controls. Venous blood samples were collected from IBD patients and healthy control subjects, and genomic DNA was extracted using commercially available kit (Qiagen, CA, USA). In order to detect TNF-α (-308G/A), TNF-β (+252A/G), IL-10 (-1082G/A), (-819C/T), and (-592C/A) polymorphisms, the *TNF-α*, *TNF-β*, and *IL-10* genes were amplified using an amplification refractory mutation systems PCR methodology. Analysis of data showed that the frequencies of alleles and genotype of TNF-α (-308G/A), TNF-β (+252A/G), and IL-10 (-1082G/A), (-819C/T), and (-592C/A) polymorphisms differ between IBD patients and control subjects. Our study clearly indicated that the TNF-α (-308G/A), TNF-β (+252A/G), and IL-10 (-1082 G/A) polymorphisms are associated significantly with the risk of IBD susceptibility while other two, IL-10-819C/T and IL-10-592C/A, polymorphisms are not associated with IBD in Saudi population. However, well-designed epidemiological as well as genetic association studies with large sample size among different ethnicities should be performed in order to have better understanding of this relationship.

Keywords: tumor necrosis factor, interleukin-10, polymorphism, inflammatory bowel disease, Saudis, Crohn's disease, ulcerative colitis

1. Introduction

The inflammatory bowel diseases (IBDs), encompassing Crohn's disease (CD, OMIM 266600) and ulcerative colitis (UC, OMIM 191390), are chronic inflammatory disorders of the gastrointestinal tract. The incidence and prevalence of IBD have been increasing with time in different regions around the world, indicating its emergence as a global disease [1–5]. Available literature indicates that IBD is a complex and multifactorial disease though the exact etiology is still not clear. However, it has been suggested that immune dysregulation caused by genetic and/or environmental factors plays an important role in the etiology of IBD [6–8]. IBD appears to be caused by overly aggressive T-cell responses directed against environmental factors and/or a subset of commensal bacteria/pathogens that inhabit the distal ileum and colon of genetically susceptible hosts. Patients with long-lasting IBD, both UC and CD, have been at increased risk of developing colorectal cancer, and CD patients are at increased risk of small intestine cancer [9].

The incidence of IBD is higher in North American and European populations compared with those in Asian and African, reflecting the role of both environmental and genetic factors. The rising prevalence of various autoimmune and inflammatory conditions in developed countries has been attributed to hygiene hypothesis, and they are thought to result from the lack of early exposure to select microbial agents due to stringent sanitation conditions [10]. The changes in dietary and intestinal microbial milieu have been suggested to play a key pathogenic role in the etiology of IBD, though the exact environmental factors responsible for changing IBD prevalence are not clearly defined [11]. Intriguingly, the characteristics of Western and Asian IBD patients differ in epidemiology, phenotype, and genetic susceptibility [12–15] highlighting ethnic variations. Various epidemiological and population-based studies have indicated that genetic factors contribute to the pathogenesis of IBD [16–18].

According to Jump and Levine [19], cytokines act as key signal in the intestinal immune system and participate in the disruption of the physiological inflammation of the gut. They are produced mainly by immune cells as small peptide proteins and facilitate communication between cells, by stimulating the proliferation of antigen-specific effector cells, and mediate the local and systemic inflammation in an autocrine, paracrine, and endocrine pathways [20]. A critical role is played by innate immune system in IBD pathology, and several cytokines secreted by activated dendritic cells (DC) and macrophages actively regulate the inflammatory response in IBD.

The production of cytokines can be affected by genetic polymorphisms within the coding and promoter regions of cytokine genes [21, 22]. Therefore, a genetic predisposition for the high or low production of a particular cytokine may affect disease susceptibility and clinical outcome [23, 24].

The IBD is believed to be caused by immunogenic responses against environmental factors and/or microbes inhabiting distal ileum and colon of genetically susceptible hosts. Inflammatory response in IBD is an important feature and proinflammatory cytokine; tumor necrosis factor-alpha (TNF) has been indicated to play a key role in the initiation and propagation of IBD. Increased expressions of TNF-α have been reported in peripheral phagocytes and intestinal tissues of IBD patients. High levels of TNF-α have also been documented in the serum of IBD patients [25–27]. Moreover, monoclonal antibodies against TNF-α have been effectively used to decrease inflammation in IBD [28]. Variations in levels/expression of TNF due to its genetic polymorphism have been linked with pathogenic role of this cytokine in various autoimmune and inflammatory diseases and thus have been regarded to be an appropriate target for management of diseases by interfering with the inflammatory responses.

In view of the important immunoregulatory roles of TNF-α and TNF-β, they are considered as subject of interest for studies in IBD. TNF-α is produced mainly by monocytes and activated macrophages while TNF-β is produced mainly by activated T cells. Both *TNF-α* (OMIM 191160) and *TNF-β* (MIM153440) genes are located on chromosome 6 within the MHC III region and show close linkage to the HLA class I (*HLA-B*) and class II (*HLA-DR*) genes. It has been shown by various studies on monozygotic twins and first-degree relatives that 60% of variation in the production capacity of TNF-α is genetically determined [29]. A number of polymorphisms within the promoter region of *TNF-α* and the intron 1 polymorphism of *TNF-β,* in particular have been associated with variations in the serum levels of TNF-α [30, 31] One of the best described single nucleotide polymorphisms (SNPs) is located at nucleotide position -308 within the *TNF-α* promoter region (rs1800629) and affects a consensus sequence for a binding site of transcription factor AP-2 [32]. TNF-α (-308) promoter polymorphism leads to a less common allele-A (allele 2), which has been associated with increased TNF-α production in vitro [33, 34] and higher rate of TNF-α transcription than wild-type GG genotype [35, 36]. This polymorphism has been linked to increased susceptibility to several chronic metabolic degenerative, inflammatory and autoimmune diseases [37–41].

Of interest, G/A polymorphism at nucleotide position -308 within the human TNF-α promoter region is associated with elevated TNF levels, disease susceptibility, and poor prognosis in several diseases [42–45]. Adenine at position -308 makes the TNF-α promoter a much more powerful transcription activator than guanine [42].

TNF-β +252A/G (rs909253) polymorphism affects a phorbol ester-responsive element. The presence of G at +252 position refers to the less frequent mutant allele known as TNF-β * 1 (allele-1), which is associated with higher TNF-α and TNF-β production [42, 46].

TNF-β resembles to TNF-α in terms of several biological activities including apoptosis and gives rise to a similar proinflammatory response and has been shown to play a critical role in pathogenesis of many diseases. TNF-β has also been shown to contribute to the susceptibility of several inflammatory/autoimmune diseases. Association of TNF-β +252 A/G polymorphism has been reported with various autoimmune disorders including Gravis' disease [47] idiopathic membranous glomerulonephritis, IgA nephropathy, insulin-dependent diabetes mellitus [48], myasthenia gravis [49], asthma diathesis [50], SLE with nephritis [51], systemic sclerosis [52], plaque psoriasis [53], rheumatoid arthritis [54], and type 1 diabetes [55]. Recently, TNF-β +252 A/G polymorphism is reported to be associated with both susceptibility to and mortality from sepsis [56].

A few studies have been undertaken to determine the association of TNF-α polymorphisms and IBD in different parts of the world [57–59]. The results of these studies on association of TNF-α polymorphism with IBD are not consistent, and variations have been reported [60]. These variations might be due to genetic differences in populations or systemic variations in the ancestry of IBD patients and control subjects involved in the studies [27]. Moreover, differences have been found in the characteristics, epidemiology, phenotype, and genetic susceptibility to IBD in Western and Asian populations [15, 16]. Therefore, studies involving these unique features in different ethnic populations will help not only identifying the pathophysiology but also understanding the etiology of IBD.

No research has been done on the association between TNF-β polymorphism and IBD. TNF-α and TNF-β are closely related cytokines, and both are involved in the expression of TNF-α and in a suggested mechanism for autoimmune/inflammatory diseases; therefore, the joint analysis of polymorphisms in *TNF-α* and *TNF-β* genes will provide further insight into the pathogenesis of IBD and help in developing effective therapeutic agents. Saudi population is ideal for such genetic association studies because of the fact that it is a closed and isolated society with quite high rate of consanguinity. So, we studied and evaluated the possible association of alleles and genotypes of TNF-α (-308G/A) and TNF-β (+252A/G) polymorphisms with the susceptibility risk to IBD in this population.

On the other hand, interleukin-10 (IL-10) is an anti-inflammatory cytokine and can inhibit the synthesis of proinflammatory cytokines, such as interferon-γ, IL-2, IL-3, and tumor necrosis factor-α (TNF-α), produced by macrophages and regulatory T cells [61]. IL-10 is responsible for various functions. It shifts the Th1/Th2 balance by downregulating the Th1 responses and by suppression of proinflammatory cytokines [62]. Several studies have shown that serum IL-10 levels are significantly lower in IBD patients than in normal controls, suggesting that altered IL-10 levels may be involved in the pathogenesis of IBD and may be an IBD biomarker. IL-10 is capable of depressing the activated immune system. It has been reported that IL-10 knockout mice develop colitis when they are kept in unsterile environment [63], and the inflammation is reduced after administration of IL-10 in vivo and in vitro models [64]. Moreover, the production of IL-10 has been found to be impaired in severe cases of IBD [65, 66].

IL-10 suppresses CD4+ T helper, Th1, clones (which secrete IL-2, interferon-γ, and TNF-α) and promotes the immunomodulatory T helper, Th2, clones (which secrete IL-4, IL-10, and IL-13). The secretion of cytokines is responsible for regulating the balance between Th1 and Th2 cells which is critical for immunoregulation. In case of reduced capacity of T cells to produce IL-10 in response to a stimulus, Th1 responses continue with the breakdown of peripheral tolerance and are potential to develop autoimmunity [67].

IL-10 is a multifunctional cytokine mainly produced by immune cells, such as T cells, monocytes, appropriately stimulated macrophages, some subsets of dendritic cells (DCs), and B cells [68]. Non-immune cell sources of IL-10 also exist, including keratinocytes, epithelial cells, and some tumor cells [69, 70]. The human *IL-10* gene is located on chromosome 1q32.1 and contains five exons. Recently, IL-10 has been identified as an important player in the development of immunological and inflammatory responses involving in the pathogenesis of various diseases including IBD [71–73].

Several single nucleotide polymorphisms (SNPs) have been reported in the proximal and distal regions of the *IL-10* gene, out of which three promoter polymorphisms (rs18000896-1082A/G, rs1800871-819T/C, and rs1800872-592A/C) are involved in IL-10 transcription rate and directly affect its production level and expression [74–77]. The -1082G, -819C, and -592C (GCC) alleles have been associated with elevated levels of IL-10 production [78], while ACC and ATA haplotypes show intermediate and low *IL-10* gene transcription, respectively [79]. These IL-10 gene polymorphisms are reported to be associated with susceptibility/development to various inflammatory disorders [40, 80–82]. However, data are limited and inconsistent and therefore do not allow drawing unequivocal conclusions.

Studies on the *IL-10* promoter polymorphisms and IBD susceptibility have also been inconsistent [71, 83–89]. Some studies have found an associations between *IL-10* polymorphism and IBD [71, 86, 87, 90], whereas other studies were unable to find any association between IBD and the *IL-10* promoter polymorphisms [83, 84, 88, 91]. In this study, we evaluated the association of five polymorphism in *IL-10*, *TNF-α*, and *TNF-β* genes with susceptibility risk of IBD in Saudi patients.

2. Methods

2.1. Subjects

Study groups consisted of 379 Saudi subjects including 179 IBD patients and 200 age- and sex-matched healthy controls visiting Gastroenterology Clinic of Prince Sultan Military Medical City (PSMMC), Riyadh. IBD patients included 20 cases of familial forms and 159 cases of sporadic forms. Of these patients, 95 were diagnosed to suffer with CD (57 men, 38 women) aged 17–65 years (mean age 32 years), while 84 patients with UC (34 men, 50 women) aged 22–68 years (mean age 34 years). Control group consisted of 120 men and 80 women matched for age and ethnicity (Saudi). Control subjects were screened for any history of IBD, diabetes, rheumatoid arthritis, systemic lupus erythematosus, or other autoimmune/inflammatory diseases and excluded if found positive. The diagnoses of CD and UC were based on conventional endoscopic, radiological, and histological criteria [92]. Demographic and clinical data were collected and used for exclusion and inclusion as described elsewhere [93]. This study was approved by the research and ethical committee of PSMMC, and written informed consent was obtained from all subjects to participate in this study.

2.2. Polymerase chain reaction (PCR) amplification

Venus blood (3 ml) was collected from all the participants, and genomic DNA was extracted using a commercially available kit (Qiagen, CA, USA). To detect polymorphisms at position -308 and intron 1 +252 of the TNF-α and TNF-β genes, respectively, and at position -592, -819 and -1082 of IL-10 gene, the amplification of TNF-α, TNF-β, and IL-10 genes was performed using an amplification refractory mutation systems PCR methodology described elsewhere [39, 93]. PCR amplification was carried out in PuReTaq Ready-to-Go PCR Beads (GE Healthcare, Buckinghamshire, UK) as described earlier [82]. The allele and genotype frequencies of all 5 polymorphisms were evaluated in IBD patients and controls. Hardy-Weinberg equilibrium was determined using Hardy-Weinberg Equilibrium Calculator for 2 Alleles. (http//www.had2know.com/academics/hardy-weinberg-equilibrium calculator-2alleles.html)

2.3. Statistical analysis

The difference between the frequency distribution of various alleles and genotypes in patients and controls was analyzed by Fisher's exact test using the CalcFisher software (http://www.jstatsoft.org/v08/i21/paper), and the *P*-values ≤ 0.05 were considered as significant. The odd ratio interpreted as *relative risk* (RR) indicated the strength of the association of disease with respect to a particular allele/genotype and was calculated according to the method of Woolf as outlined by Schallreuter et al. [94]. The RR was calculated using the following formula only for those alleles and genotype, which were increased or decreased in IBD patients as compared to normal Saudis.

$$RR = \frac{a \times d}{b \times c} \tag{1}$$

where "a" indicates number of patients expressing the allele or genotype, "b" number of patients without allele or genotype expression, "c" number of controls expressing the allele or genotype, and "d" number of controls without allele or genotype expression.

The etiologic fraction (EF) is the hypothetical genetic component of the disease. Values >0.00–0.99 are significant. EF is calculated for positive associations where value of RR is >1 using the following formula [95]:

$$EF = \frac{(RR - 1)f}{RR}, \text{where } f = \frac{a}{a + c} \tag{2}$$

Preventive fraction (PF) shows the hypothetical protective effect of one allele/genotype for a disease. PF is calculated for negative associations where RR is <1 using following formula [95]. Values >0.00–0.99 indicate the protective effect of an allele/genotype against the manifestation of disease.

$$PF = \frac{(1 - RR)f}{RR(1 - f) + f}, \text{where } f = \frac{a}{a + c} \tag{3}$$

3. Results

The representative gel pictures of amplification of different genotypes for TNF-α (-308G/A) and TNF-β (+252A/G) are shown in **Figures 1** and **2**.

Allelic frequencies and genotype distributions of TNF-α (-308G/A) and TNF-β (+252A/G) polymorphisms were different in patients and controls. The allele frequencies of both patients and

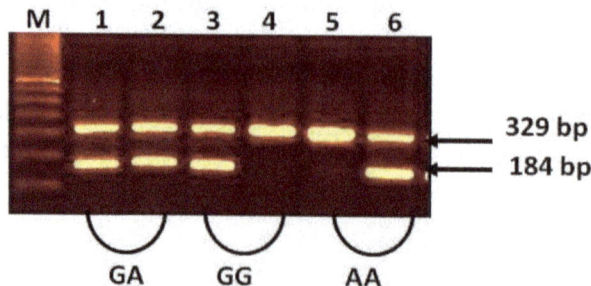

Figure 1. Shows the amplification of TNF-α (-308G/A) alleles (G and A). Lane M: 100-bp DNA marker, lanes 1 and 3: amplification of allele G, lanes 2 and 6: amplification of allele A, 184-bp band for target DNA, 329-bp band for internal control.

controls were in Hardy-Weinberg equilibrium. The frequencies of genotype GA and allele A were significantly higher, while those of genotypes (GG and AA) and allele A of TNF-α (-308G/A) were lower in IBD patients as compared to controls (**Table 1**). Allele A and genotype GA were susceptible to the IBD ($P < 0.001$), while allele G and genotype GG were protective against IBD ($P < 0.001$) in Saudi patients.

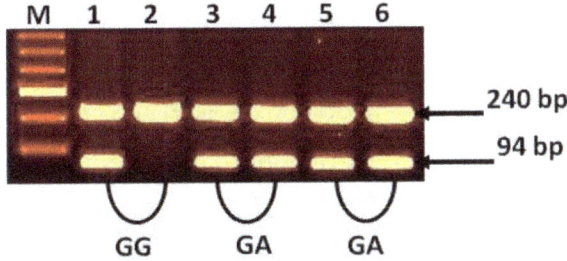

Figure 2. Shows the amplification of TNF-β (+252A/G) alleles (A and G). Lane M: 100-bp DNA marker, lanes 1, 3, and 5: amplification of allele G, lanes 4 and 6: amplification of allele A, 94-bp band for target DNA, 240-bp band for internal control.

Genotype/allele	IBD (n = 179)		Control (n = 200)		P-value	RR	EF*/PF
	n	%	n	%			
GG	5	2.79	110	55	0.00001♣	0.235	0.123
GA	173	96.65	76	38	0.0001♣	47.044	0.080*
AA	1	0.56	14	7	0.0009♣	0.075	0.449
G-allele	183	51.12	296	74	0.0001♣	0.367	0.397
A-allele	175	48.88	104	26	0.0001♣	2.722	0.396*

EF = Etiologic fraction, PF = preventive fraction.
♣Statistically significant.
*data for EF

Table 1. Genotype and allele frequencies of TNF-α (-308G/A) polymorphism in IBD patients and matched controls.

Because of the fact that two forms of IBD are characterized by different clinical pictures, it is reasonable to perform genetic association studies on homogenous group of patients; therefore, the genotyping results were stratified into UC and CD. However, similar association with TNF-α (-308G/A) polymorphism was noticed in the two groups. The genotype GA and allele A were significantly associated with CD and UC susceptibility in our population (**Table 2** and **Figure 1**). Allele A and genotype GA were susceptible to the UC and CD ($Ps < 0.01$), while allele G and genotype GG were protective ($Ps < 0.01$) in Saudi patients with UC and CD.

The association of TNF-α (-308G/A) polymorphism with UC, CD, or IBD in various ethnic populations worldwide has been summarized in **Table 3**. The association is not consistent, and

Genotype/allele	CD (95) n (%)	UC (84) n (%)	Control (200) n (%)
GG	3 (3.16)*	2 (2.38)*	110 (55)
GA	91 (95.79)*	82 (97.62)*	76 (38)
AA	1 (1.05)*	0 (0.0)*	14 (7)
G-allele	97 (51.05)*	86 (51.19)*	296 (74)
A-allele	93 (48.95)*	82 (48.81)*	104 (26)

*P value <0.05 compared to the frequency in controls.

Table 2. Genotype and allele frequencies of TNF-α (-308G/A) polymorphism in UC and CD patients.

ethnic variations are evident in the type or/and degree of association of TNF-α (-308G/A) polymorphism and IBD, UC, or CD susceptibility/severity or response to therapy.

On the other hand, studies on TNF-β gene polymorphism showed that the frequency of GG at position +252 of intron 1 was significantly higher in IBD as compared to controls, while the frequency of GA genotype was also higher in patient group but the difference was not statistically significant. The difference in the distribution of allele A and allele G was also not statistically significant in IBD and control groups albeit the frequency of mutant allele G is higher in IBD patients (**Table 4**).

The stratification of TNF-β gene polymorphism results for IBD patients into UC and CD showed that the distribution of genotypes GG and GA was different in UC as compared to controls indicating that the genotype GG is susceptible and GA protective only for UC but not for CD as almost similar distribution of genotypes and allele frequencies of TNF-β -intron 1 +252 polymorphism was found among the CD and controls (**Table 5** and **Figure 2**).

The frequency distribution of alleles and genotypes of both TNF-α and-β polymorphisms is not affected by gender or type of IBD (familial or sporadic) (**Tables 6** and **7**).

The representative gel pictures of amplification of different genotypes for IL-10 G (-1082)A, IL-10 C (-819)T, and IL-10 C (-592)A are shown in **Figures 3–5**.

The results of three promoter polymorphism of IL-10 gene are summarized in **Tables 8–12**. The genotype GG of IL10 (-1082) was significantly higher (P = 0.02) in IBD patients (15.08%) than control group (7.50%). Contrarily, the genotype AA was found to be significantly lower (P = 0.02) in IBD patients (9.50%) as compared to controls (17.50%). On the other hand, the heterozygous GA genotype was almost same in patients and controls (P = 0.99) (**Table 8**).

Upon stratification of genotyping results into CD and UC, we noticed that frequency of genotypes and alleles of IL-10 G (-1082)A differed significantly between CD patients and controls. Frequencies of genotype GG and allele G were higher in CD patients while those of genotype AA and allele A lower in CD patients as compared to controls. On the other hand, no significant different was found in the frequencies of alleles and genotypes between UC and controls (**Table 9**).

The frequency of -819 CC genotype was 33.52% in the IBD patients compared to 41.50% in controls, while CT was 38.12% in IBD patients as compared to 48.50% in controls. The frequency of homozygous TT genotype was similar in both IBD and control samples (10.61 vs. 10.00%). The frequencies of all genotypes of IL-10 (819C/T) polymorphism did not differ

Ethnicity/population	Type of association with IBD	Reference
American	UC susceptibility	[96]
*Asian	Associated with UC	[59]
*Asian	Associated with UC and CD	[58]
*Asian	Associated with UC susceptibility	[97]
Belgian	No association with CD treatment	[98]
Belgian	Associated with CD behavior	[99]
Brazilian	Associated with severity of CD	[60]
Canadian	No association with CD	[27]
Canadian	No association with IBD	[100]
*Caucasians	Better response to TNF blockers	[101]
Czech	Associated with IBD	[102]
Dutch	No association with IBD	[103]
English	IBD susceptibility	[104]
*European	No association with UC	[97]
*European	Associated with UC and CD	[58]
German	No association with IBD	[105]
Han Chinese	Association with UC susceptibility	[106]
Han Chinese	Association with UC susceptibility	[57]
Hungarian	IBD susceptibility	[107]
Indian	No association with IBD	[108]
Iranian	No association with IBD	[109]
Iranian	No association with IBD	[110]
Irish	No association with IBD	[83]
Israeli	No association with granulomas in CD	[111]
Italian	Associated with therapy	[112]
Japanese	UC susceptibility	[113]
Korean	Association with CD susceptibility	[114]
Korean	Association with CD susceptibility	[115]
Mexican-Mestizo	UC susceptibility	[116]
Portuguese	Pathological profiles of CD	[117]
Russian	UC susceptibility	[118]
Saudis	IBD susceptibility	[93]
Spanish	No association with CD	[114]
Spanish	No association with UC	[119]
Turkish	No association with IBD susceptibility	[120]
Turkish	Association with UC susceptibility	[121]

*meta–analysis

Table 3. Association of TNF-a 308G/A polymorphism in UC, CD, or IBD in various ethnic populations worldwide.

Genotype/allele	IBD (n = 179)		Control (n = 200)		*P*-value	RR	EF*/PF
	n	%	n	%			
GG	39	21.79	28	14	0.05♣	1.711	0.241*
GA	120	67.04	148	74	0.14	0.714	0.151
AA	20	11.17	24	12	0.87	0.922	0.037
G-allele	198	55.31	204	51	0.24	1.189	0.078*
A-allele	160	44.69	196	49	0.24	0.841	0.078

EF = Etiologic fraction, PF = preventive fraction.
♣Statistically significant.
*data for EF

Table 4. Genotype and allele frequencies of TNF-β (+252A/G) polymorphism in IBD patients and matched controls.

Genotype/allele	CD (n = 95) n (%)	UC (n = 84) n (%)	Control (n = 200) n (%)
GG	16 (16.84)	23 (27.38)*	28 (14)
GA	69 (72.63)	51 (60.72)*	148 (74)
AA	10 (10.53)	10 (11.90)	24 (12)
G-allele	101 (53.16)	97 (57.74)	204 (51)
A-allele	89 (46.84)	71 (42.26)	196 (49)

*P value <0.05 compared to the frequency in controls.

Table 5. Genotype and allele frequencies of TNF-β (+252A/G) polymorphism in CD and UC patients.

Genotype/allele	Male (n = 89)		Female (n = 90)		*P*-value
	n	%	n	%	
GG	23	25.84	16	17.78	0.209
GA	57	64.05	63	70.00	0.429
AA	9	10.11	11	12.22	0.813
G-allele	103	57.87	95	52.78	0.340
A-allele	75	42.13	85	47.22	0.340

N = number of subjects.

Table 6. Genotype and allele frequencies of TNF-β (+252A/G) polymorphism in IBD male and female patients.

Genotype/allele	Familial (n = 22)		Sporadic (n = 157)		P-value
	n	%	n	%	
GG	4	18.18	35	22.29	0.780
GA	15	68.18	105	66.88	1.000
AA	3	13.64	17	10.83	0.717
G-allele	23	52.27	175	55.73	0.746
A-allele	21	47.73	139	44.27	0.746

Table 7. Genotypes and alleles of TNF-β (+252A/G) polymorphism in familial and sporadic IBD patients.

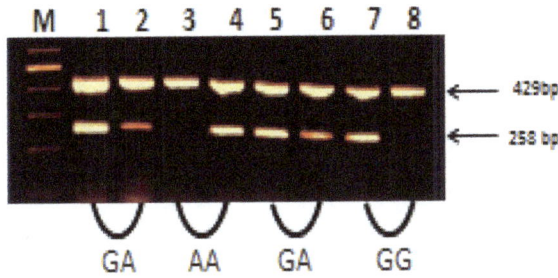

Figure 3. Shows the amplification of IL-10-1082G/A genotypes (GG, GA, and AA). Lane M: 100-bp DNA marker, lanes 1, 5, and 7: amplification of allele G, lanes 2,4, and 6: amplification of allele A, 258-bp band for target DNA, 429-bp band for internal control.

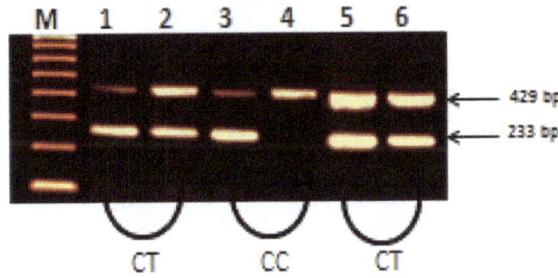

Figure 4. Shows the amplification of IL-10-819C/T genotypes (CT and CC). Lane M: 100-bp DNA marker, lanes 1, 3, and 5: amplification of allele C, lanes 2 and 6: amplification of allele T, 233-bp band for target DNA, 429-bp band for internal control.

significantly in patients and control groups. The allelic frequencies were also not different in patient and control groups (**Table 10**).

Upon stratification of subjects in to CD and UC, no significant difference was found in distribution of alleles and genotypes between patients and controls (**Table 11**).

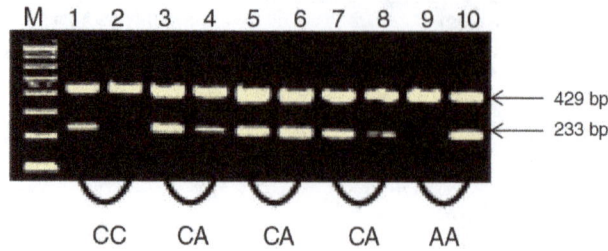

Figure 5. Shows the amplification of IL-10-592C/A genotypes (CC, CA, and AA). Lane M: 100-bp DNA marker, lanes 1, 3, 5, and 7: amplification of allele C, lanes 4, 6, 8, and 10: amplification of allele A, 233-bp band for target DNA, 429-bp band for internal control.

Genotype/allele	IBD (n = 179)		Control (n = 200)		P-value	RR	EF*/PF
	n	%	n	%			
GG	27	15.08	15	7.50	0.02♣	2.19	0.347*
GA	135	75.42	150	75.00	0.99	1.02	0.009*
AA	17	9.50	35	17.50	0.02♣	0.49	0.253
G-allele	189	52.79	180	45.00	0.03♣	1.36	0.135*
A-allele	169	47.21	220	55.00	0.03♣	0.73	0.138

EF = Etiologic fraction, PF = Preventive fraction.
♣Statistically significant.
*data for EF.

Table 8. Genotype and allele frequencies of (-1082G/A) IL-10 variants in IBD and matched controls.

Genotype/allele	CD (95) n (%)	UC (84) n (%)	Control (200) n (%)
GG	17 (17.90)*	10 (11.90)	15 (7.5)
GA	73 (76.84)	62 (73.81)	150 (75.0)
AA	5 (5.26)*	12 (14.29)	35 (17.50)
G-allele	107 (56.32)*	82 (48.81)	180 (45.0)
A-allele	83 (43.68)*	86 (51.19)	220 (55.0)

*P value <0.05 compared to the frequency in controls.

Table 9. Genotype and allele frequencies of (-1082G/A) IL-10 variants polymorphism in UC and CD patients.

Similarly, the frequencies of alleles and genotypes of IL-10(-592C/A) polymorphism were not significantly different in IBD patient and controls (**Table 12**).

Upon stratification of subjects into CD and UC, no significant difference was found in distribution of IL-10(-592C/A) alleles and genotypes between patients and controls (**Table 13**)

Genotype/allele	IBD (n = 179)		Control (n = 200)		P-value	RR	EF*/PF
	n	%	n	%			
CC	60	33.52	83	41.50	0.11	0.91	0.039
CT	100	55.87	97	48.50	0.18	1.34	0.128*
TT	19	10.61	20	10.00	0.86	1.06	0.027*
C-allele	220	61.45	263	65.75	0.22	0.83	0.085
T-allele	138	38.55	137	34.25	0.22	1.20	0.084*

*data for EF

Table 10. Genotype and allele frequencies of (819C/T) IL-10 variants in IBD and matched controls.

Genotype/Allele	CD (95) n (%)	UC (84) n (%)	Control (200) n (%)
CC	31 (32.63)	29 (34.52)	83 (41.50)
CT	53 (55.79)	47 (55.95)	97 (48.50)
TT	11 (11.58)	8 (9.53)	20 (10.00)
C-allele	115 (60.53)	105 (62.5)	263 (65.75)
T-allele	75 (39.47)	63 (37.5)	137 (34.25)

Table 11. Genotype and allele frequencies of (819C/T) IL-10 variants polymorphism in UC and CD patients.

Genotype/allele	IBD (n = 179)		Control (n = 200)		P-value	RR	EF*/PF
	n	%	n	%			
CC	60	33.52	83	41.50	0.11	0.91	0.039
CA	100	55.87	97	48.50	0.18	1.34	0.128*
AA	19	10.61	20	10.00	0.86	1.06	0.027*
C-allele	220	61.45	263	65.75	0.22	0.83	0.085
A-allele	138	38.55	137	34.25	0.22	1.20	0.084*

*data for EF

Table 12. Genotype and allele frequencies of (-592C/A) IL-10 variants in IBD and matched controls.

The association of IL-10 promoter polymorphism with UC, CD, or IBD in various ethnic population worldwide has been summarized in **Table 14**. The association is not consistent, and ethnic variations are evident in the type polymorphism and IBD, UC, or CD susceptibility.

Genotype/allele	CD (95) n (%)	UC (84) n (%)	Control (200) n (%)
CC	31 (32.63)	29 (34.52)	83 (41.50)
CA	53 (55.79)	47 (55.95)	97 (48.50)
AA	11 (11.58)	8 (9.53)	20 (10.00)
C-allele	115 (60.53)	105 (62.5)	263 (65.75)
T-allele	75 (39.47)	63 (37.5)	137 (34.25)

Table 13. Genotype and allele frequencies of (592C/A) IL-10 variants polymorphism in UC and CD patients.

Ethnicity/population	IL-10 polymorphism	Type of association with IBD	Reference
Australian	1082 G/A, 592 C/A	CD susceptibility	[84]
Canadian	1082 G/A, 819 C/T, 592 C/A	No association with IBD	[100]
Canadian	819 C/T	Associated with CD	[87]
*Caucasian	1082 G/A, 819 C/T	Associated with IBD susceptibility	[89]
*Caucasian	592 C/A	No association with IBD	[89]
Caucasian	1082 G/A	Associated with IBD	[38]
*Mixed	819 C/T, 519 C/A	Associated with UC	[88]
*Mixed	1082 G/A	No association with CD or UC	[88]
Mixed	1082 G/A, 819 C/T, 592 C/A	Associated with CD phenotype	[73]
*Mixed	1082 G/A	Associated with CD, No association with UC	[122]
New Zealand population	1082 G/A	Associated with CD,	[72]
Indian	1082 G/A, 819 C/T, 592 C/A	No association with IBD	[123]
Mexican	1082 G/A, 592 C/A	Associated with IBD susceptibility	[90]
Danish	1082 G/A, 819 C/T, 592 C/A	No association with IBD	[124]
Tunisian	Promoter polymorphism	Associated with CD	[125]
Turkish	1082 G/A	No association with IBD	[120]
Spanish	1082 G/A, 819 C/T, 592 C/A	No association with UC or CD	[126]
Spanish	1082 G/A	Associated with CD	[71]
Hungarian	1082 G/A	No association with CD	[127]
Korean	Promoter polymorphism	No association with IBD	[114]
German	1082 G/A, 592 C/A	No association with IBD	[91]
Italian	1082 G/A	Associated with UC	[86]
Italian	819 C/T	No association with UC	[86]

*Meta-analysis.

Table 14. Association of IL-10 promoter polymorphisms in UC, CD, or IBD in various ethnic populations worldwide.

4. Discussion

TNF-α being a key cytokine in the inflammatory response of IBD plays an important role in the digestive and systemic manifestations of the disease. Available literature on the TNF-α (-308G/A) polymorphism shows its importance in the pathogenesis of CD and UC [58–60]. From the outgoing results, it is clear that allele A and genotype GA of TNF-α (-308G/A) polymorphism are associated with IBD susceptibility in Saudi population. Our results are in accordance with the earlier reports from other populations. This polymorphism has been shown to affect the UC and CD susceptibility in Asians and Europeans. The allele A of TNF-α (-308G/A) is associated with UC susceptibility in Japanese and Han Chinese patients [57, 106, 113]. The genotype GA is a risk factor for UC in Asians, whereas homozygous genotype AA is risk for both UC and CD in European patients [58]. A meta-analysis besides supporting the association of TNF-α (308G/A) polymorphism with IBD in Asians suggested that genetic polymorphisms vary in Asians from Caucasians [59].

On the other hand, some reports support the association of TNF-α (-308G/A) polymorphism with the severity of IBD. TNF-α (-308G/A) polymorphism is reported to be significantly associated with the severity of CD and/or UC in Irish [83], Czech [102], Italian [112], Caucasian patients from New Zealand [128], and Brazilian patients [60]. However, it is not clear whether it is directly involved in pathophysiology of IBD or serve merely as markers in Linkage disequilibrium with susceptibility genes [83].

Moreover, the carriers of allele A are at greater risk of pancolitis and more likely to require bowel resection in UC and CD [102, 112]. The CD patients with allele A were reported to be more resistant to steroids compared with non-carriers. The CRP levels in UC and CD patients carrying allele A were found to be higher and reported to modify the disease phenotype, influence its activity, and lead to a more intense inflammatory response [112].

The increased inflammation, higher levels of C-reactive protein (CRP), TNF-α, and interleukin-1ß have been associated with the A-containing genotypes of TNF-α (-308G/A) polymorphism in the active phase of IBD [98, 99, 107, 129]. The higher frequency of allele A of TNF-α (308G/A) was found in anti-neutrophil cytoplasmic antibodies (ANCA)-positive than ANCA-negative IBD patients, which may have influences on the susceptibility IBD or the behavior of IBD [114].

On the other hand, homozygous genotype AA of TNF-α (-308) has been associated with susceptibility to CD in Portuguese patients, and it has been suggested that TNF-α (-308G/A) polymorphism is responsible for displaying distinct clinicopathological profiles in Portuguese CD patients [117].

However, contrary reports are also available in the literature. The lower frequency of allele A of TNF-α (-308G/A) has been reported in North European Caucasian and Korean patients with CD or UC as compared to healthy controls [103]. Although the frequency of allele G was reported to be slightly higher in Iranian Azeri Turkish IBD patients, it did not reach statistical significance [110]. Further, no association of TNF-α(-308G/A) polymorphism with IBD susceptibility was found in Australian [82], Brazilian [60, 130], Canadian [100], Chinese [106, 131],

Czech [132], French [133], Indian [108], Korean [115], Newfoundland [27], Spanish [126], and Turkish [120] populations. The reason for these differences in the TNF-α genetic associations with IBD etiology might be the variations in sample size, genotyping methods, and/or ethnicity itself as frequencies of alleles and genotypes of TNF-α (-308G/A) also vary in different ethnic healthy populations worldwide [39] (**Table 3**).

Our genotyping results for TNF-β (+252A/G) polymorphism showed that genotype GG was significantly associated with IBD susceptibility. Our results also indicated that genotype GA was slightly lower in IBD patient than the controls, but the difference did not reach statistical significance. However, when the results were stratified into CD and UC, it became evident that this polymorphism was associated only with UC but not with CD in Saudi population (**Table 4**, **Figure 2**). In contrast, some earlier reports suggested that the TNF-β (+252) polymorphism is not associated with CD or UC in Chinese, French, Korean, and Spanish patients [57, 106, 115, 119, 133]. It is possible that the TNF-β (+252A/G) polymorphism may be indirectly associated with IBD as it has been suggested to influence the expression/production of TNF-α [42].

Muro et al. [134] reported that the inflammatory response in IBD is effected by the changes in TNF-α and TNF-β levels and IBD patients are commonly treated with TNF-α inhibitors. Moreover, TNF-α gene polymorphisms are reported to affect the gene expression level of TNF-α, and a particular TNF-α genotype may influence the response of IBD patients treated with TNF-α inhibitors as mutated allele A of TNF-α(-308) and allele G of TNF-β(+252) polymorphisms have been associated with greater TNF-α transcription [35, 36, 42, 135].

Our study on Saudi IBD patients suggested a significant association between allele and genotype frequency of TNF-α (-308G/A) and TNF-β (+252A/G) polymorphisms and IBD susceptibility in Saudi population. It is evident from outgoing discussion that ethnicity plays a very important role in genetic association of TNF-α and TNF-β polymorphism with IBD. It is also inferred that the both the polymorphism may have synergistic effect on the susceptibility and may work in tandem to influence the etiology of IBD in Saudi population. The outcome of present study will not only help in the prognosis of IBD in Saudi population but also provide guideline for the treatment with anti-TNF therapy as individuals with different genotypes of TNF-α (-308G/A) respond differently to anti-TNF-α treatment [136, 137]. However, further studies are required involving other ethnic populations to strengthen these findings.

The genotyping results for IL-10-1082 G/A polymorphism indicated that genotype -1082GG and allele G are susceptible to IBD (RR = 2.19, EF = 0.347, RR = 1.36, EF = 0.135, respectively), while genotype AA and allele A are resistant to IBD (RR = 0.49, PF = 0.0.253, RR = 0.73, PF = 0.138, respectively). Upon stratification of genotyping results into CD and UC, we noticed that genotype GG and allele G of -1082 G/A polymorphism were associated with CD susceptibility, while genotype AA and allele A might be protective for CD. On the other hand, no significant association was found either with alleles or genotypes of -1082 G/A polymorphism and UC in Saudi patients. These results are in accordance with the various reports, which also indicted an association of IL-10-1082G/A polymorphism susceptibility to IBD [89, 122]. A meta-analysis including 18 case-control studies provided evidence for the association between IL-10-1082G/A polymorphism and susceptibility of CD [122]. Another met-analysis including 15 studies demonstrated clear association between the IL-10-1082G/A polymorphisms and the risk of IBD [89]. The allele G of -1082G/A polymorphism has been associated with the IBD, and higher serum levels of IL-10 concentration have been reported in IBD patients than in the controls [72, 90]. Earlier studies with CD patients also indicated that IL-10-1082 G/A polymorphisms contribute to susceptibility to CD [71] and -1082G allele was significantly increased in patients with CD than controls [73] while A allele of the IL-10-1082G/A was associated with decreased IL-10 production in CD patients and controls [78].

Contrary to these, some studies reported that there are no significant differences in the allele and genotype frequencies of the IL-10-1082G/A polymorphism between IBD patients and controls in various populations [88, 91, 120]. Klein et al. [91] reported that IL-10-1082G/A polymorphism is not demonstrably involved in the predisposition of IBD in German cohort. Similarly, no association between Turkish IBD patients and IL-10-1082G/A was found [120]. A meta-analysis by Zou et al. [88] observed that IL-10-1082G/A polymorphism is not associated with IBD. These data provide evidence that the effect of IL-10 gene polymorphisms on cytokine production differs in CD, UC patients, and controls in various populations.

Further, our results indicated that IL-10-1082G/A polymorphism is not associated with UC susceptibility in Saudi patients. These are in accordance with earlier reports indicating no association of IL-10-1082G/A polymorphisms with susceptibility of UC [88, 122]. Mendoza et al. [138] reported that IL-1082G allele is not associated with the phenotype of UC patients in Madrid's Spanish population.

On the other hand, IL-10-1082 G/A polymorphism has been reported to influence susceptibility to UC [38, 86, 126]. A gender effect has been reported, with women of AG/AA genotypes of IL-10-1082 G/A, having a higher risk of developing UC at a younger age and is related to the lower IL-10 production associated with the -1082A allele and to the IL10 downregulating effect of estrogens [86]. A mild influence of -1082 G allele in UC appearance has also been reported by Castro-Santos et al. [126]. In a stratified analysis, a highly significant association between the -1082 AA genotype and the steroid dependency was observed in IBD, and it was suggested that carriage of the -1082 AA genotype (low producer) is a relevant risk factor for developing steroid-dependent IBD. Tagore et al. [38] suggested that individuals genetically predisposed to produce less IL-10 are at a higher risk of developing IBD, and the frequency of the high IL-10 producer allele (-1082 G) is decreased in the whole IBD group and in the UC patients compared with normal.

The two other polymorphisms of IL-10 gene (IL-10-819C/T and IL-10-592C/A) are not associated with the susceptibility of IBD as the frequency distribution of genotypes and alleles of these two polymorphisms did not differ significantly between controls and IBD patient groups. The stratification of our results in to CD and UC patients also indicated that IL-10-819C/T and IL-10-592C/A polymorphisms are associated with neither with CD nor UC susceptibility in our patients. Similarly, Castro-Santos et al. [126] did not find any association between IL-10 (-812 C/T and -592 C/A) polymorphisms and UC or CD susceptibility. A recent meta-analysis demonstrated no significant association between the -592C/A polymorphism and IBD, CD, or UC, but a clear association with IL-10-819C/T polymorphism [89], while several other report showed that these polymorphisms are associated with IBD risk [72, 87, 88, 90, 139].

These differences in the association of IL-10-819C/T and IL-10-592C/A polymorphisms with CD or UC can be attributed to ethnic variations.

The exact mechanism by which IL-10 affects the susceptibility/pathogenesis of IBD is far from clear. It participates in the regulation of the immune response at several levels [69]. IL-10 regulates the inflammatory response, by inhibiting proinflammatory Th1 cytokines production [140].

IL-10 cytokine downregulates the expression of major histocompatibility complex (MHC) of class I and II molecules [141, 142]. It also has potent stimulatory effects on B lymphocytes, resulting in increased production of immunoglobulin and DNA replication [141]. The immune-stimulating effects of IL-10 have also been reported. IL-10 is shown to induce activated B cells to secrete large amounts of IgG, IgA, and IgM and in combination with IL-4 which results in the secretion of four immunoglobulin isotypes. The increased levels of IL-10 play a role in the amplification of humoral responses in some diseases [141].

Sanchez-Munoz et al. [143] suggested that the intestinal inflammation in IBD is controlled by a complex interplay of innate and adaptive immune mechanisms. Cytokines determine T-cell differentiation of Th1, Th2, T regulatory, and Th17 cells in IBD, and cytokines levels regulate the development, recurrence, and exacerbation of the inflammatory process in IBD. The dysregulation of T cells, or an over-production of effector T cells, results in the development and exacerbation of IBD [144]. Thus, the antigen-presenting cells (APCs), Th1, Th2, T regulatory cells, and Th17 and their cytokine products play an important role in the etiology of IBD [8]. These cellular interactions are modulated by pro- or anti-inflammatory cytokines (such as TNF-α, INF-γ, IL-1, IL-6, IL-4, IL-5, IL10, TGF-β, IL-13, IL-12, IL-18, IL-23) [145]. Although many common responses in IBD are mediated by cytokines, how cytokines determine the nature of the immune response in IBD may be quite different among different IBD forms [146].

A highly significant increase in IL-10 mRNA levels in T lymphocytes and in IL-10-positive cells in the colons of UC patients has been reported by Melgar et al. [147]. Moreover, IL-10 production by regulatory T cells has also been implicated as important factor in IBD [148]. Another regulatory B cells subtype called Bregs may also take part in UC etiology by producing IL-10 [149]. The significance of IL-10 produced by B cells has been indicated in IBD patients and animal models also [150, 151]. The Bregs can be responsible for the suppression and/or recovery from acquired immune-mediated inflammations by IL-10 and TGF-β1 in IBD [143, 149]. However, the exact mechanism is still far from clear and needs to be investigated.

5. Conclusion

Our study dealing with the five polymorphisms of proinflammatory and anti-inflammatory cytokine genes in Saudi IBD patients clearly indicates that the TNF-α (-308G/A), TNF-β (+252A/G), and IL-10 (-1082 G/A) polymorphisms are associated significantly with the risk of IBD susceptibility while other two, IL-10-819C/T and IL-10-592C/A, polymorphisms are not associated with IBD in Saudi population. However, due to several limitations in the present study, it is suggested that well-designed epidemiological as well as genetic association studies with large sample size among different ethnicities should be performed in order to have better understanding of this relationship.

Acknowledgment

The authors would like to thank S. Sadaf Rizvi and Mohammad Al-Asmari for their help in laboratory work.

Author details

Abdulrahman Al-Robayan[1], Misbahul Arfin[2], Ebtissam Saleh Al-Meghaiseeb[1], Reem Al-Amro[1] and Abdulrahman K Al-Asmari[2]*

*Address all correspondence to: abdulrahman.alasmari@gmail.com

1 Department of Gastroenterology, Prince Sultan Military Medical City, Riyadh, Saudi Arabia

2 Research Centre, Prince Sultan Military Medical City, Riyadh, Saudi Arabia

References

[1] Cosnes J, Gower-Rousseau C, Seksik P, Cortot A. Epidemiology and natural history of inflammatory bowel diseases. Gastroenterology. 2011; 140: 1785–1794.

[2] Fadda MA, Peedikayil MC, Kagevi I, Kahtani KA, Ben AA, Al HI, Sohaibani FA, Quaiz MA, Abdulla M, Khan MQ, Helmy A. Inflammatory bowel disease in Saudi Arabia: a hospital-based clinical study of 312 patients. Ann Saudi Med. 2012; 32: 276–282.

[3] Gunisetty S, Tiwari S, Bardia A, Phanibhushan M, Satti V, Habeeb M, Khan A. The epidemiology and prevalence of Ulcerative colitis in the South of India. O J Immunol. 2012; 2: 144–148.

[4] Molodecky NA, Soon IS, Rabi DM, et al. Increasing incidence and prevalence of the inflammatory bowel diseases with time, based on systematic review. Gastroenterology. 2012; 142: 46–54.

[5] Zeng Z, Zhu Z, Yang Y, Ruan W, Peng X, Su Y, Peng L, Chen J, Yin Q, Zhao C, Zhou H, Yuan S, Hao Y, Qian J, Ng SC, Chen M, Hu P. Incidence and clinical characteristics of inflammatory bowel disease in a developed region of Guangdong Province, China: a prospective population-based study. J Gastroenterol Hepatol. 2013; 28: 1148–1153.

[6] Podolsky DK. Inflammatory bowel disease. N Engl J Med. 2002; 347: 417–429.

[7] Strober W, Fuss I, Mannon P. The fundamental basis of inflammatory bowel disease. J Clin Invest. 2007; 117: 514–52.

[8] Xavier RJ, Podolsky DK. Unravelling the pathogenesis of inflammatory bowel disease. Nature. 2007; 448: 427–434.

[9] Jussila A, Virta LJ, Pukkala E, Färkkilä MA. Mortality and causes of death in patients with inflammatory bowel disease: a nationwide register study in Finland. J Crohns Colitis. 2014; 8: 1088–1096.

[10] Gent AE, Hellier MD, Grace RH, Swarbrick ET, Coggon D. Inflammatory bowel disease and domestic hygiene in infancy. Lancet. 1994; 343: 766–767.

[11] Matricon J, Barnich N, Ardid D. Immunopathogenesis of inflammatory bowel disease. Self Nonself. 2010; 1: 299–309.

[12] Yang SK, Hong WS, Min YI, Kim HY, Yoo JY, Rhee PL, Rhee JC, Chang DK, Song IS, Jung SA, Park EB, Yoo HM, Lee DK, Kim YK. Incidence and prevalence of ulcerative colitis in the Songpa-Kangdong District, Seoul, Korea, 1986–1997. J Gastroenterol Hepatol. 2000; 15: 1037–1042.

[13] Ling KL, Ooi CJ, Luman W, Cheong WK, Choen FS, Ng HS. Clinical characteristics of ulcerative colitis in Singapore, a multiracial city-state. J Clin Gastroenterol. 2002; 35: 144–148.

[14] Inoue N, Tamura K, Kinouchi Y, Fukuda Y, Takahashi S, Ogura Y, Inohara N, Núñez G, Kishi Y, Koike Y, Shimosegawa T, Shimoyama T, Hibi T. Lack of common NOD2 variants in Japanese patients with Crohn's disease. Gastroenterology. 2002; 123: 86–91.

[15] Leong RW, Lau JY, Sung JJ. The epidemiology and phenotype of Crohn's disease in the Chinese population. Inflamm Bowel Dis. 2004; 10: 646–651.

[16] Kim ES, Kim WH. Inflammatory bowel disease in Korea: epidemiological, genomic, clinical, and therapeutic characteristics. Gut Liver. 2010; 4: 1–14.

[17] Yun J, Xu CT, Pan BR. Epidemiology and gene markers of ulcerative colitis in the Chinese. World J Gastroenterol. 2009; 15: 788–803.

[18] Waterman M, Xu W, Stempak JM, et al. Distinct and overlapping genetic loci in Crohn's disease and ulcerative colitis: correlations with pathogenesis. Inflamm Bowel Dis. 2011; 17: 1936–1942.

[19] Jump RL, Levine AD. Mechanisms of natural tolerance in the intestine: implications for inflammatory bowel disease. Inflamm Bowel Dis. 2004; 10(4): 462–478.

[20] Neuman MG. Immune dysfunction in inflammatory bowel disease. Transl Res. 2007; 149 (4): 173–186.

[21] Hoffmann SC, Stanley EM, Darrin Cox E, Craighead N, DiMercurio BS, Koziol DE, Harlan DM, Kirk AD, Blair PJ. Association of cytokine polymorphic inheritance and in vitro cytokine production in anti-CD3/CD28-stimulated peripheral blood lymphocytes. Transplantation. 2001; 72(8): 1444–1450.

[22] Melk A, Henne T, Kollmar T, Strehlau J, Latta K, Offner G, Jhangri GS, Ehrich JH, Von Schnakenburg C. Cytokine single nucleotide polymorphisms and intrarenal gene expression in chronic allograft nephropathy in children. Kidney Int. 2003; 64(1): 314–320.

[23] Hotoleanu C, Popp R, Trifa AP, Nedelcu L, Dumitrascu DL. Genetic determination of irritable bowel syndrome. World J Gastroenterol. 2008; 14(43): 6636–6640.

[24] van der Veek PP, van den Berg M, de Kroon YE, Verspaget HW, Masclee AA. Role of tumor necrosis factor-alpha and interleukin-10 gene polymorphisms in irritable bowel syndrome. Am J Gastroenterol. 2005; 100(11): 2510–2516.

[25] Plevy SE, Landers CJ, Prehn J, et al. A role for TNF-alpha and mucosal T helper-1 cytokines in the pathogenesis of Crohn's disease. J Immunol. 1997; 159: 6276–6282.

[26] Komatsu M, Kobayashi D, Saito K, et al. Tumor necrosis factor-alpha in serum of patients with inflammatory bowel disease as measured by a highly sensitive immuno-PCR. Clin Chem. 2001; 47: 1297–1301.

[27] Zipperlen K, Peddle L, Melay B, Hefferton D, Rahman P. Association of TNF-alpha polymorphisms in Crohn disease. Hum Immunol. 2005; 66: 56–59.

[28] Deleporte A, Viennot S, Dupont B, et al. Efficacy of anti-TNF-alpha monoclonal antibodies in inflammatory bowel disease treatment. Int J Interferon Cytokine Mediator Res. 2013; 5: 11–31.

[29] Westendorp RG, Langermans JA, Huizinga TW, Elouali AH, Verweij CL, Boomsma DI, Vandenbroucke JP. Genetic influence on cytokine production and fatal meningococcal disease. Lancet. 1997; 349(9046): 170–173.

[30] Sharma S, Sharma A, Kumar S, Sharma SK, Ghosh B. Association of TNF haplotypes with asthma, serum IgE levels, and correlation with serum TNF-alpha levels. Am J Respir Cell Mol Biol. 2006; 35: 488–495.

[31] Sharma S, Ghosh B, Sharma SK. Association of TNF polymorphisms with sarcoidosis, its prognosis and tumour necrosis factor (TNF)-alpha levels in Asian Indians. Clin Exp Immunol. 2008; 151: 251–259.

[32] Abraham LJ, Kroeger KM. Impact of the -308 TNF promoter polymorphism on the transcriptional regulation of the TNF gene: relevance to disease. J Leukoc Biol. 1999; 66: 562–566.

[33] Braun N, Michel U, Ernst BP, Metzner R, Bitsch A, Weber F, Riechmann P. Gene polymorphism at position -308 of the tumor-necrosis-factor-alpha (TNF-alpha) in multiple sclerosis and its influence on the regulation of TNF-alpha production. Neurosci Lett. 1996; 215: 75–78.

[34] Wilson AG, Gordon C, di Giovine FS, de Vries N, van de Putte LB, Emery P, Duff GW. A genetic association between systemic lupus erythematosus and tumor necrosis factor alpha. Eur J Immunol. 1994; 24: 191–195.

[35] Wilson AG, Symons JA, McDowell TL, McDevitt HO, Duff GW. Effects of a polymorphism in the human tumor necrosis factor alpha promoter on transcriptional activation. Proc Natl Acad Sci USA. 1997; 94: 3195–3099.

[36] Jeong P, Kim EJ, Kim EG, Byun SS, Kim CS, Kim WJ. Association of bladder tumors and GA genotype of -308 nucleotide in tumor necrosis factor-alpha promoter with greater tumor necrosis factor-alpha expression. Urology. 2004; 64: 1052–1056.

[37] Cuenca J, Perez C, Aguirre A, Schiattino I, Aguillon JC. Genetic polymorphism at position -308 in the promoter region of the tumor necrosis factor (TNF): implications of its allelic distribution on susceptibility or resistance to diseases in the Chilean population. Biological Res. 2001; 34: 237–241.

[38] Tagore A, Gonsalkorale WM, Pravica V, Hajeer AH, McMahon R, Whorwell PJ, Sinnott PJ, Hutchinson IV. Interleukin-10 (IL-10) genotypes in inflammatory bowel disease. Tissue Antigens. 1999; 54(4): 386–390.

[39] Al-Rayes H, Al-Swailem R, Albelawi M, Arfin M, Al-Asmari A, Tariq M. TNF-α and TNF-β gene polymorphism in Saudi Rheumatoid Arthritis patients. Clin Med Insights Arthritis Musculoskelet Disord. 2011; 4: 55–63.

[40] Al-Okaily F, Arfín M, Al-Rashidi S, Al-Balawi M, Al-Asmari A. Inflammation-related cytokine gene polymorphisms in Behçet's disease. J Inflamm Res. 2015; 8: 173–180.

[41] Al-Mohaya MA, Al-Harthi F, Arfin M, AL-Asmari A. TNF-α, TNF-β and IL-10 gene polymorphism and association with oral lichen planus risk in Saudi patients. J Appl Oral Sci. 2015; 23(3): 295–301.

[42] Messer G, Spengler U, Jung MC, et al. Polymorphic structure of the tumor necrosis factor (TNF) locus: an Ncol Polymorphism in the first intron of the human TNF-beta gene correlates with a variant amino acid in position 26 and a reduced level of TNF-beta production. J Exp Med. 1991; 173: 209–219.

[43] Wilson AG, Di Giovine FS, Blakemore AIF, Duff GW. Single base polymorphism in the human tumor necrosis factor alpha (TNF-α) gene detectable by Nco1 restriction of PCR product. Hum Mol Gen. 1992; 1: 353.

[44] Galbratith GM, Pendey JP. Tumor necrosis factor alpha (TNF-alpha) gene polymorphism in alopecia areata. Hum Genet. 1995; 96: 433–436.

[45] Patino-Gracia A, Sotillo-Pineiro E, Modesto C, Sierrasesumaga L. Analysis of the human tumour necrosis factor-alpha(TNF α) gene promoter polymorphisms in children with bone cancer. J Med Genet. 2000; 37: 789–792.

[46] Abraham LJ, French MAH, Dawkins RL. Polymorphic MHC ancestral haplotypes affect the activity of tumour necrosis factor-alpha. Clin Exp Immunol. 1993; 92: 14–18.

[47] Kula D, Jurecka-Tuleja B, Gubala E, Krawczyk A, Szpak S, Jarzab M. Association of polymorphism of LT alpha and TNF genes with Graves disease. Folia Histochem Cytobiol. 2001; 39 Suppl 2: 77–78.

[48] Medcraft J, Hitman GA, Sachs JA, Whichelow CE, Raafat I, Moore RH. Autoimmune renal disease and tumour necrosis factor beta gene polymorphism. Clin Nephrol. 1993; 40: 63–68.

[49] Zelano G, Lino MM, Evoli A, Settesoldi D, Batocchi AP, Torrente I, Tonali PA. Tumor necrosis factor beta gene polymorphism in myasthenia Gravis. Eur J Immunogenet. 1998; 25: 403–408. ISSN 0960-7420.

[50] Albuquerque RV, Hayden CM, Palmer LJ, Laing IA, Rye PJ, Gibson NA, Burton PR, Goldblatt J, Lesouef PN. Association of polymorphism within the tumour necrosis factor (TNF) genes and childhood asthma. Clin Exp Allergy. 1998; 28: 578–584. ISSN 0954-7894.

[51] Lu LY, Cheng HH, Sung PK, Tai MH, Yeh JJ, Chen A. Tumor necrosis factor –beta +252A polymorphism is associated with systemic lupus erythematosus in Taiwan. J Formos Med Assoc. 2005; 104: 563–570. ISSN 0929-6646.

[52] Pandey JP, Takeuchi F. TNF-alpha and TNF-beta gene polymorphism in systemic sclerosis. Hum Immunol. 1999; 60: 1128–1130. ISSN 0198-8859.

[53] Vasku V, Vasku A, Izakovicova Holla L, Tschoplova S, Kankova K, Benakova N, Semradova V. Polymorphism in inflammation genes (angiotensinogen, TAP1 and TNF-beta) in Psoriasis. Arch Dermatol Res. 2000; 292: 531–534. ISSN 0340-3696.

[54] Takeuchi F, Nabeta H, Hong GH, Kawasugi K, Mori M, Matsuta K, Kuwata S, Murayama T, Nakano K. The genetic contribution of the TNFa11 microsatellite allele and the TNFb +252*2 allele in Japanese RA. Clin Exp Rheumatol. 2005; 23: 494–498. ISSN 0392-856X.

[55] Boraska V, Zeggini E, Groves CJ, Rayner NW, Skrabic V, Diakite M, Rockett KA, Kwiatkowski D, McCarthy MI, Zemunik T. Family based analysis of tumor necrosis factor and lymphotoxin-alpha Tag polymorphism with type 1 diabetes in the population of South Croatia. Hum Immunol. 2009; 70: 195–199. ISSN 0198-8859.

[56] Tiancha H, Huiqin W, Jiyong J, Jingfen J, Wei C. Association between lymphotoxin-α intron +252 polymorphism and sepsis: a meta analysis. Scand J Infect Dis. 2011; 43: 436–447. ISSN 0036-5548.

[57] Cao Q, Zhu Q, Wu ML, Hu WL, Gao M, Si JM. Genetic susceptibility to ulcerative colitis in the Chinese Han ethnic population: association with TNF polymorphisms. Chin Med J (Engl). 2006; 119: 1198–1203.

[58] Fan W, Maoqing W, Wangyang C, et al. Relationship between the polymorphism of tumor necrosis factor-α-308 G>A and susceptibility to inflammatory bowel diseases and colorectal cancer: a meta-analysis. Eur J Hum Genet. 2011; 19: 432–437.

[59] Ng SC, Tsoi KK, Kamm MA, et al. Genetics of inflammatory bowel disease in Asia: systematic review and meta-analysis. Inflamm Bowel Dis. 2012; 18: 1164–1176.

[60] Santana G, Bendicho MT, Santana TC, Reis LB, Lemaire D, Lyra AC. The TNF-α -308 polymorphism may affect the severity of Crohn's disease. Clinics (Sao Paulo). 2011; 66: 1373–1377.

[61] Maynard CL, Weaver CT. Diversity in the contribution of interleukin- 10 to T-cell-medi-ated immune regulation. Immunol Rev. 2008; 226: 219–233.

[62] Thio CL. Host genetic factors and antiviral immune responses to hepatitis C virus. Clin Liver Dis. 2008; 12: 713–726.

[63] Kuhn R, Lohler J, Rennick D, Rajewsky K, Muller W. Interleukin-10-deficient mice develop chronic enterocolitis. Cell. 1993; 75: 263–274.

[64] Ishizuka K, Sugimura K, Homma T, Matsuzawa J, Mochizuki T, Kobayashi M, Suzuki K, Otsuka K, Tashiro K, Yamaguchi O, Asakura H. Influence of interleukin-10 on the inter-leukin-1 receptor antagonist/interleukin-1 beta ratio in the colonic mucosa of ulcerative colitis. Digestion. 2001; 63(Suppl 1): 22–27.

[65] Correa I, Veny M, Esteller M, Piqué JM, Yagüe J, Panés J, Salas A. Defective IL-10 production in severe phenotypes of Crohn's disease. J Leukoc Biol. 2009; 85(5): 896–903.

[66] Schreiber S, Heinig T, Thiele HG, Raedler A. Immunoregulatory role of interleukin 10 in patients with inflammatory bowel disease. Gastroenterology. 1995; 108: 1434–1444.

[67] Mitchell SA, Grove J, Spurkland A, Boberg KM, Fleming KA, Day CP, Schrumpf E, Chapman RW. European study group of primary sclerosing cholangitis. Association of the tumour necrosis factor alpha -308 but not the interleukin 10-627 promoter polymor-phism with genetic susceptibility to primary sclerosing cholangitis. Gut. 2001; 49(2): 288–294.

[68] Fillatreau S, Gray D, Anderton SM. Not always the bad guys: B cells as regulators of autoimmune pathology. Nat Rev Immunol. 2008; 8(5): 391–397.

[69] Moore KW, de Waal Malefyt R, Coffman RL, O'Garra A. Interleukin-10 and the interleu-kin-10 receptor. Annu Rev Immunol. 2001; 19: 683–765.

[70] Williams LM, Ricchetti G, Sarma U, Smallie T, Foxwell BM. Interleukin-10 suppression of myeloid cell activation—a continuing puzzle. Immunology. 2004; 113(3): 281–292.

[71] Fernandez L, Martinez A, Mendoza JL, Urcelay E, Fernandez-Arquero M, Garcia-Paredes J, et al. Interleukin-10 polymorphisms in Spanish patients with IBD. Inflamm Bowel Dis. 2005; 11: 739–743.

[72] Wang AH, Lam WJ, Han DY, Ding Y, Hu R, Fraser AG, Ferguson LR, Morgan AR. The effect of IL-10 genetic variation and interleukin 10 serum levels on Crohn's disease susceptibility in a New Zealand population. Hum Immunol. 2011; 72(5): 431–435.

[73] Almeida NP, Santana GO, Almeida TC, Bendicho MT, Lemaire DC, Cardeal M, Lyra AC. Polymorphisms of the cytokine genes TGFB1 and IL10 in a mixed-race population with Crohn's disease. BMC Res Notes. 2013; 6: 387.

[74] D'Alfonso S, Rampi M, Rolando V, Giordano M, Momigliano-Richiardi P. New poly-morphisms in the IL-10 promoter region. Genes Immun. 2000; 1: 231–233.

[75] Mormann M, Rieth H, Hua TD, Assohou C, Roupelieva M, Hu SL, et al. Mosaics of gene variations in the interleukin-10 gene promoter affect interleukin-10 production depending on the stimulation used. Genes Immun. 2004; 5: 246–255.

[76] Eskdale J, Gallagher G, Verweij CL, Keijsers V, Westendorp RG, Huizinga TW. Interleukin 10 secretion in relation to human IL-10 locus haplotypes. Proc Natl Acad Sci USA. 1998; 95(16): 9465–9470.

[77] Liang L, Zhao YL, Yue J, Liu JF, Han M, Wang H, Xiao H. Interleukin-10 gene promoter polymorphisms and their protein production in pleural fluid in patients with tuberculosis. FEMS Immunol Med Microbiol. 2011; 62(1): 84–90.

[78] Koss K, Satsangi J, Fanning GC, Welsh KI, Jewell DP. Cytokine (TNF alpha, LT alpha and IL-10) polymorphisms in inflammatory bowel diseases and normal controls: differential effects on production and allele frequencies. Genes Immun. 2000; 1: 185–190.

[79] Turner DM, Williams DM, Sankaran D, Lazarus M, Sinnott PJ, Hutchinson IV. An investigation of polymorphism in the interleukin-10 gene promoter. Eur J Immunogenet. 1997; 24: 1–8.

[80] Lesiak A, Zakrzewski M, Przybyłowska K, Rogowski-Tylman M, Wozniacka A, Narbutt J. Atopic dermatitis patients carrying G allele in -1082 G/A IL-10 polymorphism are predisposed to higher serum concentration of IL-10. Arch Med Sci. 2014; 10 (6): 1239–1243.

[81] Wang NG, Wang DC, Tan BY, Wang F, Yuan ZN. TNF-α and IL10 polymorphisms interaction increases the risk of ankylosing spondylitis in Chinese Han population. Int J Clin Exp Pathol. 2015; 8(11): 15204–15209. eCollection 2015.

[82] Al-Asmary S, Kadasah S, Arfin M, TariqM, Al-Asmari A. Genetic variants of Interleukin - 10 gene promoter are associated with schizophrenia in Saudi patients: a case control study. North Am J Med Sci. 2014; 6: 558–565.

[83] Balding J, Livingstone WJ, Conroy J, Mynett-Johnson L, Weir DG, Mahmud N, Smith OP. Inflammatory bowel disease: the role of inflammatory cytokine gene polymorphisms. Mediators Inflamm. 2004; 13(3): 181–187.

[84] Fowler EV, Eri R, Hume G, Johnstone S, Pandeya N, Lincoln D, et al. TNFalpha and IL10 SNPs act together to predict disease behaviour in Crohn's disease. J Med Genet. 2005; 42: 523–528.

[85] Franke A, Balschun T, Karlsen TH, Hedderich J, May S, Lu T, et al. Replication of signals from recent studies of Crohn's disease identifies previously unknown disease loci for ulcerative colitis. Nat Genet. 2008; 40: 713–715.

[86] Tedde A, Laura PA, Bagnoli S, Congregati C, Milla M, Sorbi S, et al. Interleukin-10 promoter polymorphisms influence susceptibility to ulcerative colitis in a gender-specific manner. Scand J Gastroenterol. 2008; 43: 712–718.

[87] Amre DK, Mack DR, Morgan K, Israel D, Lambrette P, Costea I, Krupoves A, Fegury H, Dong J, Grimard G, Deslandres C, Levy E, Seidman EG. Interleukin 10 (IL-10) gene variants and susceptibility for paediatric onset Crohn's disease. Aliment Pharmacol Ther. 2009; 29(9): 1025–1031.

[88] Zou L, Wang L, Gong X, Zhao H, Jiang A, Zheng S. The association between three promoter polymorphisms of IL-10 and inflammatory bowel diseases (IBD): a meta-analysis. Autoimmunity. 2014; 47(1): 27–39.

[89] Lv H, Jiang Y, Li J, Zhang M, Shang Z, Zheng J, Wu X, Liu P, Zhang R, Yu H. Association between polymorphisms in the promoter region of interleukin-10 and susceptibility to inflammatory bowel disease. Mol Biol Rep. 2014; 41(3): 1299–1310.

[90] Garza-González E, Pérez-Pérez GI, Mendoza-Ibarra SI, Flores-Gutiérrez JP, Bosques-Padilla FJ. Genetic risk factors for inflammatory bowel disease in a North-eastern Mexican population. Int J Immunogenet. 2010; 37(5): 355–359.

[91] Klein W, Tromm A, Griga T, Fricke H, Folwaczny C, Hocke M, Eitner K, Marx M, Runte M, Epplen JT. The IL-10 gene is not involved in the predisposition to inflammatory bowel disease. Electrophoresis. 2000; 21(17): 3578–3582.

[92] Lennard-Jones JE. Classification of inflammatory bowel disease. Scand J Gastroenterol Suppl. 1989; 170: 2–6; discussion 16–9.

[93] Al-Meghaiseeb ES, Al-Robayan AA, Al-Otaibi MM, Arfin M, Al-Asmari AK. Association of tumor necrosis factor-α and -β gene polymorphisms in inflammatory bowel disease. J Inflamm Res. 2016; 9: 133–140.

[94] Schallreuter KU, Levenig C, Kühnl P, Löliger C, Hohl-Tehari M, Berger J. Histocompatibility antigens in vitiligo: Hamburg study on 102 patients from northern Germany. Dermatology. 1993; 187: 186–192.

[95] Svejgaard A, Platz P, Ryder LP. HLA and disease 1982—a survey. Immunol Rev. 1983; 70: 193–218.

[96] Garrity-Park MM, Loftus EV Jr, Bryant SC, Sandborn WJ, Smyrk TC. Tumor necrosis factor-alpha polymorphisms in ulcerative colitis-associated colorectal cancer. Am J Gastroenterol. 2008; 103(2): 407–415.

[97] Lu Z, Chen L, Li H, Zhao Y, Lin L. Effect of the polymorphism of tumor necrosis factor-alpha-308 G/A gene promoter on the susceptibility to ulcerative colitis: a meta-analysis. Digestion. 2008; 78(1): 44–51.

[98] Louis E, Vermeire S, Rutgeerts P, et al. A positive response to infliximab in Crohn disease: association with a higher systemic inflammation before treatment but not with -308 TNF gene polymorphism. Scand J Gastroenterol. 2002; 37: 818–824.

[99] Louis E, Peeters M, Franchimont D, et al. Tumor necrosis factor (TNF) gene polymorphism in Crohn's disease (CD): influence on disease behavior? Clin Exp Immunol. 2000; 119: 64–68.

[100] Cantor MJ, Nickerson P, Bernstein CN. The role of cytokine gene polymorphisms in determining disease susceptibility and phenotype in inflammatory bowel disease. Am J Gastroenterol. 2005; 100: 1134–1142.

[101] Song GG, Seo YH, Kim JH, Choi SJ1, Ji JD, Lee YH. Association between TNF-α (-308 A/ G, -238 A/G, -857 C/T) polymorphisms and responsiveness to TNF-α blockers in spondyloarthropathy, psoriasis and Crohn's disease: a meta-analysis. Pharmaco-genomics. 2015; 16(12): 1427–1437.

[102] Sykora J, Subrt I, Didek P, et al. Cytokine tumor necrosis factor-alpha A promoter gene polymorphism at position -308 G–>A and pediatric inflammatory bowel disease: implications in ulcerative colitis and Crohn's disease. J Pediatr Gastroenterol Nutr. 2006; 42: 479–487.

[103] Bouma G, Xia B, Crusius JB, et al. Distribution of four polymorphisms in the tumor necrosis factor (TNF) genes in patients with inflammatory bowel disease (IBD). Clin Exp Immunol. 1996; 103: 391–396.

[104] Shetty A, Forbes A. Pharmacogenomics of response to anti-tumor necrosis factor therapy in patients with Crohn's disease. Am J Pharmacogenomics. 2002; 2(4): 215–221.

[105] Martin K, Radlmayr M, Borchers R, Heinzlmann M, Folwaczny C. Candidate genes co-localized to linkage regions in inflammatory bowel disease. Digestion. 2002; 66(2): 121–126.

[106] Song Y, Wu KC, Zhang L, et al. Correlation between a gene polymorphism of tumor necrosis factor and inflammatory bowel disease. Chin J Dig Dis. 2005; 6: 170–174.

[107] Vatay A, Bene L, Kovacs A, et al. Relationship between the tumor necrosis factor alpha polymorphism and the serum C-reactive protein levels in inflammatory bowel disease. Immunogenetics. 2003; 55: 247–252.

[108] Mittal RD, Manchanda PK, Bid HK, Ghoshal UC. Analysis of polymorphisms of tumor necrosis factor-alpha and polymorphic xenobiotic metabolizing enzymes in inflammatory bowel disease: study from northern India. J Gastroenterol Hepatol. 2007; 22: 920–924.

[109] Naderi N, Farnood A, Dadaei T, Habibi M, Balaii H, Firouzi F, Mahban A, Soltani M, Zali M. Association of tumor necrosis factor alpha gene polymorphisms with inflammatory bowel disease in Iran. Iran J Public Health. 2014; 43(5): 630–636.

[110] Bonyadi M, Abdolmohammadi R, Jahanafrooz Z, Somy MH, Khoshbaten M. TNF-alpha gene polymorphisms in Iranian Azeri Turkish patients with inflammatory bowel diseases. Saudi J Gastroenterol. 2014; 20: 108–112.

[111] Dalal I, Karban A, Wine E, Eliakim R, Shirin H, Fridlender M, Shaoul R, Leshinsky-Silver E, Levine A. Polymorphisms in the TNF-alpha promoter and variability in the granulomatous response in patients with Crohn's disease. Pediatr Res. 2006; 59(6): 825–828.

[112] Cucchiara S, Latiano A, Palmieri O, et al. Polymorphisms of tumor necrosis factor alpha but not MDR1 influence response to medical therapy in pediatric-onset inflammatory bowel disease. J Pediatr Gastroenterol Nutr. 2007; 44: 171–179.

[113] Sashio H, Tamura K, Ito R, et al. Polymorphisms of the TNF gene and the TNF receptor super family member 1B gene are associated with susceptibility to ulcerative colitis and Crohn's disease, respectively. Immunogenetics. 2002; 53: 1020–1027.

[114] Kim TH, Kim BG, Shin HD, et al. Tumor necrosis factor-alpha and interleukin-10 gene polymorphisms in Korean patients with inflammatory bowel disease. Korean J Gastroenterol. 2003; 42: 377–386.

[115] Yang SK, Lee SG, Cho YK, Lim J, Lee I, Song K. Association of TNF-a/LTA polymorphisms with Crohn's disease in Koreans. Cytokine. 2006; 35: 13–20.

[116] Yamamoto-Furusho JK, Uscanga LF, Vargas-Alarcón G, Rodríguez-Pérez JM, Zuñiga J, Granados J. Polymorphisms in the promoter region of tumor necrosis factor alpha (TNF-alpha) and the HLA-DRB1 locus in Mexican mestizo patients with ulcerative colitis. Immunol Lett. 2004; 95(1): 31–35.

[117] Ferreira AC, Almeida S, Tavares M, et al. NOD2/CARD15 and TNFA, but not IL1B and IL1RN, are associated with Crohn's disease. Inflamm Bowel Dis. 2005; 11: 331–339.

[118] Livzan MA, Makeĭkina MA. Prognostic factors of ulcer colitis flow. Eksp Klin Gastroenterol. 2013; 8: 17–23.

[119] Papo M, Quer JC, Gutierrez C, et al. Genetic heterogeneity within ulcerative colitis determined by an interleukin-1 receptor antagonist gene polymorphism and antineutrophil cytoplasmic antibodies. Eur J Gastroenterol Hepatol. 1999; 11: 413–420.

[120] Celik Y, Dagli U, Kiliç MY, et al. Cytokine gene polymorphisms in Turkish patients with inflammatory bowel disease. Scand J Gastroenterol. 2006; 41: 559–565.

[121] Gök İ, Uçar F, Ozgur O. Inflammatory cytokine gene polymorphism profiles in Turkish patients with ulcerative colitis. Med Glas (Zenica). 2015; 12(1): 33–39.

[122] Zhu H, Lei X, Liu Q, Wang Y. Interleukin-10-1082A/G polymorphism and inflammatory bowel disease susceptibility: a meta-analysis based on 17,585 subjects. Cytokine. 2013; 61(1): 146–153.

[123] Ahirwar DK, Kesarwani P, Singh R, Ghoshal UC, Mittal RD. Role of tumor necrosis factor-alpha (C-863A) polymorphism in pathogenesis of inflammatory bowel disease in Northern India. J Gastrointest Cancer. 2012; 43(2): 196–204.

[124] Andersen V, Ernst A, Christensen J, Østergaard M, Jacobsen BA, Tjønneland A, Krarup HB, Vogel U. The polymorphism rs3024505 proximal to IL-10 is associated with risk of ulcerative colitis and Crohn's disease in a Danish case-control study. BMC Med Genet. 2010; 11: 82.

[125] Marrakchi R, Moussa A, Ouerhani S, Bougatef K, Bouhaha R, Messai Y, Rouissi K, Khadimallah I, Khodjet-el-Khil H, Najar T, Benammar-Elgaaeid A. Interleukin 10

promoter region polymorphisms in inflammatory bowel disease in Tunisian population. Inflamm Res. 2009; 58(3): 155–160.

[126] Castro-Santos P, Suarez A, Lopez-Rivas L, Mozo L, Gutierrez C. TNF alpha and IL-10 gene polymorphisms in inflammatory bowel disease. Association of -1082 AA low producer IL-10 genotype with steroid dependency. Am J Gastroenterol. 2006; 101: 1039–1047.

[127] Klausz G, Molnár T, Nagy F, Gyulai Z, Boda K, Lonovics J, Mándi Y. Polymorphism of the heat-shock protein gene Hsp70-2, but not polymorphisms of the IL-10 and CD14 genes, is associated with the outcome of Crohn's disease. Scand J Gastroenterol. 2005; 40 (10): 1197–1204.

[128] Ferguson LR, Huebner C, Petermann I, et al. Single nucleotide polymorphism in the tumor necrosis factor-alpha gene affects inflammatory bowel diseases risk. World J Gastroenterol. 2008; 14: 4652–4661.

[129] Gonzalez S, Rodrigo L, Martinez-Borra J, et al. TNF-alpha -308A promoter polymorphism is associated with enhanced TNF-alpha production and inflammatory activity in Crohn's patients with fistulizing disease. Am J Gastroenterol. 2003; 98: 1101–1106.

[130] Queiroz DM, Oliveira AG, Saraiva IE, et al. Immune response and gene polymorphism profiles in Crohn's disease and ulcerative colitis. Inflamm Bowel Dis. 2009; 15: 353–358.

[131] Han Z, Li C, Han S, et al. Meta-analysis: polymorphisms in TNF-alpha gene promoter and Crohn's disease. Aliment Pharmacol Ther. 2010; 32: 159–170.

[132] Hradsky O, Lenicek M, Dusatkova P, et al. Variants of CARD15, TNFA and PTPN22 and susceptibility to Crohn's disease in the Czech population: high frequency of the CARD15 1007fs. Tissue Antigens. 2008; 71: 538–547.

[133] Heresbach D, Ababou A, Bourienne A, et al. Polymorphism of the microsatellites and tumor necrosis factor genes in chronic inflammatory bowel diseases. Gastroenterol Clin Biol. 1997; 21: 555–561.

[134] Muro M, López-Hernández R, Mrowiec A. Immunogenetic biomarkers in inflammatory bowel diseases: role of the IBD3 region. World J Gastroenterol. 2014; 20: 15037–15048.

[135] Brinkman BM, Giphart MJ, Verhoef A, Kaijzel EL, Naipal AM, Daha MR, Breedveld FC, Verweij CL. Tumor necrosis factor alpha-308 gene variants in relation to major histocompatibility complex alleles and Felty's syndrome. Hum Immunol. 1994; 41: 259–266.

[136] Peyrin-Biroulet L. Anti-TNF therapy in inflammatory bowel diseases: a huge review. Minerva Gastroenterol Dietol. 2010; 56: 233–243.

[137] Lopez A, Billioud V, Peyrin-Biroulet C, Peyrin-Biroulet L. Adherence to anti-TNF therapy in inflammatory bowel diseases: a systematic review. Inflamm Bowel Dis. 2013; 19: 1528–1533.

[138] Mendoza JL, Urcelay E, Lana R, Martínez A, Taxonera C, de la Concha EG, Díaz-Rubio M. Polymorphisms in the interleukin-10 gene and relation to phenotype in patients with ulcerative colitis. Rev Esp Enferm Dig. 2006; 98(2): 93–100.

[139] Shiotani A, Kusunoki H, Kimura Y, Ishii M, Imamura H, Tarumi K, Manabe N, Kamada T, Hata J, Haruma K. S100A expression and interleukin-10 polymorphisms are associated with ulcerative colitis and diarrhea predominant irritable bowel syndrome. Dig Dis Sci. 2013; 58(8): 2314–2323.

[140] Fiorentino DF, Zlotnik A, Vieira P, Mosmann TR, Howard M, Moore KW, O'Garra A. IL-10 acts on the antigen-presenting cell to inhibit cytokine production by Th1 cells. J Immunol. 1991; 146(10): 3444–3451.

[141] Rousset F, Garcia E, Defrance T, Vezzio N, Peronne C, Hsu DH, Kastelein R, Moore KW, Banchereau J. Interleukin 10 is a potent growth and differentiation factor for activated human B lymphocytes. Proc Natl Acad Sci USA. 1992; 89: 1890–1893.

[142] Tsuruma T, Yagihashi A, Torigoe T, Sato N, Kikuchi K, Watanabe N, Hirata K. Interleukin-10 reduces natural killer sensitivity and downregulates MHC class I expression on H-ras-transformed cells. Cell Immunol. 1998; 184(2): 121–128.

[143] Sanchez-Munoz F, Dominguez-Lopez A, Yamamoto-Furusho JK. Role of cytokines in inflammatory bowel disease. World J Gastroenterol. 2008; 14(27): 4280–4288.

[144] Leon F, Smythies LE, Smith PD, Kelsall BL. Involvement of dendritic cells in the pathogenesis of inflammatory bowel disease. Adv Exp Med Biol. 2006; 579: 117–132.

[145] Papadakis KA, Targan SR. Role of cytokines in the pathogenesis of inflammatory bowel disease. Annu Rev Med. 2000; 51: 289–298.

[146] Ince MN, Elliott DE. Immunologic and molecular mechanisms in inflammatory bowel disease. Surg Clin North Am. 2007; 87(3): 681–696.

[147] Melgar S, Yeung MM, Bas A, Forsberg G, Suhr O, Oberg A, Hammarstrom S, Danielsson A, Hammarstrom ML. Over-expression of interleukin 10 in mucosal T cells of patients with active ulcerative colitis. Clin Exp Immunol. 2003; 134(1): 127–137.

[148] Latinne D, Fiasse R. New insights into the cellular immunology of the intestine in relation to the pathophysiology of inflammatory bowel diseases. Acta Gastroenterol Belg. 2006; 69(4): 393–405.

[149] Mizoguchi A, Bhan AK. A case for regulatory B cells. J Immunol. 2006; 176(2): 705–710.

[150] Mizoguchi A, Mizoguchi E, Takedatsu H, Blumberg RS, Bhan AK. Chronic intestinal inflammatory condition generates IL-10-producing regulatory B cell subset characterized by CD1d upregulation. Immunity. 2002; 16(2): 219–230.

[151] Goetz M, Atreya R, Ghalibafian M, Galle PR, Neurath MF. Exacerbation of ulcerative colitis after rituximab salvage therapy. Inflamm Bowel Dis. 2007; 13(11): 1365–1368.

11

Interleukin 23 in IBD Pathogenesis

Ahmet Eken and Mohamed Oukka

Abstract

Interleukin-23 (IL-23) is a cytokine that belongs to the IL-12 cytokine family that is produced mainly by antigen-presenting cells. IL-23 receptor is expressed by various innate and adaptive immune cells, including group 3 innate lymphoid cells (ILC3), neutrophils, γδ T cells, Th17 and natural killer T (NKT) cells. IL-23 regulates various functions of the responding cells critical for host protective responses but is also implicated in many chronic inflammatory diseases including inflammatory bowel diseases (IBD). IL-23 receptor signaling components and downstream effector cytokines IL-17A/F, interferon-gamma (IFN-γ), IL-22, granulocyte macrophage colony–stimulating factor (GMCSF) have been shown to impact IBD-like disease development in various animal models; therapeutic approaches targeting the IL-23 pathway in IBD are in clinical trials. In this chapter, we attempt to review the literature on IL-23–mediated IBD pathogenesis. We did this by gathering the current information about the individual IL-23–producing and IL-23–responsive cells as to how they contribute to IBD pathology through various inflammatory mediators.

Keywords: IL-23, p19, Th17, ILC3

1. Introduction

1.1. IL-23 cytokine

Interleukin-23 (IL-23) is a heterodimeric cytokine that belongs to the IL-12 family cytokines and shares both ligand and receptor subunits with IL-12. IL-23 heterodimer is made up of p19 (IL-23A) and the shared beta chain, p40 (IL12β) subunit which also dimerizes with IL-12p35 and makes up IL-12 cytokine. Due to the shared use of p40, studies performed via the manipulation of p40 prior to the discovery of IL-23 suggested causality between many chronic inflammatory conditions and the IL-12/Th1 axis. With the genetic and immunologic studies that targeted individual subunits of IL-12 and IL-23 in mice, a critical causal role for IL-23 in inflammatory bowel disease (IBD) pathogenesis has been established.

1.2. General features of IL-23 protein structure

Human p19 is a four-α-helix protein with 70% similarity with its mouse ortholog. It is encoded by its gene located on chromosome 12q13.2 which is composed of four exons and three introns. p19 protein contains five cysteine residues and several O-glycosylation but no N-glycosylation sites. Human p40 gene, however, is located on chromosome 11q1.3. It is made up of eight exons and seven introns. p40 has homology with soluble class I cytokine receptor chains such as IL-6Rα, and it is composed of three domains (D1-3). p40 is N-glycosylated and can form homodimers. p19 protein by itself does not have any known biological role. Both p40 and p19 has to be produced within the same cell for the generation of biologically active IL-23 hetero-dimers [1]. The heterodimeric interaction between the p19 and p40 subunits is stabilized by a disulfide bond between p19 residue Cys54 and p40 Cys177 [2].

1.3. Cellular sources of IL-23

IL-23 is expressed and secreted by professional antigen-presenting cells (APCs), chiefly dendritic cells, macrophages and monocytes. Epithelial cells were also shown to contribute to IL-23 production. These include keratinocytes [3], intestinal epithelial cells [4] and glomerular podocytes (epithelial cells in the Bowman's capsule especially during nephrotoxic serum (NTS) nephritis (NTN)) [5]. Furthermore, human fibroblast-like synoviocytes (*ex vivo* and *in vivo*) and human colon subepithelial myofibroblasts were shown to produce IL-23p19 upon IL-1β and TNF-α all of which suggest that non-hematopoietic sources may also contribute to IL-23 production to some extent, given the right stimulation [6, 7].

Different subsets of DCs exist, defined by their developmental origin, tissue location and surface markers [8, 9]. Stimulation with select ligands induces IL-23 production by CD11c$^+$ conventional DCs, pDCs or *ex vivo*-generated BMDC (mice) to varying degrees. The exact source of IL-23 *in vivo* among DC subsets during steady state, infection or chronic inflammation has been queried in various reports and, it appears, may be context dependent. Conventional DCs (cDCs) rely on transcription factor Zbtb46 and include CD8$^+$, CD4$^+$, CD4$^-$CD8$^-$ subsets in the lymphoid organs, and Langerhans cells in the skin, and interstitial single positive CD103$^+$ or CD11b$^+$ DCs in the connective tissues; CD11b$^+$CD103$^+$, CD11b$^-$CD103$^+$, CD11b$^+$CD103$^-$ as well as DN DC subsets are present in the gut [10]. CD11b$^+$ CD103$^+$ DCs were shown to be dependent on Notch2 and IRF4, and during *Citrobacter rodentium* infection, this subset was reported to be the primary source of IL-23 [10–12]. CD11b$^-$ fraction of CD103$^+$ DCs, which relies on Batf3 was shown to be dispensable for *C. rodentium* immunity [12]. Others also reported CD11b$^+$CD103$^+$ population as the main IL-23 source upon exposure to TLR5 ligand flagellin [13]. In the lung, CD11b$^+$ but not CD103$^+$ DCs were reported to be the major IL-23 source [10].

Siddiqui et al. showed that, in the context of intestinal inflammation (during T-cell transfer colitis and anti-CD40-induced colitis), E-cadherin$^+$ CD11b$^+$ DCs increase, and these cells are potent IL-23 producers. Despite the expression of CD103 by E-cadherin$^+$ DCs in the steady state, during inflammation, the investigators reported loss of CD103 expression, and inflammatory E-cadherin[+]CD11b[+] DCs were proposed to develop from Gr-1[+] monocyte precursors [14].

Besides the reports implicating CD103[+] DCs' role in IL-23 production, another study by Longman et al., however, reported that CX3CR1[+] phagocytes not CD103[+] DCs are the main IL-23 producer in mice [15]. Also in humans, they showed that CX3CR1[+]CD14[+] monocyte/macrophages, rather than CD103[+] DCs, produced more IL-23 upon various Toll-like receptors (TLR) ligands. These are in line with previous reports which showed elevated macrophages (CD14[+] CD68[+] also CD205[+]) with increased IL-23 production in the intestines of IBD patients [16]. Similarly, in *Helicobacter hepaticus*/anti-IL-10R model of murine colitis, CD103[+] DCs were shown to be dispensable and produced low amounts of IL-23; the major source of IL-23 was MHCII[+] Ly6C[+] monocytes, CXCR1High F4/80[+] macrophages and CX3CR1intLy6C[low] macrophages/DC population [17]. Thus, in summary, the results regarding the source of IL-23 are divergent; information regarding IL-23 production by different APC subsets in the human intestine is incomplete (**Figure 1**).

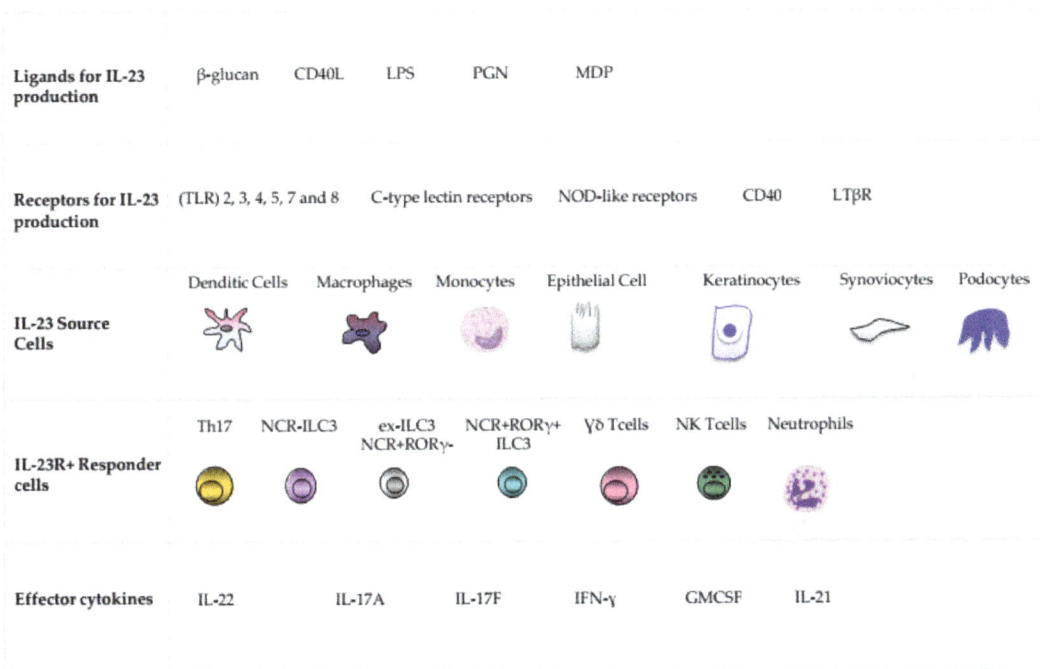

Ligands for IL-23 production	β-glucan	CD40L	LPS	PGN	MDP			
Receptors for IL-23 production	(TLR) 2, 3, 4, 5, 7 and 8		C-type lectin receptors	NOD-like receptors		CD40	LTβR	
IL-23 Source Cells	Denditic Cells	Macrophages	Monocytes	Epithelial Cell		Keratinocytes	Synoviocytes	Podocytes
IL-23R+ Responder cells	Th17	NCR-ILC3	ex-ILC3 NCR+RORγ-	NCR+RORγ+ ILC3	Yδ Tcells	NK Tcells	Neutrophils	
Effector cytokines	IL-22	IL-17A	IL-17F	IFN-γ	GMCSF	IL-21		

Figure 1. IL-23 inducers, producers and responders.

1.4. IL-23 stimulatory ligands

Microbiota (and pathogen-associated molecular patterns [PAMPs]) play an essential role in IL-23 production. As such, while IL-23 is constitutively expressed in the terminal ileum of SPF-housed mice, its expression is drastically reduced in the germ-free animals [18]. Pattern recognition receptors (PRR) link extracellular signals to p19 and p40 production [19,

20]. Stimulation of C-type lectin receptors, select Toll-like receptors (TLR), and CD40 by their corresponding ligands leads to IL-23 production [21]. β-glucan stimulation of APCs through C-type lectin receptor dectin-1 activates p19, p40 and p35 production (both IL-12 and IL-23) [22]. The ligand used here is curdlan, which is a pure β-glucan. β-glucan when combined with R848 (TLR7/8 ligand) or Pam2C (TLR2/6 ligand) also further increases IL-23 production [23]. TLR2 stimulation with peptidoglycan (PGN) alone, a gram-positive bacterial cell wall component, also induces preferential IL-23 production over IL-12 by DCs. LPS, a TLR4 ligand, can also induce IL-23p19 production, though not as potent as TLR2 ligand PGN [24]. The involvement of TLR4 in IL-23 production was shown using WT and LPS-deficient bacterial strains [25]. Bacterial nucleotide oligomerization domain 2 (NOD2)-ligand muramyl dipetide (MDP) can synergize with TLR2, TLR3, TLR4 ligands (PGN, dsRNA, LPS, respectively) and induces IL-23 production [26]. MDP can also synergize with TLR7/8 ligand R848 to promote IL-23 production [23]. TLR5 ligand flagellin also promotes IL-23 production [13]. It must be noted that DC type used in the abovementioned studies (BMDC, moDC or CD11c⁺) is important and may result in differential degrees of IL-23 expression in response to abovementioned ligands.

CD40L stimulation of intestinal DCs preferentially stimulates IL-23 production and this induction is much higher compared with moDCs or splenic DCs [27]. Thus, not only microbial signals, but also those coming from T cells can regulate IL-23 production.

Prostaglandin E2 (PGE2), by engaging the G-protein coupled receptors E prostanoid 2 and EP4, also stimulates IL-23 production [28]. Similarly, extracellular nucleotides can signal through purinergic P2Y receptor for IL-23 production [29].

Non-hematopoietic cells also can express IL-23p19. IL-1β and TNF-α stimulation induces IL-23p19 production by synoviocytes [6]. LPS stimulation of TLR4 or ligation of agonistic antibody to LTβR in the colon epithelial cell line stimulates IL-23 production [4]. Similarly, colon epithelial cells, *in situ*, were shown to produce IL-23 in an LTβR-dependent fashion.

1.5. IL-23 gene expression

IL-23 expression is induced through various MAPKs including p38, JNK and ERK [30], as well as NFκB. The p40 gene expression is regulated at the transcriptional level by binding of NFκB, CCAAT/enhancer-binding protein (C/EBP), ets-2, PU.1, IRF1, IRF2, IRF5, IRF8 and activator protein 1 (AP-1) to the promoter region of p40 [31–34] upon stimulation with various ligands. The murine and human p19 promoter was also shown to contain three NFκB binding sites [30]. Two of these binding sites have been shown to be involved in TLR-mediated activation of p19 transcription. Smad3, AP-1 and activating transcription factor-2 (ATF-2) transcription factors were also shown to bind p19 promoter and positively regulate IL-23p19 expression. There are two binding sites for 2 interferon regulatory factor (IRF) genes, IRF3 and IRF7 in both human and murine p19 promoters. IRF3 was reported to be a positive regulator of p19 expression, and thus, its absence was shown to lead to the downregulation of p19 [35].

1.6. IL-23 responsive cells

IL-23 receptor is expressed by both innate and adaptive immune cells. Group 3 ILCs (ILC3), dendritic cells, macrophages/monocytes, $\gamma\delta$ T cells, and more recently, neutrophils were among the innate cells that were shown to respond to IL-23. Among IL-23R$^+$ adaptive immune cells are Th17, Th22 and some iNKT cells [36].

1.6.1. Th17 cells

The most studied IL-23 responsive cells are Th17 cells. IL-23 is needed for the maintenance/maturation and expansion of Th17 cells in humans and mice and is dispensable for their initial differentiation from naïve CD4$^+$ T cells. The maintenance of Th17 identity relies on IL-23-mediated induction of *Rorc, Il23r* and *Il17* expression [19]. Th17 cells also require IL-23 to fully acquire a pathogenic character [37]. In fact, several laboratories showed that Th17 cells are very weak inducers of EAE, a mouse model of human MS, unless they are generated in the presence of IL-23 or they express IL-23R. IL-23 exposure programs Th17 cells transcriptionally to have a unique effector cytokine profile compared to nonpathogenic Th17 cells which are not exposed to IL-23. Unlike nonpathogenic Th17 cells, which express only IL-17, IL-23-activated pathogenic Th17 cells express IFN-γ and GMCSF in addition to the IL-17. Various lines of evidence suggest that Th17 cells, and hence IL-23R signaling, is critical for the development of chronic inflammatory conditions such as Crohn's disease, ulcerative colitis, psoriasis, rheumatoid arthritis (RA) and systemic lupus erythematous (SLE) in addition to MS.

1.6.2. Group 3 ILCs

Rorγt$^+$ Group 3 innate lymphoid cells (ILC3s) are a heterogeneous population of cells which have an irreplaceable function in protective immunity against extracellular pathogens in the gastrointestinal mucosa. ILC3s have also been recently implicated in the pathogenesis of inflammatory bowel diseases (IBD) [38–40]. ILC3s express IL-23R and depend on IL-23 for their production of various effector cytokines including IL-22, IFN-γ and IL-17, which take part in the abovementioned processes.

1.6.3. $\gamma\delta$ T cells

A fraction of $\gamma\delta$ T cells ubiquitously express IL-23R and produce IL-22, IL-21 and IL-17 upon IL-23 stimulation [41]. Skin and mucosal surfaces, particularly intestinal intraepithelial compartment, contain more $\gamma\delta$ T cells than other microenvironments. These cells are involved in protective immunity against various pathogens. Studies in mouse models of various chronic inflammatory diseases revealed that $\gamma\delta$ T cells may take part in the pathogenesis of IBD, psoriasis, MS and rheumatoid arthritis (RA) via their effector cytokines [41].

1.6.4. Antigen-presenting cells

Data regarding expression of IL-23R by APCs are scarce but do exist. Rorγt was reported to be expressed by CD45$^+$CD11b$^+$ cells, but these cells were found to be CD11c$^-$Gr1$^-$ initially. However, this study focused more on LTi cells not APCs. Sakhina Begum-Haque reported the presence of Rorγt+ DCs in the context of EAE in the CNS [42]. More recently, Karthaus et al. profiled nuclear receptor expression in murine DCs from various tissues and reported expression of RORγ in pLN and SPLN-resident DCs, and some expression was even observed in BMDC [43]. MLN-resident DCs expressed much higher RORγ message. Conventional DCs expressed more mRNA message than pDCs. Protein levels, however, were not quantified in this work. Short Rorc isoform Rorγt was also not examined. In line with these studies, we reported GFP+ CD11b+ myleoid cells in our IL-23R GFP reporter mice [36]. A better character-ization at the protein and functional level of IL-23R and Rorγt is needed to decipher the role of IL-23R in APC function and chronic inflammation.

1.6.5. Neutrophils

Neutrophils in both humans and mice were shown to express IL-23R, Rorγt, IL-17A and IL-22 and respond to IL-23. Due to their prompt recruitment to the sites of infection and abundance, they can limit the infections [44] and the damage associated with chronic inflammation [45].

1.6.6. NKT and other cells

A fraction of NK1.1− invariant Natural killer T cells (iNKT) express Rorγt, IL-23R and, in response to IL-23, produce IL-17 and IL-22. Rorγt+ iNKT cells are present in the peripheral lymph nodes. IL-23R signaling appears to be important for maintaining the number of such iNKT cells in humans [46]. How IBD pathology is regulated via IL-23-dependent response of iNKT is unclear [47, 48].

A group of CD3+ CD4−CD8− Rag-dependent T cells were also reported to express IL-23R [49]. Such cells have been shown to increase in number in an IL-23-dependent manner during systemic lupus erythematosus and ankylosing spondylitis murine models.

1.7. IL-23 receptor signaling and down-stream inflammatory mediators

IL-23 signals through its heterodimeric receptor (IL-23R) that is composed of two subunits: IL-12Rβ1, which is shared by IL-12 receptor complex, and IL-23R, which is the unique subunit. The p19 subunit of IL-23 heterodimer interacts with IL-23R, whereas the p40 subunit interacts with IL-12Rβ1 chain. In both humans and mice, IL-23R locus is positioned proximal to IL-12Rβ2 on chromosomes 1 and 6, respectively, and thus is believed to evolve through a gene duplication process [50]. IL-23R is conserved among amniotes and the unique IL-23R subunit protein is made up of 629 and 659 amino acids in humans and mice, respectively. Mouse and human IL-23R has 84% similarity. IL-23R sequence is also highly similar to IL-12Rβ2 and gp130.

IL-23 receptor signals through JAK kinases and STAT transcription factors. IL-23 binding of IL-23R activates of Jak2 and Tyk2, which then phosphorylate the receptor, creating docking sites for the recruitment of STAT proteins. STAT1, 3, 4, 5 are subsequently phosphorylated by activated Jak2 and Tyk2 kinases. The major transcription factor activated by IL-23 stimulation is STAT3. Pathways activated upon IL-23 binding to its receptor include the P38 MAPK pathway, PI3K-Akt and NFκ-B pathway [51–53]. IL-23 signaling activates transcription of various effector cytokine genes including IL-17A, IL-17F, IL-22 and IFN-γ whose roles in IBD will be reviewed in the sections below.

1.8. IL-23 receptor signaling is involved in IBD in murine models and human studies

Various lines of evidence from murine studies built a pathogenic role for IL-23 signaling in IBD pathogenesis. Using $p19^{-/-}$, $p35^{-/-}$ and $p40^{-/-}$ mice and neutralizing antibodies against p19, p35 and p40, IL-23p19, but not IL-12p35, was demonstrated to be necessary for the development of spontaneous colitis in IL-10$^{-/-}$ mice [54]. Similarly, innate colitis induced by *H. hepaticus* in both Rag$^{-/-}$ or Rag sufficient hosts [55, 56] as well as adaptive T-cell colitis induced in Rag$^{-/-}$ mice via transfer of CD45RB^{high} naïve T cells [54–56] or CD45RB^{low} IL-10$^{-/-}$ memory T cells [54] were all dependent on IL-23p19 but not p35. Moreover, p19 KO mice were shown to be resistant to development of chemically induced colitis via DSS treatment [57]; conversely, IL-23p19 overexpression in mice resulted in enteropathy [58]. Similar to its ligand, IL-23 receptor is required for the development of adoptive naïve CD4$^+$ T-cell–induced colitis [59], chemically induced DSS-driven colitis in the presence of adaptive immune cells [57] and innate cell-driven colitis induced via anti-CD40 treatment [60] in mice.

Data obtained from the studies with human IBD patients regarding the ligand as well as IL-23 receptor strongly suggest a role for this pathway in IBD development. In this regard, IL-23 was found to be elevated in the intestinal tissue of IBD patients [16]. Similarly, IL-23R mRNA was upregulated in individual lymphocytes (NK$^+$, CD4$^+$, CD8$^+$ cells) obtained from both lamina propria and peripheral blood of CD and UC patients [61, 62]. Sophisticated genome wide association studies revealed IL-23R and downstream signaling molecules JAK2, TYK2, STAT3 variants as risk or resistance factors for CD and UC [63, 64]. Some of the identified variants have been studied. rs11209026 (or R381Q) SNP was discovered as a protective variant for CD [63] and UC [65] in Jewish and non-Jewish cohorts which was later shown to be a loss of function mutation in IL-23R [66, 67]. Arg-381 is located in the cytoplasmic domain of IL-23R protein and is well conserved among species, whereas Gln-381 allele is less frequent [63]. A later study demonstrated that CD8$^+$ and memory CD4$^+$ T cells purified from Gln-381 IL23R allele carriers produced less IL-17 and IL-22 in response to IL-23 stimulation, and that R381Q carriers contain fewer circulating Th17 and Tc17 cells compared to healthy Arg-381 carriers [68]. Peripheral blood mononuclear cells (PBMC) from individuals with R381Q variant also produce less IL-17 in response to the *Borrelia burgdorferi*, a potent inducer of Th17 responses [69]. Moreover, R381Q IL-23R transfected cell lines displayed reduced STAT3 phosphorylation compared with control IL-23R. These reports collectively provide a mechanistic explanation for the resistance to CD and UC of R381Q SNP allele. Other protective variants against Crohn's include p.Arg86Gln, p.Gly149Arg and p.Val362Ile [70]. The last two also protect from UC. Mechanistically how they affect IL-23R signaling remains unknown. p.Gly149Arg affects a highly conserved extracellular domain of IL-23R, whereas p.Arg86Gln and p.Val362Ile are variants in the poorly conserved domains [71]. These SNPs are believed to reduce IL-23R activity, but experimentally this has yet to be shown.

Risk variants of IL-23R for CD were also described [63]. They are thought to be gain of function mutations. rs10889677 is one such variant with a transversion in the 3' UTR of IL-23R where an A in the wild-type allele is mutated to C. This mutation was shown to abolish a regulatory pathway directed by miRNA Let-7e and Let-7f, which consequently resulted in elevated IL-23R mRNA and protein production in human PBMC and CD4$^+$ T cells [72].

Other SNPs in SAT3 (rs381676, rs744166 and rs11871801), in JAK2 (rs10758669), and in TYK2 have been described. However, mechanisms of action of these variants with regard to their impact on IL-23R signaling requires further study [73, 74].

2. IL-23-producing cells in IBD pathogenesis

Antigen-presenting cells are the primary source of IL-23. Thus, mutations in any of the genes responsible in the IL-23 production pathway by APCs would potentially have consequences for IBD pathogenesis. Indeed, examples of such defects in the literature exist. An example of a link between PRR and dysregulated IL-23 production was observed in individuals with NOD2 variant 1007fsinsC [75]. As described above, NOD2 is a cytosolic PRR that detects bacterial cell wall component, and three variants of this receptor were found in 40% of CD patients in western countries [76]. Recently, NOD2 was shown to crosstalk with TLR2 pathway to regulate IL-23 expression by dendritic cells via mobilizing miRNAs. miR-29 expression was shown to be augmented by this crosstalk, which directly targets IL-12p40 mRNA and indirectly IL-23p19. DCs with homozygous or heterozygote NOD2 variant 1007fsinsC from CD patients thus have defective miR-29, and consequently augmented IL-23 expression [75].

Susceptibility and protective variants of CARD9 have been discovered [77, 78]. CARD9 works downstream of β-glucan receptor dectin-1 and regulates IL-23 production. It is, however, unclear whether these variants are loss or gain of function mutations, but it is likely that these variants may lead to dysregulated IL-23 production by APC.

In some mouse IBD models, APCs were manipulated to determine their impact on pathogenesis. In DSS-induced chemical colitis, depletion of CD11c$^+$ DCs via DT injections in CD11c DTR mice during disease confers protection, whereas depletion before disease exacerbates the pathology [79–81]. Direct depletion of DCs during T-cell–induced colitis has not been performed although IL-23 production has been traced back to these cells in various IL-23-dependent colitis models and IL-23 neutralization or genetic deletion systems have been utilized along with targeting of various costimulatory molecules expressed by DCs. Nevertheless, transfer of E-cadherin$^+$ BMDCs which express IL-23 exacerbates T-cell–induced colitis [14].

Deletion of monocytes via CCR2 gene targeting or anti-CCR2 antibodies also confers protection from DSS-induced colitis [82, 83].

The importance of APC-derived IL-23 in murine colitis models based on infection has been documented by selective targeting of DCs, macrophages and monocytes [15, 17, 84], all pointing to the significance of APC-derived IL-23.

3. IL-23 responsive cells in IBD pathogenesis

In this section, "how IL-23 responsive cells drive or prevent IBD pathology" will be discussed. Although IL-23R-expressing cells are manifold, effector cytokines produced upon IL-23 signaling are similar or identical by these innate and adaptive immune cells. The current literature regarding how each IL-23-dependent cytokine coming exclusively from a defined IL-23R+ cell impact IBD pathology will be reviewed. A summary of the IL-23R positive cells are shown in **Figure 2**.

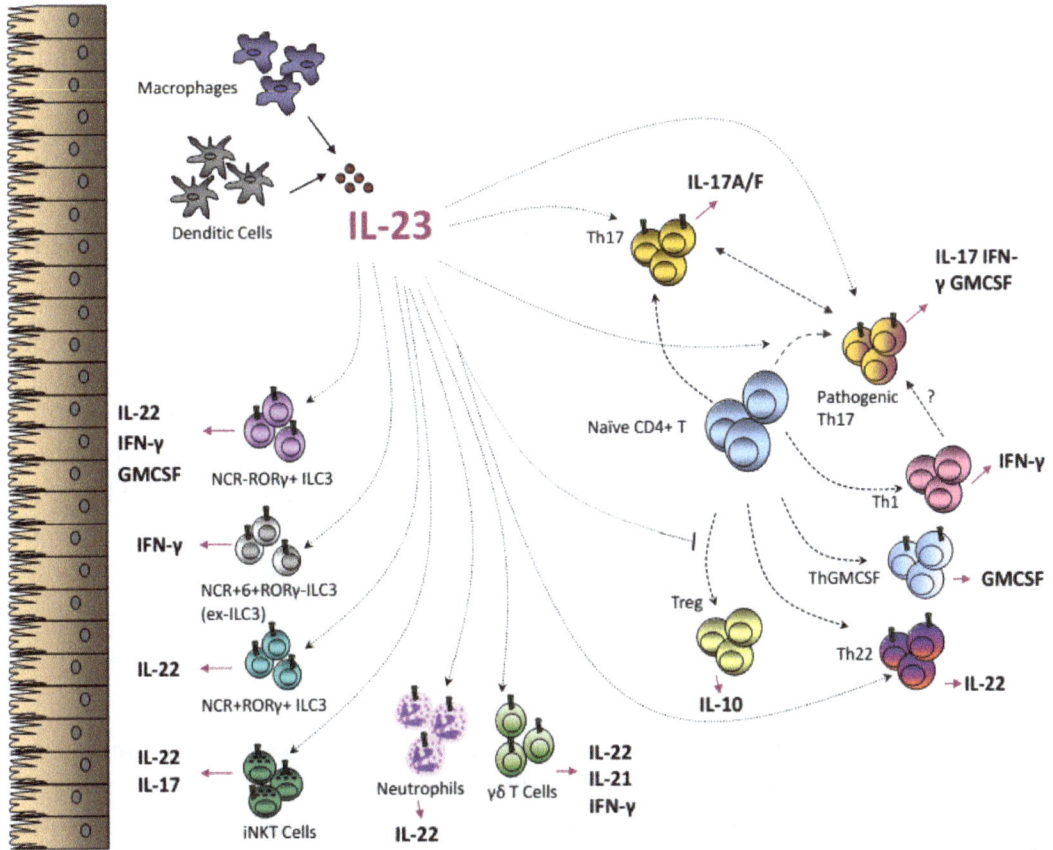

Figure 2. Summary of action of IL-23 on its target cells. IL-23 acts on both innate and adaptive immune cells to promote inflammation during IBD.

3.1. Th17 cells in IBD

3.1.1. IL-17A and F

IL-17 A and F are closely related (50% homology) Th17 signature cytokines that are produced in an IL-23-dependent manner. IL-17A and IL-17F are made of homodimers, however, IL-17A/ F heterodimers also form. All of the combinations are recognized by the same heterodimeric receptor composed of IL-17RA and IL-17RC subunits [19]. Both cytokines were expressed at high levels in the intestines of CD patients [62, 85–87]. Because these cytokines stimulate production of various inflammatory mediators by epithelial or endothelial cells that recruit neutrophils, monocytes and dendritic cells their involvement as pathogenic molecules were studied in IBD context [88, 89]. IL-17A neutralization in DSS model resulted in exacerbation of colitis with higher CD4+ T-cell infiltrates and CD11b+ granulocyte-monocyte infiltrates [90]. IL-17KO mice recapitulated this phenotype [91]. Similar to the chemically induced colitis, adaptive colitis induced by naïve CD4+ T cells also developed more aggressively when $il17^{-/-}$ or $il17r^{-/-}$ T cells transferred as compared with WT T cells [92]. This protective role of IL-17 in murine models has been confirmed in Crohn's disease patients. Monoclonal anti-IL-17A secukinumab treatment exacerbated the disease, and adverse effects (high incidences of fungal infection) have been reported [93]. Recently, it was shown that IL-17 is critical for epithelial homeostasis and that the absence of IL-17A during colitis induced by DSS treatment further decreases epithelial integrity and barrier function, resulting in bacterial translocation across the intestinal epithelial barrier [94]. The same phenomenon of IL-17-dependent regulation of epithelial barrier function was reported by Maxwell et al. in a colitis model which was induced in *Abcb1a*-deficient mice upon *Helicobacter bilis* infection [95] which may provide a mechanistic explanation to protective role of IL-17A/F.

In some models of murine IBD, IL-17A and F demonstrated a pathogenic character. In this regard, IL-17FKO mice developed milder DSS-induced colitis compared with WT mice [91]. IL-17A neutralization also improved colitis in a T-cell transfer model in which colitis was induced by IL-17F$^{-/-}$ CD4+CD25$^-$ T cells (Naïve + memory) [96]. Furthermore, Yen et al. had demonstrated a pathogenic role for IL-17A in CD4+ T-cell transfer colitis induced by IL-10$^{-/-}$ T cells [54]. Lastly, deletion of IL-17RA, receptor for both IL17 and F (but also for IL-17C), or blocking of signaling via IL-17RA IgG in WT mice conferred protection from in TNBS-induced colitis [97].

3.1.2. IFN-γ

IFN-γ is a Th1 cytokine. However, Th17 cells and ILC3s also produce it when stimulated with IL-23. IL-17A expression by T cells is not required for naïve T-cell–driven colitis; in fact, its neutralization in IBD patients does not ameliorate the disease as described above. However, Th17 cells are needed for the pathogenesis of IBD in several murine models as RORγT [87], STAT3 [98], IL-23 [99], and IL-23R [59] manipulation by genetic and biochemical means alters the disease course. These data point to the involvement of other Th17-derived cytokines in colitogenesis. In fact, in naïve T-cell transfer-induced adaptive cell–driven coltitis, anti-CD40 or *Hepaticus*-induced innate colitis models, IL-23-dependent IFN-γ produced by either Th17 or innate ILC3 cells was shown to play a pathogenic role [38, 100]. IFN-γ in this context was shown to regulate myeloid inflammatory cell recruitment (neutrophils, monocytes and eosinophils) to the tissue [60, 101, 102]. In both CD4+ T-cell transfer and *H. hepaticus*-driven murine adaptive models of IBD, Th17 cells that produce IFN-γ+IL-17A+ together have been described. These double producer cells were eliminated when donor T cells lack IL-23R in the T-cell–transfer colitis model, and colitis scores are improved [103]. IFN-γ+IL-17A+ double producers increase in colitic mouse intestine. Independently-performed fate map studies have shown that IFN-γ^+IL-17A$^+$ double producers can further turn RORγT expression off and gradually turn into "alternative" Th1 cells through a process promoted by IL-23 and IL-12 [59, 104, 105]. It is unclear as yet what the relative contribution of Th17/Th1 double producers or alternative Th1 cells or the conventional Th1 cells to IBD pathogenesis are and if it applies to humans.

Besides acting as an inflammatory cytokine, IFN-γ was also shown to regulate IEC survival proliferation through Wnt inhibitor Dkk, which ultimately negatively impacts intestinal epithelial barrier function [106, 107]. Whether epithelial integrity is regulated by IFN-γ of Th17, or ILC3 origin is also unclear.

3.1.3. GMCSF

Granulocyte macrophage colony-stimulating factor (GMCSF) is a hematopoietic growth factor produced by various immune cells such as activated T and B cells, monocytes/macrophages, neutrophils, eosinophils and ILC3s, as well as other sources such as endothelial cells, fibroblasts epithelial cells, mesothelial cells, chondrocytes, Paneth cells and tumor cells [108]. It was shown that GMCSF is produced by Th17 cells in a Rorγt and IL-23-dependent fashion [109, 110]. More importantly, independent studies revealed that GMCSF is required for classical EAE development in mice, especially by activating microglia or mobilizing inflammatory myeloid lineages to the inflammation site [109, 110]. Studies from Fiona Powrie's lab more recently showed that IL-23-dependent production of GMCSF also contributes to the pathogenesis of colitis in naïve CD4$^+$ T-cell transfer- and *Hepaticus*-induced models of murine IBD [111, 112]. In both models, GMCSF was shown to promote eosinophil recruitment and activation in the colon which was needed for pathogenesis. On the other hand, work including with human cells proposed that a distinct lineage of Th cells is programmed to produce only GMCSF and that they constitute the major fraction GMCSF$^+$ Th cells (Though GMCSF$^+$IFN-γ^+ or GMCSF$^+$IL-17A$^+$ cells are also reported) [113]. STAT5 and IL-7 or IL-2 may be important in differentiation or activation of GMCSF$^+$ cells [114, 115]. It is noteworthy that STAT5$^{-/-}$ CD4 T cells are still able to induce colitis [114]. Thus, though GMCSF may have a role in IBD development, how much of that comes through IL-23-dependent pathway or from Th17 cells is unclear and more cell-specific deletion of GMCSF is needed to address this question.

3.1.4. IL-22

IL-22 is an alpha-helical cytokine which belongs to IL-10 family cytokine. Th17, Th22 and $\gamma\delta$ T cells [19], neutrophils [45] and ILC3s produce IL-22 cytokine in response to IL-23 stimulation [116]. IL-22 signals through a heterodimeric cytokine composed of the specific IL-22R1 and IL-10Rβ subunits. Although IL-22 is mostly produced by cells of the hematopoietic lineage, IL-22 receptor is expressed by the non-hematopoietic compartment which includes epithelial cells in the skin, lung and intestines, liver and kidney [117]. IL-22 is needed in the mucosal surfaces for the containment of microbial flora at an arms distance of epithelia. IL-22 stimulates production of various antimicrobial proteins and peptides (Reg3β and γ, β-defensins, S100A7-9 etc.) as well chemokines and cytokines (CXCL1$^-$, 5, 9, IL-6, G-CSF) [116]. Thus, it is also crucial for host defense against various pathogens including *C. rodentium* [118]. IL-22 promotes mucus production by goblet cells; acts as a growth factor and stimulates epithelial regeneration [118, 119].

IL-22 levels are elevated in the mucosal tissue of both UC and CD patients [120]. As with other Th17- specific cytokines, both protective and colitogenic roles for IL-22 have been described in murine IBD models. Sugimoto et al. were the first to demonstrate that IL-22 could improve murine IBD pathology. They observed a reduction in IL-22 levels after the disease onset in their spontaneous colitis murine model compared with control animals which developed disease due to a T-cell receptor defect (*Tcra*$^{-/-}$mouse) and went after IL-22 [121]. Using this model and DSS-induced colitis, these investigators showed that IL-22 overexpression improved colitis, and its neutralization via IL-22BP (the soluble receptor) or antibody, delayed recovery from colitis. Although the exact source of IL-22 in this work remained less defined due to the possible innate sources (γδ T cells, ILC3, neutrophils), during naïve CD4$^+$ T-cell transfer-induced colitis, IL-22 coming from exclusively Th17 cells were shown to be protective. This was shown by the transfer of IL-22$^{-/-}$ naïve CD4$^+$ T-cell transfer into *Rag*$^{-/-}$ mice which developed exacerbated colitis compared to that of WT T cells [122]. ILC3 also contribute to intestinal IL-22 production, as such IL-23R$^{-/-}$ Rag1$^{-/-}$ mice develop exacerbated colitis upon naïve CD4$^+$ T-cell transfer compared with control Rag1$^{-/-}$ hosts. IL-23R deficient Rag1KO mice had far less IL-22 in their intestines than control Rag1KO mice even after naïve T-cell transfer, showing that indeed ILC3 contribution to IL-22 is significant [60]. So, regardless of the cellular source, reduction in IL-22 levels impacted IBD development/recovery in naïve T-cell–induced colitis. IL-22-mediated protection from colon inflammation was demonstrated by targeting molecules responsible for the induction of IL-22 in different contexts. When AhR signaling was activated via its ligand Ficz, which increased IL-22 production, less colitis developed in TNBS, DSS and CD4$^+$ naïve T-cell–induced mice model; Ficz-dependent protection was reversed by neutralization of IL-22 [123, 124]. In all these models, IL-22 was believed to promote epithelial barrier regeneration. Conversely in its absence, epithelial barrier was breached and could not be repaired [122]. IL-22 receptor signaling activates STAT3; research shows that deletion of STAT3 in IL-22 responsive epithelial cells impairs IL-22-mediated intestinal epithelial repair which was demonstrated in a DSS-induced model [125]. This study revealed an important role for IL-22-induced mucin in IL-22-mediated protection from colitis.

IL-22 was also shown to drive colitis in noninfectious and infection-induced T-cell–dependent colitis models [126, 127]. Kamanaka et al. developed a T-cell–dependent colitis model by adoptive transfer of IL-10 unresponsive IL-10dn$^-$ CD45RB^{low} CD25$^-$ CD4$^+$ memory T cells into *Rag*$^{-/-}$ hosts. The colitis developed in this model was IL-22-dependent (exclusively of TH17/Th22 origin), as such IL-22$^{-/-}$ CD45RB^{low} CD25$^-$ CD4$^+$ memory T cells did not induce colitis compared with IL-22. It is noteworthy that colitis in this model, unlike the naïve T-cell transfer model, does not cause ulcers, but rather is characterized by mucosal thickening and hyperplasia consistent with proliferative potential of IL-22 [127]. *Toxoplasma gondii* infection-induced colitis in B6 mice has also been shown to be IL-22 driven (through its effects on MMP-2), thus IL-22 deletion ameliorated colitis in this context [128].

3.2. ILC3, γδ T and NKT cells in IL-23R-mediated pathology

3.2.1. Group3 ILCs

Group 3 ILCs (ILC3) are Rorγ$^+$ innate cells that respond to IL-23 and are enriched in mucosal surfaces [129]. Although very rare in the circulation, in the intestinal lamina propria, Rorγ$^+$ ILC3s are enriched and constitute up to 8% of lymphocytes and ~70% of ILCs in the murine intestinal LP [39]. ILC3s include fetal LTi cells and adult ILC3s [130]. Various adult ILC3s were described in humans and in mice based on the expression of natural cytotoxicity receptors and cytokine production. These include (1) IL-22 producing NCR$^+$ ILC3 [131] which are also called ILC22, NK22, NKR-LTi or NCR22 [132]; (2) NCR$^-$IL-17A$^+$IFN-γ$^+$ double producing ILC3 [38] and (3) NCR$^-$IL-17A$^+$ ILC3s [133, 134] in mice [135]. Fetal and adult ILC3 were shown to differ in their CCR6 expression. Fetal LTi cells express higher CCR6, whereas adult ILC3s appear to be CCR6 low and accumulate after birth in a microbiota-dependent fashion. CCR6$^-$ adult ILC3s were also reported to rely on AhR and ligands acquired through diet [135]. All the ILC3 cells depend on Rorγt for their development and express IL-23R and produce Th17 cytokines in response to the IL-23, although the combination of cytokines differ with the microbial signal and ILC3 type.

Regardless of our incomplete understanding of their ontogeny, ILC3s have been shown to take part in the pathogenesis of IBD-like diseases in many murine models in the past 5 years. More importantly, not only Th17 cells but also CD3$^-$ ILC3s were reportedly elevated in the intestinal tissue of both UC and CD patients; they also contributed to elevated IL-22, IL-17A/F and IL-26 levels in tissue of IBD patients [136].

3.2.1.1. ILC3-derived IL-17 and IFN-γ

Although IL-17A neutralization trials failed at achieving a clinical benefit to IBD patients, IL-17A, particularly of ILC3 origin, has been shown to promote IBD-like pathogenesis in murine models. This was shown to be the case in *H. hepaticus*-induced colitis in Rag$^{-/-}$ mice, shown by Buonocore et al. in their landmark paper [38, 55, 56]. In this innate model, IL-17A$^+$ IFN-γ$^+$ ILC3 numbers elevated and neutralization of either cytokine alone or together ameliorated colitis. Additionally, deletion of ILC3 by crossing Rag$^{-/-}$ mice to Rorc$^{-/-}$ animals or ILC3 depletion via anti-Thy1 antibodies make them resistant to colitis induced by *H. hepaticus*. Pathogenicity of IL-17A was also reported in another innate colitis model, the *Tbx21$^{-/-}$Rag2$^{-/-}$* (TRUC) mice. TRUC mice develop spontaneous colitis in a microbe-dependent fashion (which has recently been shown to be *H. Typhlonius*-dependent) [137]. Interestingly, colitis in this model is TNF-α-dependent until the age of 12 weeks after which blockade of TNF-α is ineffective. Through neutralization of IL-23 or IL-17A or blockade of IL-7R signaling, it was shown that ILC3s have been shown to drive colitis in this model via IL-17A. Both TNF-α and IL-6 appear to enhance the disease by enhancing IL-23 production or its signaling [133, 134].

In both *H. Hepaticus*-induced colitis and anti-CD40-induced colitis models (both of which are IL-23 mediated) ILC3-derived IFN-γ drives pathogenesis, and as such, IFN-γ neutralization in these models ameliorated colitis [27, 38, 100]. ILC3s indeed produce IFN-γ when stimulated with IL-23 [60]. Similar to Th17 cells, ILC3 cells have been reported to be plastic cells. Vonarbourg et al.'s studies revealed that that RORγT⁺NKp46⁻ ILC3s (NCR⁻ILC3), upon exposure to IL-12 and IL-15, upregulate NK cell marker NKp46 giving rise to NCR⁺ILC3 *in vivo*. These cells subsequently downregulate RORγT and assume a Th1 or NK such as phenotype and called RORγt-NKR LTi. (currently considered as ILC1) [100]. These ex-ILC3s were shown to produce IFN-γ and were argued to be the major source of IFN-γ and the driver of colitis in the anti-CD40-induced colitis model. The plasticity of ILC3s has also been described in humans [138, 139]. In the presence of IL-12 and IL-2, human CD3⁻CD127⁺c-kit⁺ NKp44⁺ ILC3s downregulate Roγt and IL-23R; upregulate T-bet and then produce IFN-γ. These ex-ILC3s are categorized as non-NK ILC1 [138]. More recently, the ILC3-to ILC1 conversion has been shown to be a reversible process regulated by different subsets of antigen-presenting cell, presumably depending on the microbes or other external signals [139]. Elevated percentages of ILC1 have been reported in Crohn's disease-inflamed intestine [140], as well as in humanized mice treated with DSS [138]. However, causality with the disease, or whether their contribution is significant for pathogenesis in humans is also unclear given the scarcity of their number [136].

3.2.1.2. ILC3-derived IL-22 in IBD

ILC3s also produce IL-22 in response to the IL-23. Both pathogenic [60, 102] and protective [57, 141, 142] roles have been described for IL-22 that is coming from exclusively ILC3s. Deletion of ILC3s by crossing *Rag⁻/⁻* mice to *Rorc⁻/⁻* renders double KO mice more susceptible to DSS-induced colitis and also delays the recovery [57, 141]. Similarly, IL-22-deficient B6 mice or IL-23R⁻/⁻ *Rag⁻/⁻* mice develop more severe intestinal damage in response to the DSS challenge which are reversible by recombinant IL-22-Fc injections [57]. IL-22 is needed for the healing of epithelia upon DSS-induced damage. However, too much of it in certain context may also promote colitis characterized by hyperplasia and mucosal thickening and myeloid inflammatory cell recruitment [119, 125]. We and others have shown this pathogenic effect of IL-22 using the innate cell-mediated colitis model induced by anti-CD40 injections. Neutralization of IL-22 in *Rag⁻/⁻* mice ameliorated colitis, conversely, restoring IL-22 expression in *IL-23R⁻/⁻Rag⁻/⁻* animals (which are protected from colitis), brought colitis back [60, 102]. How IL-22 mediates colitis is not entirely clear, but our data suggest that IL-22 may modulate IL-10, IFN-γ levels and neutrophil recruitment [60].

Protective effects of IL-22 may also be due to impact on microbial flora. Recent studies suggested that IL-22 may contribute to protection from IBD by restricting growth of certain genera of bacteria in the steady state [143]. A study by Zenewicz et al. revealed that intestine of *Il-22⁻/⁻* mice differs in representation of 14 different genera compared with WT mice and is more susceptible to DSS-induced colitis. More importantly, this susceptibility is transmissible to WT mice through co-housing of WT with *il22* KO mice, which points to functions of IL-22 independent of epithelial regeneration [143]. Supporting this view, another study using *AhR⁻/⁻Rorc⁻/⁺* mice demonstrated that reduced IL-22 levels in the murine intestine allows overgrowth of SFB, which consequently promotes Th17 differentiation [144]. Thus *AhR⁻/⁻Rorc⁻/⁺* mice develop spontaneous colitis owing to hyper-Th17 responses.

3.2.1.3. ILC3-derived GMCSF in IBD

Both human and mouse ILC3s form IBD patient intestine and murine intestine, respectively, were shown to produce GMCSF in an IL-23-dependent manner [101, 102]. Similar to adaptive cell-induced colitis models, during anti-CD40-induced colitis ILC3 contributed to GMCSF substantially, and its blockade via neutralizing antibodies blocked colitogenesis [101, 102]. GMCSF-dependent recruitment of myeloid effector cells (eosinophils-monocytes) may be the underlining mechanism for the pathogenic effects as described in adaptive cell-induced colitis models [111, 112]. GMCSF, however, was also shown to impact ILC3 motility out of crypto-patches, which may additionally contribute to its pathogenic role during innate cell-induced colitis [101].

3.2.2. γδ T cells

γδ T cells are nonconventional T cells with innate features and comprise 1–5% of lymphocytes in mice and human blood. Their numbers go up to 50% of lymphocytes in skin and mucosal tissues [145]. γδ T cells express Rorγt and IL-23R and are another source of IL-17 and IL-22, which can be produced both in IL-23-dependent and independent manner. In peripheral blood as well the intestines [146–148] of active IBD patients, elevated percentage and absolute number of γδ T cells were reported. Both tissue protective and pro-inflammatory roles in murine IBD models have been described for γδ T cells. In this regard, $Tcr\delta^{-/-}$ mice developed more severe DSS-induced colitis accompanied by reduced regeneration and epithelial tissue repair [149, 150]. Depletion of γδ T cells also exacerbated TNBS-induced colitis in rats [151]. A recent study showed that this protective effect (of γδ T cells) was mediated through IL-22 and further enhanced by retinoic acid (RA) which induced RA receptor binding to IL-22 promoter [152]. More recently, γδ T cells were shown to be the major IL-17A source during acute DSS-induced colitis. In this model, IL-17 production was reported to be mostly IL-23 independent and regulated epithelial permeability through instructing localization of occluding, a tight junction protein [94].

Studies in some murine IBD models implicated γδ T cells as the contributor to pathology. Colitis in $Tcra^{-/-}$ mice, which resembles to UC and spontaneously develops in a microbiota-dependent fashion, improved up on genetic deletion of γδ T cells [147]. In also a T-cell transfer model, γδ T cells enhanced colitis [153]. $Tcr\beta\delta^{-/-}$ mice developed less colitis compared with $Tcr\delta^{+/+}$ mice upon naïve CD4+ T-cell transfer. Cotransfer of IL-17+ CCR6+ γδ T cells but not CCR6- IFN-γ+ γδ T cells with naïve T cells restored colitis in this model through potentiating Th17 and Th1 cells [153]. In another murine spontaneous colitis model which develops due to CD4+ T-cell--specific deletion of phosphoinositide-dependent protein kinase 1 (Pdk1), γδ T cells were shown to be required for colitogenesis [154].

3.2.3. NKT cells

Type I NKT (iNKT) cells are characterized by their invariant T-cell receptor α-chain which is detectable by α-galactosylceramide loaded CD1d tetramers [155]. A population of NK1.1⁻ iNKT cells were shown to express RORγT and IL-23R [47, 48] and produce IL-17. These

RORγT + iNKT cells, when costimulated with IL-23 and IL1β, induce production of large amounts of IL-22 and IL-17 [47, 48]. Some studies documented a reduction in type I iNKT cells in the blood and intestinal tissue of CD and UC patients [156] (see the review for detailed role of iNKT in IBD [155]). Because iNKT cells produce IL-4, IL-13 and can promote Th2-responses, they have been experimentally shown to play a protective role in various murine IBD models including DSS [157, 158], TNBS [159], naïve CD4+ T-cell transfer [160] and *T. gondii* induced [161, 162] models of colitis. However, exactly how IL-23–dependent production of IL-22 or IL-17 by iNKT cells confers protection or impacts IBD pathogenesis has not been fully elucidated.

3.2.4. Neutrophils

Some fractions of murine neutrophils (~20%) express Rorγt and IL-23R; even higher factions of human neutrophils (75%) have been shown to respond to IL-23 and produce IL-17A and IL-22 [163, 164]. A recent study demonstrated that during DSS-induced colitis, neutrophils significantly contribute IL-22 production; as such IL-22 WT neutrophil transfer improves colitis [45]. Neutrophils are recruited to intestine during T-cell transfer colitis and *Hepaticus*-induced colitis as well. Their neutralization in one study did not suggest any pathogenic role in these models [111]. It is unclear how neutrophils would impact intestinal pathology in other innate and T-cell–dependent colitis models.

4. Therapeutic approaches targeting IL-23 signaling in IBD

With the motivation from studies described above and the commonality of IL-23 signaling across a number of autoimmune/chronic inflammatory conditions, several companies have targeted IL-23 signaling pathway components with various means for therapeutic intervention in multiple inflammatory diseases including IBD. Most of these antagonists are monoclonal human or humanized antibodies that target specific (p19) or common (p40) subunits of IL-23 (**Table 1**). Others target downstream effector cytokines or cytokine receptors induced by IL-23 signaling such as IL-17A, IL-17F, IL-22 or IL-17RA. Few of those attempt to block IL-23 signaling and Th17 arm by inhibiting the transcription factors regulating IL-23 or IL-23R production via blockade with apilimod and Rorc inhibitors, respectively. Some of therapeutics are currently in use for conditions other than IBD; others are in the development–discovery stage, and some have been discontinued due to lack of efficacy or adverse effects (review by [165, 166]. **Table 1** gives a summary of the therapies directly targeting IL-23.

Ustekinumab is the only FDA-approved IL-23/IL-12 blocker that is currently used for treatment of psoriasis and psoriatic arthritis. It is a neutralizing fully human monoclonal antibody against the common p40 subunit. Several clinical trials are assessing its effectiveness against a list of autoimmune conditions. Ustekinumab phase III trials for Crohn's disease and ankylosing spondylitis showed promising results [167–169]. Ustekinumab is also being tested for atopic dermatitis and rheumatoid arthritis. Multiple Sclerosis patients, however, did not benefit from Ustekinumab for unknown reasons [170]. Briakinumab is also a p40-specific monoclonal antibody developed by Abbott, but due to cardiac problems associated with its use, it did not make to the market [171]. Since Ustekinumab blocks both IL-12 and IL-23, the Th17 and Th1 arm of the helper T cells are affected together. IL-23p19-specific monoclonal antibodies which will exclusively target Th17 arm and spare Th1 lineage may be more beneficial for the long-term use. Although both Th1 and Th17 cells are implicated in many autoimmune conditions (Psoriasis, IBD, MS), the Th1 arm of the helper cells are crucial for immunity against intracellular pathogens and tumors, and thus selective targeting of Th17 may help to reduce the risk of certain infections or developing tumors during long-term use of immunosuppression.

Drug	Target	Company	Status	Disease
Ustekinumab	p40 (IL-12p40; IL-23p40) mAb human	Centocor Ortho Biotech and Janssen Research	Approved Approved Phase III Phase I Phase II Phase II Phase II Phase II Discontinued	Plaque psoriasis Psoriatic arthritis Crohn's disease CVID-dependent enteropathy Ankylosing spondylitis; Sarcoidosis atopic dermatitis; rheumatoid arthritis Multiple sclerosis
Briakinumab	p40 (IL-12p40; IL-23p40) mAb human	Abbott	Discontinued Discontinued Discontinued	Psoriasis Crohn's disease Multiple sclerosis
Guselkumab	IL-23 p19 antagonist mAb human	Janssen Research	Phase III	Psoriasis
BI 655066	IL-23 p19 antagonist mAb humanized	BoehringerIngelheim	Phase II	Crohn's disease; psoriasis
Tildrakizumab	IL-23 p19 antagonist mAb human	Schering-Plough/Merck	Phase III	Psoriasis
MP-196	IL-23p19 antagonist mAb	Effimune	–	Autoimmune disease
FM-303	IL-23p19 antagonist mAb	Femta Pharmaceuticals	Discovery	Inflammatory bowel disease
AMG 139	IL-23p19 mAb human	Amgen, AstraZeneca	PhaseII	Crohn's disease; psoriasis
IL-23 Adnectin	IL-23R	Bristol-Myers Squibb	Discovery	Immune disorder
Anti-IL-23 immunotherapy	IL-23R	Peptinov SAS	Discovery	Inflammatory disease
LY3074828	IL-23 p19 antagonist mAb humanized	Eli Lilly	Phase I	Psoriasis
Apilimod (STA-5326)	Blocks NFKB translocation, IL-12, IL-23 production	Synta Pharmaceuticals	Discontinued	Psoriasis; rheumatoid arthritis; common immunodeficiency

Adapted and modified from Tang and Iwakura [165] and Patel and Kuchroo [166].

Table 1. Identified interleukin-23 receptor (IL-23R) antagonists.

Guselkumab, Tildrakizumab, BI655066, AMG 139, MP-196 are monoclonal anti-p19 neutralizing antibodies that are now actively being tested by different companies for psoriasis at different phases (ClinicalTrials.gov). BI 655066 is additionally being tested on CD patients in a phase II trial. With positive results from psoriasis cases, the remaining p19 blockers are very likely to be extended to trials with Crohn's disease patients soon.

In addition to the IL-23 itself, several other downstream effector cytokines of IL-23R signaling pathway are being targeted with monoclonal antibodies to treat autoimmune diseases. Monoclonal antibodies against IL-17A, IL-17F, IL-17RA proved to be very effective treating psoriasis in various trials [166, 172]. However, secukinumab (anti-IL-17A) trial did not benefit CD patients [93], thus due to lack of any improvement with IL-17A neutralization brodaluzumab (IL-17RA antibody) development and trials were terminated [173]. As described in previous sections, recent studies suggest an important role to IL-17A intestinal barrier function which may be essential for the containment of microbiota. Thus, its removal may exacerbate the condition in IBD [94, 95].

IL-22 is another IL-23 regulated cytokine which went through clinical trials (ClinicalTrials.gov). Fezakinumab (ILV-094) is a monoclonal human IL-22 antibody and has been tested in psoriasis and RA with no results being revealed. Due to its involvement in various IBD models, IL-22 antibodies are also a likely candidate to through clinical trials in CD patients.

There are Rorc inhibitors that are being tested in healthy volunteers (VTP-43472 and JTE-151). They inhibit both Rorγ and Rorγt *ex vivo* and *in vivo* results are not yet available [166].

IL-23 receptor signals through JAK2/TYK2 kinases. Several JAK2 inhibitors are in clinical trials for treatment of cancer and autoimmune disease. Ruxolitinib is a JAK1/JAK2 inhibitor approved by FDA for myelofibrosis and is now being tested in RA and psoriasis patients. Baricitinib is another Jak1/Jak2 inhibitor in Phase II clinical trials in RA patients. Lastly, lestaurtinib is a JAK2 inhibitor and is in Phase II trials on psoriasis patients. These molecules (ClinicalTrials.gov) are eventually likely to be tested on IBD patients.

Author details

Ahmet Eken[1,2] and Mohamed Oukka[3,4*]

*Address all correspondence to: moukka@u.washington.edu

1 Medical Biology, Faculty of Medicine, Erciyes University, Kayseri, Turkey

2 Betül-Ziya Eren Genome and Stem Cell Research Center, Kayseri, Turkey

3 Center for Immunity and Immunotherapies, Seattle Children's Research Institute, Seattle, WA, USA

4 Department of Immunology, University of Washington, Seattle, WA, USA

References

[1] Oppmann B, Lesley R, Blom B, et al. Novel p19 protein engages IL-12p40 to form a cytokine, IL-23, with biological activities similar as well as distinct from IL-12. Immunity; 2000; 13: 715–25.

[2] Lupardus PJ, Garcia KC. The structure of interleukin-23 reveals the molecular basis of p40 subunit sharing with interleukin-12. J Mol Biol; 2008. 382: 931–41.

[3] Piskin G, Sylva-Steenland RMR, Bos JD, et al. In vitro and in situ expression of IL-23 by keratinocytes in healthy skin and psoriasis lesions: enhanced expression in psoriatic skin. J Immunol; 2006. 176: 1908–15.

[4] Macho-Fernandez E, Koroleva EP, Spencer CM, et al. Lymphotoxin beta receptor signaling limits mucosal damage through driving IL-23 production by epithelial cells. Mucosal Immunol; 2015. 8: 403–13.

[5] Goto K, Kaneko Y, Sato Y, et al. Leptin deficiency down-regulates IL-23 production in glomerular podocytes resulting in an attenuated immune response in nephrotoxic serum nephritis. Int Immunol; (2016) 28 (4): 197–208 Epub ahead of print 13 November 2015. doi:10.1093/intimm/dxv067.

[6] Liu F-L, Chen C-H, Chu S-J, et al. Interleukin (IL)-23 p19 expression induced by IL-1beta in human fibroblast-like synoviocytes with rheumatoid arthritis via active nuclear factor-kappaB and AP-1 dependent pathway. Rheumatology (Oxford); 2007. 46: 1266–73.

[7] Zhang Z, Andoh A, Yasui H, et al. Interleukin-1beta and tumor necrosis factor-alpha upregulate interleukin-23 subunit p19 gene expression in human colonic subepithelial myofibroblasts. Int J Mol Med; 2005. 15: 79–83.

[8] O'Keeffe M, Mok WH, Radford KJ. Human dendritic cell subsets and function in health and disease. Cell Mol Life Sci; 2015. 72: 4309–25.

[9] Varol C, Vallon-Eberhard A, Elinav E, et al. Intestinal lamina propria dendritic cell subsets have different origin and functions. Immunity; 2009. 31: 502–12.

[10] Schlitzer A, McGovern N, Teo P, et al. IRF4 transcription factor-dependent CD11b[+] dendritic cells in human and mouse control mucosal IL-17 cytokine responses. Immunity; 2013. 38: 970–83.

[11] Lewis KL, Caton ML, Bogunovic M, et al. Notch2 receptor signaling controls functional differentiation of dendritic cells in the spleen and intestine. Immunity; 2011. 35: 780–91.

[12] Satpathy AT, Briseño CG, Lee JS, et al. Notch2-dependent classical dendritic cells orchestrate intestinal immunity to attaching-and-effacing bacterial pathogens. Nat Immunol; 2013. 14: 937–48.

[13] Kinnebrew MA, Buffie CG, Diehl GE, et al. Interleukin 23 production by intestinal CD103[(+)]CD11b[(+)] dendritic cells in response to bacterial flagellin enhances mucosal innate immune defense. Immunity; 2012. 36: 276–87.

[14] Siddiqui KRR, Laffont S, Powrie F. E-cadherin marks a subset of inflammatory dendritic cells that promote T cell-mediated colitis. Immunity; 2012. 32: 557–67.

[15] Longman RS, Diehl GE, Victorio DA, et al. CX$_3$CR1[+] mononuclear phagocytes support colitis-associated innate lymphoid cell production of IL-22. J Exp Med; 2014. 211: 1571–83.

[16] Kamada N, Hisamatsu T, Okamoto S, et al. Unique CD14 intestinal macrophages contribute to the pathogenesis of Crohn disease via IL-23/IFN-gamma axis. J Clin Invest; 2008. 118: 2269–80.

[17] Arnold IC, Mathisen S, Schulthess J, et al. CD11c[(+)] monocyte/macrophages promote chronic Helicobacter hepaticus-induced intestinal inflammation through the production of IL-23. Mucosal Immunol; 2016 Mar;9(2): 352–63. Epub ahead of print 5 August 2015. doi:10.1038/mi.2015.65.

[18] Becker C, Wirtz S, Blessing M, et al. Constitutive p40 promoter activation and IL-23 production in the terminal ileum mediated by dendritic cells. J Clin Invest; 2003. 112: 693–706.

[19] Korn T, Bettelli E, Oukka M, et al. IL-17 and Th17 Cells. Annu Rev Immunol; 2009. 27: 485–517.

[20] Goriely S, Neurath MF, Goldman M. How microorganisms tip the balance between interleukin-12 family members. Nat Rev Immunol; 2008. 8: 81–6.

[21] Langrish CL, McKenzie BS, Wilson NJ, et al. IL-12 and IL-23: master regulators of innate and adaptive immunity. Immunol Rev; 2004. 202: 96–105.

[22] Leibund Gut-Landmann S, Gross O, Robinson MJ, et al. Syk- and CARD9-dependent coupling of innate immunity to the induction of T helper cells that produce interleukin 17. Nat Immunol; 2007. 8: 630–8.

[23] Gerosa F, Baldani-Guerra B, Lyakh LA, et al. Differential regulation of interleukin 12 and interleukin 23 production in human dendritic cells. J Exp Med; 2008. 205: 1447–61.

[24] Re F, Strominger JL. Toll-like receptor 2 (TLR2) and TLR4 differentially activate human dendritic cells. J Biol Chem; 2001. 276: 37692–9.

[25] Kulsantiwong P, Pudla M, Boondit J, et al. Burkholderia pseudomallei induces IL-23 production in primary human monocytes. Med Microbiol Immunol; (2016) 205: 255. Epub ahead of print 12 November 2015. doi:10.1007/s00430-015-0440-z.

[26] van Beelen AJ, Zelinkova Z, Taanman-Kueter EW, et al. Stimulation of the intracellular bacterial sensor NOD2 programs dendritic cells to promote interleukin-17 production in human memory T cells. Immunity; 2007. 27: 660–9.

[27] Uhlig HH, McKenzie BS, Hue S, et al. Differential activity of IL-12 and IL-23 in mucosal and systemic innate immune pathology. Immunity; 2006. 25: 309–18.

[28] Sheibanie AF, Tadmori I, Jing H, et al. Prostaglandin E2 induces IL-23 production in bone marrow-derived dendritic cells. FASEB J; 2004. 18: 1318–20.

[29] Schnurr M, Toy T, Shin A, et al. Extracellular nucleotide signaling by P2 receptors inhibits IL-12 and enhances IL-23 expression in human dendritic cells: a novel role for the cAMP pathway. Blood; 2005. 105: 1582–9.

[30] Liu W, Ouyang X, Yang J, et al. AP-1 activated by toll-like receptors regulates expression of IL-23 p19. J Biol Chem; 2009. 284: 24006–16.

[31] Zhu C, Rao K, Xiong H, et al. Activation of the murine interleukin-12 p40 promoter by functional interactions between NFAT and ICSBP. J Biol Chem; 2003. 278: 39372–82.

[32] Wang I-M, Contursi C, Masumi A, et al. An IFN-inducible transcription factor, ifn consensus sequence binding protein (ICSBP), stimulates IL-12 p40 expression in macrophages. J Immunol; 2000. 165: 271–9.

[33] Plevy SE, Gemberling JH, Hsu S, et al. Multiple control elements mediate activation of the murine and human interleukin 12 p40 promoters: evidence of functional synergy between C/EBP and Rel proteins. Mol Cell Biol; 1997. 17: 4572–88.

[34] Masumi A, Tamaoki S, Wang I-M, et al. IRF-8/ICSBP and IRF-1 cooperatively stimulate mouse IL-12 promoter activity in macrophages. FEBS Lett; 2002. 531: 348–53.

[35] Al-Salleeh F, Petro TM. Promoter analysis reveals critical roles for SMAD-3 and ATF-2 in expression of IL-23 p19 in macrophages. J Immunol; 2008. 181: 4523–33.

[36] Awasthi A, Riol-Blanco L, Jäger A, et al. Cutting edge: IL-23 receptor gfp reporter mice reveal distinct populations of IL-17-producing cells. J Immunol; 2009. 182: 5904–8.

[37] Gaffen SL, Jain R, Garg AV, et al. The IL-23-IL-17 immune axis: from mechanisms to therapeutic testing. Nat Rev Immunol; 2014. 14: 585–600.

[38] Buonocore S, Ahern PP, Uhlig HH, et al. Innate lymphoid cells drive interleukin-23-dependent innate intestinal pathology. Nature; 2010. 464: 1371–5.

[39] Singh AK, Eken A, Fry M, et al. DOCK8 regulates protective immunity by controlling the function and survival of RORγt+ ILCs. Nat Commun; 2014. 5: 4603.

[40] Sonnenberg GF, Monticelli LA, Elloso MM, et al. CD4(+) lymphoid tissue-inducer cells promote innate immunity in the gut. Immunity; 2011. 34: 122–34.

[41] Paul S, Shilpi S, Lal G. Role of gamma-delta (γδ) T cells in autoimmunity. J Leukoc Biol; 2015. 97: 259–71.

[42] Begum-Haque S, Christy M, Wang Y, et al. Glatiramer acetate biases dendritic cells towards an anti-inflammatory phenotype by modulating OPN, IL-17, and RORγt

responses and by increasing IL-10 production in experimental allergic encephalomye-
litis. J Neuroimmunol; 2013. 254: 117–24.

[43] Karthaus N, Hontelez S, Looman MWG, et al. Nuclear receptor expression patterns in
      murine plasmacytoid and conventional dendritic cells. Mol Immunol; 2013. 55: 409–17.

[44] Werner JL, Gessner MA, Lilly LM, et al. Neutrophils produce interleukin 17A (IL-17A)
      in a dectin-1- and IL-23-dependent manner during invasive fungal infection. Infect
      Immun; 2011. 79: 3966–77.

[45] Zindl CL, Lai J-F, Lee YK, et al. IL-22-producing neutrophils contribute to antimicrobial
      defense and restitution of colonic epithelial integrity during colitis. Proc Natl Acad Sci
      U S A; 2013. 110: 12768–73.

[46] Wilson RP, Ives ML, Rao G, et al. STAT3 is a critical cell-intrinsic regulator of human
      unconventional T cell numbers and function. J Exp Med; 2015. 212: 855–64.

[47] Doisne J-M, Becourt C, Amniai L, et al. Skin and peripheral lymph node invariant NKT
      cells are mainly retinoic acid receptor-related orphan receptor (gamma)t$^+$ and respond
      preferentially under inflammatory conditions. J Immunol; 2009. 183: 2142–9.

[48] Doisne J-M, Soulard V, Bécourt C, et al. Cutting edge: crucial role of IL-1 and IL-23 in
      the innate IL-17 response of peripheral lymph node NK1.1$^-$ invariant NKT cells to
      bacteria. J Immunol; 2011. 186: 662–6.

[49] Sherlock JP, Joyce-Shaikh B, Turner SP, et al. IL-23 induces spondyloarthropathy by
      acting on ROR-γt$^+$ CD3$^+$CD4$^-$CD8$^-$ entheseal resident T cells. Nat Med; 2012. 18: 1069–
      76.

[50] Parham C, Chirica M, Timans J, et al. A receptor for the heterodimeric cytokine IL-23
      is composed of IL-12Rbeta1 and a novel cytokine receptor subunit, IL-23R. J Immunol;
      2002. 168: 5699–708.

[51] Lankford CSR, Frucht DM. A unique role for IL-23 in promoting cellular immunity. J
      Leukoc Biol; 2003. 73: 49–56.

[52] Cho M-L, Kang J-W, Moon Y-M, et al. STAT3 and NF-kappaB signal pathway is required
      for IL-23-mediated IL-17 production in spontaneous arthritis animal model IL-1
      receptor antagonist-deficient mice. J Immunol; 2006. 176: 5652–61.

[53] Floss DM, Mrotzek S, Klöcker T, et al. Identification of canonical tyrosine-dependent
      and non-canonical tyrosine-independent STAT3 activation sites in the intracellular
      domain of the interleukin 23 receptor. J Biol Chem; 2013. 288: 19386–400.

[54] Yen D, Cheung J, Scheerens H, et al. IL-23 is essential for T cell-mediated colitis and
      promotes inflammation via IL-17 and IL-6. J Clin Invest; 2006. 116: 1310–6.

[55] Kullberg MC, Jankovic D, Feng CG, et al. IL-23 plays a key role in Helicobacter
      hepaticus-induced T cell-dependent colitis. J Exp Med; 2006. 203: 2485–94.

[56] Hue S, Ahern P, Buonocore S, et al. Interleukin-23 drives innate and T cell-mediated intestinal inflammation. J Exp Med; 2006. 203: 2473–83.

[57] Cox JH, Kljavin NM, Ota N, et al. Opposing consequences of IL-23 signaling mediated by innate and adaptive cells in chemically induced colitis in mice. Mucosal Immunol; 2012. 5: 99–109.

[58] Wiekowski MT, Leach MW, Evans EW, et al. Ubiquitous transgenic expression of the IL-23 subunit p19 induces multiorgan inflammation, runting, infertility, and premature death. J Immunol; 2001. 166: 7563–70.

[59] Ahern PP, Schiering C, Buonocore S, et al. Interleukin-23 drives intestinal inflammation through direct activity on T cells. Immunity; 2010. 33: 279–88.

[60] Eken A, Singh AK, Treuting PM, et al. IL-23R$^+$ innate lymphoid cells induce colitis via interleukin-22-dependent mechanism. Mucosal Immunol; 2014. 7: 143–54.

[61] Liu Z, Yadav PK, Xu X, et al. The increased expression of IL-23 in inflammatory bowel disease promotes intraepithelial and lamina propria lymphocyte inflammatory responses and cytotoxicity. J Leukoc Biol; 2011. 89: 597–606.

[62] Kobayashi T, Okamoto S, Hisamatsu T, et al. IL23 differentially regulates the Th1/Th17 balance in ulcerative colitis and Crohn's disease. Gut; 2008. 57: 1682–9.

[63] Duerr RH, Taylor KD, Brant SR, et al. A genome-wide association study identifies IL23R as an inflammatory bowel disease gene. Science; 2006. 314(5804): 1461–63.

[64] Wellcome Trust Case Control Consortium. Genome-wide association study of 14,000 cases of seven common diseases and 3,000 shared controls. Nature. 2007; 447: 661–78.

[65] McGovern DPB, Taylor KD, Landers C, et al. MAGI2 genetic variation and inflammatory bowel disease. Inflamm Bowel Dis; 2009. 15: 75–83.

[66] Di Meglio P, Di Cesare A, Laggner U, et al. The IL23R R381Q gene variant protects against immune-mediated diseases by impairing IL-23-induced Th17 effector response in humans. PLoS One; 2011. 6: e17160.

[67] Pidasheva S, Trifari S, Phillips A, et al. Functional studies on the IBD susceptibility gene IL23R implicate reduced receptor function in the protective genetic variant R381Q. PLoS One; 2011. 6: e25038.

[68] Sarin R, Wu X, Abraham C. Inflammatory disease protective R381Q IL23 receptor polymorphism results in decreased primary CD4$^+$ and CD8$^+$ human T-cell functional responses. Proc Natl Acad Sci U S A; 2011. 108: 9560–5.

[69] Oosting M, ter Hofstede H, van de Veerdonk FL, et al. Role of interleukin-23 (IL-23) receptor signaling for IL-17 responses in human Lyme disease. Infect Immun; 2011. 79: 4681–7.

[70] Momozawa Y, Mni M, Nakamura K, et al. Resequencing of positional candidates identifies low frequency IL23R coding variants protecting against inflammatory bowel disease. Nat Genet; 2011. 43: 43–7.

[71] Kumar P, Henikoff S, Ng PC. Predicting the effects of coding non-synonymous variants on protein function using the SIFT algorithm. Nat Protoc; 2009. 4: 1073–81.

[72] Zwiers A, Kraal L, van de Pouw Kraan TCTM, et al. Cutting edge: a variant of the IL-23R gene associated with inflammatory bowel disease induces loss of microRNA regulation and enhanced protein production. J Immunol; 2012. 188: 1573–7.

[73] Franke A, McGovern DPB, Barrett JC, et al. Genome-wide meta-analysis increases to 71 the number of confirmed Crohn's disease susceptibility loci. Nat Genet; 2010. 42: 1118–25.

[74] Barrett JC, Hansoul S, Nicolae DL, et al. Genome-wide association defines more than 30 distinct susceptibility loci for Crohn's disease. Nat Genet; 2008. 40: 955–62.

[75] Brain O, Owens BMJ, Pichulik T, et al. The intracellular sensor NOD2 induces micro-RNA-29 expression in human dendritic cells to limit IL-23 release. Immunity; 2013. 39: 521–36.

[76] Cuthbert AP, Fisher SA, Mirza MM, et al. The contribution of NOD2 gene mutations to the risk and site of disease in inflammatory bowel disease. Gastroenterology; 2002. 122: 867–74.

[77] Zhernakova A, Festen EM, Franke L, et al. Genetic analysis of innate immunity in Crohn's disease and ulcerative colitis identifies two susceptibility loci harboring CARD9 and IL18RAP. Am J Hum Genet; 2008. 82: 1202–10.

[78] Rivas MA, Beaudoin M, Gardet A, et al. Deep resequencing of GWAS loci identifies independent rare variants associated with inflammatory bowel disease. Nat Genet; 2011. 43: 1066–73.

[79] Abe K, Nguyen KP, Fine SD, et al. Conventional dendritic cells regulate the outcome of colonic inflammation independently of T cells. Proc Natl Acad Sci U S A; 2007. 104: 17022–7.

[80] Berndt BE, Zhang M, Chen G-H, et al. The role of dendritic cells in the development of acute dextran sulfate sodium colitis. J Immunol; 2007. 179: 6255–62.

[81] Rutella S, Locatelli F. Intestinal dendritic cells in the pathogenesis of inflammatory bowel disease. World J Gastroenterol; 2011. 17: 3761–75.

[82] Platt AM, Bain CC, Bordon Y, et al. An independent subset of TLR expressing CCR2-dependent macrophages promotes colonic inflammation. J Immunol; 2010. 184: 6843–54.

[83] Zigmond E, Jung S. Intestinal macrophages: well educated exceptions from the rule. Trends Immunol; 2013. 34: 162–8.

[84] Bain CC, Mowat AM. Macrophages in intestinal homeostasis and inflammation. Immunol Rev; 2014. 260: 102–17.

[85] Fujino S, Andoh A, Bamba S, et al. Increased expression of interleukin 17 in inflammatory bowel disease. Gut; 2003. 52: 65–70.

[86] Saruta M, Yu QT, Avanesyan A, et al. Phenotype and effector function of CC chemokine receptor 9-expressing lymphocytes in small intestinal Crohn's disease. J Immunol; 2007. 178: 3293–300.

[87] Rovedatti L, Kudo T, Biancheri P, et al. Differential regulation of interleukin 17 and interferon gamma production in inflammatory bowel disease. Gut; 2009. 58: 1629–36.

[88] Fossiez F, Djossou O, Chomarat P, et al. T cell interleukin-17 induces stromal cells to produce proinflammatory and hematopoietic cytokines. J Exp Med; 1996. 183: 2593–603.

[89] Laan M, Cui ZH, Hoshino H, et al. Neutrophil recruitment by human IL-17 via C-X-C chemokine release in the airways. J Immunol; 1999. 162: 2347–52.

[90] Ogawa A, Andoh A, Araki Y, et al. Neutralization of interleukin-17 aggravates dextran sulfate sodium-induced colitis in mice. Clin Immunol; 2004. 110: 55–62.

[91] Yang XO, Chang SH, Park H, et al. Regulation of inflammatory responses by IL-17F. J Exp Med; 2008. 205: 1063–75.

[92] O'Connor W, Kamanaka M, Booth CJ, et al. A protective function for interleukin 17A in T cell-mediated intestinal inflammation. Nat Immunol; 2009. 10: 603–9.

[93] Hueber W, Sands BE, Lewitzky S, et al. Secukinumab, a human anti-IL-17A monoclonal antibody, for moderate to severe Crohn's disease: unexpected results of a randomised, double-blind placebo-controlled trial. Gut; 2012. 61: 1693–700.

[94] Lee JS, Tato CM, Joyce-Shaikh B, et al. Interleukin-23-independent IL-17 production regulates intestinal epithelial permeability. Immunity; 2015. 43: 727–38.

[95] Maxwell JR, Zhang Y, Brown WA, et al. Differential roles for interleukin-23 and interleukin-17 in intestinal immunoregulation. Immunity; 2015. 43: 739–50.

[96] Leppkes M, Becker C, Ivanov II, et al. RORgamma-expressing Th17 cells induce murine chronic intestinal inflammation via redundant effects of IL-17A and IL-17F. Gastroenterology; 2009. 136: 257–67.

[97] Zhang Z, Zheng M, Bindas J, et al. Critical role of IL-17 receptor signaling in acute TNBS-induced colitis. Inflamm Bowel Dis; 2006. 12: 382–8.

[98] Durant L, Watford WT, Ramos HL, et al. Diverse targets of the transcription factor STAT3 contribute to T cell pathogenicity and homeostasis. Immunity; 2010. 32: 605–15.

[99] Izcue A, Hue S, Buonocore S, et al. Interleukin-23 restrains regulatory T cell activity to drive T cell-dependent colitis. Immunity; 2008. 28: 559–70.

[100] Vonarbourg C, Mortha A, Bui VL, et al. Regulated expression of nuclear receptor RORγt confers distinct functional fates to NK cell receptor-expressing RORγt[(+)] innate lymphocytes. Immunity; 2010. 33: 736–51.

[101] Pearson C, Thornton EE, McKenzie B, et al. ILC3 GM-CSF production and mobilisation orchestrate acute intestinal inflammation. Elife; 5: e10066. Epub ahead of print January 2016. doi:10.7554/eLife.10066.

[102] Song C, Lee JS, Gilfillan S, et al. Unique and redundant functions of NKp46[+] ILC3s in models of intestinal inflammation. J Exp Med; 2015. 212: 1869–82.

[103] Ono Y, Kanai T, Sujino T, et al. T-helper 17 and interleukin-17-producing lymphoid tissue inducer-like cells make different contributions to colitis in mice. Gastroenterology; 2012. 143: 1288–97.

[104] Sujino T, Kanai T, Ono Y, et al. Regulatory T cells suppress development of colitis, blocking differentiation of T-helper 17 into alternative T-helper 1 cells. Gastroenterology; 2011. 141: 1014–23.

[105] Lee YK, Turner H, Maynard CL, et al. Late developmental plasticity in the T helper 17 lineage. Immunity; 2009. 30: 92–107.

[106] Nava P, Koch S, Laukoetter MG, et al. Interferon-gamma regulates intestinal epithelial homeostasis through converging beta-catenin signaling pathways. Immunity; 2010. 32: 392–402.

[107] Lin F-C, Young HA. The talented interferon-gamma. Adv Biosci Biotechnol; 2013. 04: 6–13.

[108] Shiomi A, Usui T. Pivotal roles of GM-CSF in autoimmunity and inflammation. Mediators Inflamm; 2015: 568543.

[109] El-Behi M, Ciric B, Dai H, et al. The encephalitogenicity of T(H)17 cells is dependent on IL-1[−] and IL-23-induced production of the cytokine GM-CSF. Nat Immunol; 2011. 12: 568–75.

[110] Codarri L, Gyülvészi G, Tosevski V, et al. RORγt drives production of the cytokine GM-CSF in helper T cells, which is essential for the effector phase of autoimmune neuroinflammation. Nat Immunol; 2011. 12: 560–7.

[111] Griseri T, Arnold IC, Pearson C, et al. Granulocyte macrophage colony-stimulating factor-activated eosinophils promote interleukin-23 driven chronic colitis. Immunity; 2015. 43: 187–99.

[112] Griseri T, McKenzie BS, Schiering C, et al. Dysregulated hematopoietic stem and progenitor cell activity promotes interleukin-23-driven chronic intestinal inflammation. Immunity; 2012. 37: 1116–29.

[113] Noster R, Riedel R, Mashreghi M-F, et al. IL-17 and GM-CSF expression are antagonistically regulated by human T helper cells. Sci Transl Med; 2014. 6: 241ra80.

[114] Sheng W, Yang F, Zhou Y, et al. STAT5 programs a distinct subset of GM-CSF-producing T helper cells that is essential for autoimmune neuroinflammation. Cell Res; 2014. 24: 1387–402.

[115] Hartmann FJ, Khademi M, Aram J, et al. Multiple sclerosis-associated IL2RA polymorphism controls GM-CSF production in human TH cells. Nat Commun; 2014. 5: 5056.

[116] Sonnenberg GF, Fouser LA, Artis D. Border patrol: regulation of immunity, inflammation and tissue homeostasis at barrier surfaces by IL-22. Nat Immunol; 2011. 12: 383–90.

[117] Wolk K, Kunz S, Witte E, et al. IL-22 increases the innate immunity of tissues. Immunity; 2004. 21: 241–54.

[118] Cash HL, Whitham CV, Behrendt CL, et al. Symbiotic bacteria direct expression of an intestinal bactericidal lectin. Science; 2006. 313: 1126–30.

[119] Brand S, Beigel F, Olszak T, et al. IL-22 is increased in active Crohn's disease and promotes proinflammatory gene expression and intestinal epithelial cell migration. Am J Physiol Gastrointest Liver Physiol; 2006. 290: G827–38.

[120] Andoh A, Zhang Z, Inatomi O, et al. Interleukin-22, a member of the IL-10 subfamily, induces inflammatory responses in colonic subepithelial myofibroblasts. Gastroenterology; 2005. 129: 969–84.

[121] Sugimoto K, Ogawa A, Mizoguchi E, et al. IL-22 ameliorates intestinal inflammation in a mouse model of ulcerative colitis. J Clin Invest; 2008. 118: 534–44.

[122] Zenewicz LA, Yancopoulos GD, Valenzuela DM, et al. Innate and adaptive interleukin-22 protects mice from inflammatory bowel disease. Immunity; 2008. 29: 947–57.

[123] Monteleone I, Rizzo A, Sarra M, et al. Aryl hydrocarbon receptor-induced signals up-regulate IL-22 production and inhibit inflammation in the gastrointestinal tract. Gastroenterology; 2011. 141: 237–48, 248.e1.

[124] Monteleone I, Pallone F, Monteleone G. Aryl hydrocarbon receptor and colitis. Semin Immunopathol; 2013. 35: 671–5.

[125] Pickert G, Neufert C, Leppkes M, et al. STAT3 links IL-22 signaling in intestinal epithelial cells to mucosal wound healing. J Exp Med; 2009. 206: 1465–72.

[126] Zheng Y, Danilenko DM, Valdez P, et al. Interleukin-22, a T(H)17 cytokine, mediates IL-23-induced dermal inflammation and acanthosis. Nature; 2007. 445: 648–51.

[127] Kamanaka M, Huber S, Zenewicz LA, et al. Memory/effector (CD45RB(lo)) CD4 T cells are controlled directly by IL-10 and cause IL-22-dependent intestinal pathology. J Exp Med; 2011. 208: 1027–40.

[128] Muñoz M, Heimesaat MM, Danker K, et al. Interleukin (IL)-23 mediates Toxoplasma gondii-induced immunopathology in the gut via matrixmetalloproteinase-2 and IL-22 but independent of IL-17. J Exp Med; 2009. 206: 3047–59.

[129] Diefenbach A, Colonna M, Koyasu S. Development, differentiation, and diversity of innate lymphoid cells. Immunity; 2014. 41: 354–65.

[130] Spits H, Artis D, Colonna M, et al. Innate lymphoid cells—a proposal for uniform nomenclature. Nat Rev Immunol; 2013. 13: 145–9.

[131] Cella M, Fuchs A, Vermi W, et al. A human natural killer cell subset provides an innate source of IL-22 for mucosal immunity. Nature; 2009. 457: 722–5.

[132] Sanos SL, Bui VL, Mortha A, et al. RORgammat and commensal microflora are required for the differentiation of mucosal interleukin 22-producing NKp46[+] cells. Nat Immunol; 2009. 10: 83–91.

[133] Powell N, Walker AW, Stolarczyk E, et al. The transcription factor T-bet regulates intestinal inflammation mediated by interleukin-7 receptor+ innate lymphoid cells. Immunity; 2012. 37: 674–84.

[134] Powell N, Lo JW, Biancheri P, et al. Interleukin 6 increases production of cytokines by colonic innate lymphoid cells in mice and patients with chronic intestinal inflammation. Gastroenterology; 2015. 149: 456–67.e15.

[135] Klose CSN, Kiss EA, Schwierzeck V, et al. A T-bet gradient controls the fate and function of CCR6-RORγt[+] innate lymphoid cells. Nature; 2013. 494: 261–5.

[136] Geremia A, Arancibia-Cárcamo CV, Fleming MPP, et al. IL-23-responsive innate lymphoid cells are increased in inflammatory bowel disease. J Exp Med; 2011. 208: 1127–33.

[137] Garrett WS, Lord GM, Punit S, et al. Communicable ulcerative colitis induced by T-bet deficiency in the innate immune system. Cell; 131: 2007. 33–45.

[138] Bernink JH, Peters CP, Munneke M, et al. Human type 1 innate lymphoid cells accumulate in inflamed mucosal tissues. Nat Immunol; 14: 2013. 221–9.

[139] Bernink JH, Krabbendam L, Germar K, et al. Interleukin-12 and -23 control plasticity of CD127[(+)] Group 1 and Group 3 innate lymphoid cells in the intestinal lamina propria. Immunity; 2015. 43: 146–60.

[140] Takayama T, Kamada N, Chinen H, et al. Imbalance of NKp44[(+)]NKp46[(-)] and NKp44[(-)]NKp46[(+)] natural killer cells in the intestinal mucosa of patients with Crohn's disease. Gastroenterology; 2010. 139: 882–92, 892.e1–3.

[141] Sawa S, Lochner M, Satoh-Takayama N, et al. RORγt[+] innate lymphoid cells regulate intestinal homeostasis by integrating negative signals from the symbiotic microbiota. Nat Immunol; 2011. 12: 320–6.

[142] Kimura K, Kanai T, Hayashi A, et al. Dysregulated balance of retinoid-related orphan receptor γt-dependent innate lymphoid cells is involved in the pathogenesis of chronic DSS-induced colitis. Biochem Biophys Res Commun; 2012. 427: 694–700.

[143] Zenewicz LA, Yin X, Wang G, et al. IL-22 deficiency alters colonic microbiota to be transmissible and colitogenic. J Immunol; 2013. 190: 5306–12.

[144] Qiu J, Guo X, Chen Z-ME, et al. Group 3 innate lymphoid cells inhibit T-cell-mediated intestinal inflammation through aryl hydrocarbon receptor signaling and regulation of microflora. Immunity; 2013. 39: 386–99.

[145] Hayday A, Tigelaar R. Immunoregulation in the tissues by gammadelta T cells. Nat Rev Immunol; 2003. 3: 233–42.

[146] McVay LD, Li B, Biancaniello R, et al. Changes in human mucosal gamma delta T cell repertoire and function associated with the disease process in inflammatory bowel disease. Mol Med; 1997. 3: 183–203.

[147] Nanno M, Kanari Y, Naito T, et al. Exacerbating role of gammadelta T cells in chronic colitis of T-cell receptor alpha mutant mice. Gastroenterology; 2008. 134: 481–90.

[148] Giacomelli R, Parzanese I, Frieri G, et al. Increase of circulating gamma/delta T lymphocytes in the peripheral blood of patients affected by active inflammatory bowel disease. Clin Exp Immunol; 1994. 98: 83–8.

[149] Chen Y, Chou K, Fuchs E, et al. Protection of the intestinal mucosa by intraepithelial gamma delta T cells. Proc Natl Acad Sci U S A; 2002. 99: 14338–43.

[150] Tsuchiya T, Fukuda S, Hamada H, et al. Role of gamma delta T cells in the inflammatory response of experimental colitis mice. J Immunol; 2003. 171: 5507–13.

[151] Hoffmann JC, Peters K, Henschke S, et al. Role of T lymphocytes in rat 2,4,6-trinitro-benzene sulphonic acid (TNBS) induced colitis: increased mortality after gammadelta T cell depletion and no effect of alphabeta T cell depletion. Gut; 2001. 48: 489–95.

[152] Mielke LA, Jones SA, Raverdeau M, et al. Retinoic acid expression associates with enhanced IL-22 production by γδ T cells and innate lymphoid cells and attenuation of intestinal inflammation. J Exp Med; 2013. 210: 1117–24.

[153] Do J, Visperas A, Dong C, et al. Cutting edge: generation of colitogenic Th17 CD4 T cells is enhanced by IL-17+ γδ T cells. J Immunol; 2011. 186: 4546–50.

[154] Park S-G, Mathur R, Long M, et al. T regulatory cells maintain intestinal homeostasis by suppressing γδ T cells. Immunity; 2010. 33: 791–803.

[155] Liao C-M, Zimmer MI, Wang C-R. The functions of type I and type II natural killer T cells in inflammatory bowel diseases. Inflamm Bowel Dis; 2013. 19: 1330–8.

[156] Grose RH, Thompson FM, Baxter AG, et al. Deficiency of invariant NK T cells in Crohn's disease and ulcerative colitis. Dig Dis Sci; 2007. 52: 1415–22.

[157] Saubermann LJ, Beck P, De Jong YP, et al. Activation of natural killer T cells by alpha-galactosylceramide in the presence of CD1d provides protection against colitis in mice. Gastroenterology; 2000. 119: 119–28.

[158] Ueno Y, Tanaka S, Sumii M, et al. Single dose of OCH improves mucosal T helper type 1/T helper type 2 cytokine balance and prevents experimental colitis in the presence of valpha14 natural killer T cells in mice. Inflamm Bowel Dis; 2005. 11: 35–41.

[159] Shibolet O, Kalish Y, Klein A, et al. Adoptive transfer of ex vivo immune-programmed NKT lymphocytes alleviates immune-mediated colitis. J Leukoc Biol; 2004. 75: 76–86.

[160] Hornung M, Farkas SA, Sattler C, et al. DX5$^+$ NKT cells induce the death of colitis-associated cells: involvement of programmed death ligand-1. Eur J Immunol; 2006. 36: 1210–21.

[161] Smiley ST, Lanthier PA, Couper KN, et al. Exacerbated susceptibility to infection-stimulated immunopathology in CD1d-deficient mice. J Immunol; 2005. 174: 7904–11.

[162] Ronet C, Darche S, Leite de Moraes M, et al. NKT cells are critical for the initiation of an inflammatory bowel response against Toxoplasma gondii. J Immunol; 2005. 175: 899–908.

[163] Taylor PR, Pearlman E. IL-17A production by neutrophils. Immunol Lett; 2016. 169: 104–5.

[164] Taylor PR, Roy S, Leal SM, et al. Activation of neutrophils by autocrine IL-17A-IL-17RC interactions during fungal infection is regulated by IL-6, IL-23, RORγt and dectin-2. Nat Immunol; 2014. 15: 143–51.

[165] Tang C, Iwakura Y. IL-23 in colitis: targeting the progenitors. Immunity; 2012. 37: 957–9.

[166] Patel DD, Kuchroo VK. Th17 cell pathway in human immunity: lessons from genetics and therapeutic interventions. Immunity; 2015. 43: 1040–51.

[167] Sandborn WJ, Feagan BG, Fedorak RN, et al. A randomized trial of Ustekinumab, a human interleukin-12/23 monoclonal antibody, in patients with moderate-to-severe Crohn's disease. Gastroenterology; 2008. 135: 1130–41.

[168] Sandborn WJ, Gasink C, Gao L-L, et al. Ustekinumab induction and maintenance therapy in refractory Crohn's disease. N Engl J Med; 2012. 367: 1519–28.

[169] Marafini I, Angelucci E, Pallone F, et al. The IL-12/23/STAT axis as a therapeutic target in inflammatory bowel disease: mechanisms and evidence in man. Dig Dis; 33(Suppl. 1): 2015. 113–9.

[170] Segal BM, Constantinescu CS, Raychaudhuri A, et al. Repeated subcutaneous injections of IL12/23 p40 neutralising antibody, ustekinumab, in patients with relapsing-remitting multiple sclerosis: a phase II, double-blind, placebo-controlled, randomised, dose-ranging study. Lancet Neurol; 2008. 7: 796–804.

[171] Gordon KB, Langley RG, Gottlieb AB, et al. A phase III, randomized, controlled trial of the fully human IL-12/23 mAb briakinumab in moderate-to-severe psoriasis. J Invest Dermatol; 2012. 132: 304–14.

[172] Lebwohl M, Strober B, Menter A, et al. Phase 3 studies comparing brodalumab with ustekinumab in psoriasis. N Engl J Med; 2015. 373: 1318–28.

[173] Mozaffari S, Nikfar S, Abdollahi M. Inflammatory bowel disease therapies discontinued between 2009 and 2014. Expert Opin Investig Drugs; 2015. 24: 949–56.

Permissions

All chapters in this book were first published in IBS&NIIBD, by InTech Open; hereby published with permission under the Creative Commons Attribution License or equivalent. Every chapter published in this book has been scrutinized by our experts. Their significance has been extensively debated. The topics covered herein carry significant findings which will fuel the growth of the discipline. They may even be implemented as practical applications or may be referred to as a beginning point for another development.

The contributors of this book come from diverse backgrounds, making this book a truly international effort. This book will bring forth new frontiers with its revolutionizing research information and detailed analysis of the nascent developments around the world.

We would like to thank all the contributing authors for lending their expertise to make the book truly unique. They have played a crucial role in the development of this book. Without their invaluable contributions this book wouldn't have been possible. They have made vital efforts to compile up to date information on the varied aspects of this subject to make this book a valuable addition to the collection of many professionals and students.

This book was conceptualized with the vision of imparting up-to-date information and advanced data in this field. To ensure the same, a matchless editorial board was set up. Every individual on the board went through rigorous rounds of assessment to prove their worth. After which they invested a large part of their time researching and compiling the most relevant data for our readers.

The editorial board has been involved in producing this book since its inception. They have spent rigorous hours researching and exploring the diverse topics which have resulted in the successful publishing of this book. They have passed on their knowledge of decades through this book. To expedite this challenging task, the publisher supported the team at every step. A small team of assistant editors was also appointed to further simplify the editing procedure and attain best results for the readers.

Apart from the editorial board, the designing team has also invested a significant amount of their time in understanding the subject and creating the most relevant covers. They scrutinized every image to scout for the most suitable representation of the subject and create an appropriate cover for the book.

The publishing team has been an ardent support to the editorial, designing and production team. Their endless efforts to recruit the best for this project, has resulted in the accomplishment of this book. They are a veteran in the field of academics and their pool of knowledge is as vast as their experience in printing. Their expertise and guidance has proved useful at every step. Their uncompromising quality standards have made this book an exceptional effort. Their encouragement from time to time has been an inspiration for everyone.

The publisher and the editorial board hope that this book will prove to be a valuable piece of knowledge for researchers, students, practitioners and scholars across the globe.

List of Contributors

Tsvetelina Velikova, Dobroslav Kyurkchiev and Ekaterina Ivanova-Todorova
Department of Clinical Laboratory and Clinical Immunology, Medical University of Sofia,
University Hospital St. Ivan Rilski, Sofia, Bulgaria

Zoya Spassova
Clinic of Gastroenterology, University Hospital St. Ivan Rilski, Medical University of Sofia, Bulgaria

Spaska Stanilova
Department of Molecular Biology, Immunology and Medical Genetics, Medical Faculty ofTrakia University, Stara Zagora, Bulgaria

Iskra Altankova
Clinical Immunology, University Hospital Lozenets, Sofia University, Sofia, Bulgaria

Victor V. Chaban
Department of Internal Medicine, Charles R. Drew University of Medicine and Science, Los Angeles, USA; Department of Medicine, University of California, Los Angeles, USA

Sumant S. Arora
Department of Medicine, University of Alabama at Birmingham, Montgomery Residency Program, Montgomery, Alabama, USA

Talha A. Malik
Department of Medicine-Gastroenterology and Department of Epidemiology, University of Alabama at Birmingham, Birmingham, Alabama, USA

Elsa M. Eriksson, Kristina I. Andrén and Henry T. Eriksson
Department of Functional Gastroenterology, Sahlgrenska University Hospital, Göteborg, Sweden

Lin Hai Kurahara, Keizo Hiraishi, Yaopeng Hu, Miho Sumiyoshi and Ryuji Inoue
Department of Physiology, Fukuoka University School of Medicine, Fukuoka University, Fukuoka, Japan

Kunihiko Aoyagi
Department of Gastroenterology, Fukuoka University School of Medicine, Fukuoka University, Fukuoka, Japan

Mihaela Fadgyas Stanculete
Department of Neurosciences, Discipline of Psychiatry and Pediatric Psychiatry, University of Medicine and Pharmacy "Iuliu Hațieganu", Cluj-Napoca, Romania
Second Psychiatric Clinic, Emergency County Hospital Cluj, Cluj-Napoca, Romania

Mònica Aguilera and Silvia Melgar
APC Microbiome Institute, University College Cork, National University of Ireland, Cork, Ireland

Alexandra Chira and Dan Lucian Dumitrascu
2nd Medical Clinic, Department of Internal Medicine, "Iuliu Hatieganu" University of Medicine and Pharmacy Cluj-Napoca, Romania

Romeo Ioan Chira
1st Medical Clinic, Department of Internal Medicine, Div. Gastroenterology, "Iuliu Hatieganu"
University of Medicine and Pharmacy Cluj-Napoca, Romania

Fernando de la Portilla, Ana M. García-Cabrera, Rosa M. Jiménez-Rodríguez and Maria L. Reyes
Department of General and Digestive Surgery, Colorectal Surgery Unit, "Virgen del Rocío" University Hospital/IBiS/CSIC/University of Seville, Seville, Spain

Damian García-Olmo
Department of Surgery (Fundacion Jimenez Diaz), Universidad Autonoma de Madrid, Spain

Abdulrahman Al-Robayan, Ebtissam Saleh Al-Meghaiseeb and Reem Al-Amro
Department of Gastroenterology, Prince Sultan Military Medical City, Riyadh, Saudi Arabia

Misbahul Arfin and Abdulrahman K Al-Asmari
Research Centre, Prince Sultan Military Medical City, Riyadh, Saudi Arabia

Ahmet Eken
Medical Biology, Faculty of Medicine, Erciyes University, Kayseri, Turkey
Betül-Ziya Eren Genome and Stem Cell Research Center, Kayseri, Turkey

Mohamed Oukka
Center for Immunity and Immunotherapies, Seattle Children's Research Institute, Seattle, WA, USA
Department of Immunology, University of Washington, Seattle, WA, USA

Index

www.ingramcontent.com/pod-product-compliance
Lightning Source LLC
Chambersburg PA
CBHW061939190326
41458CB00009B/2783